National Incident Management System

Dr.
Dr. Hank T. Christen, Jr., EdP, MPA
Christian E. Callsen, Jr., LP
Geoffrey T. Miller, AS, EMT-P
Paul M. Maniscalco, MPA, MS, EMT-P
Graydon C. Lord, MS, NREMT-P
Neal J. Dolan, BS, MCJ, NREMT-P

Principles and Practice

Second Edition

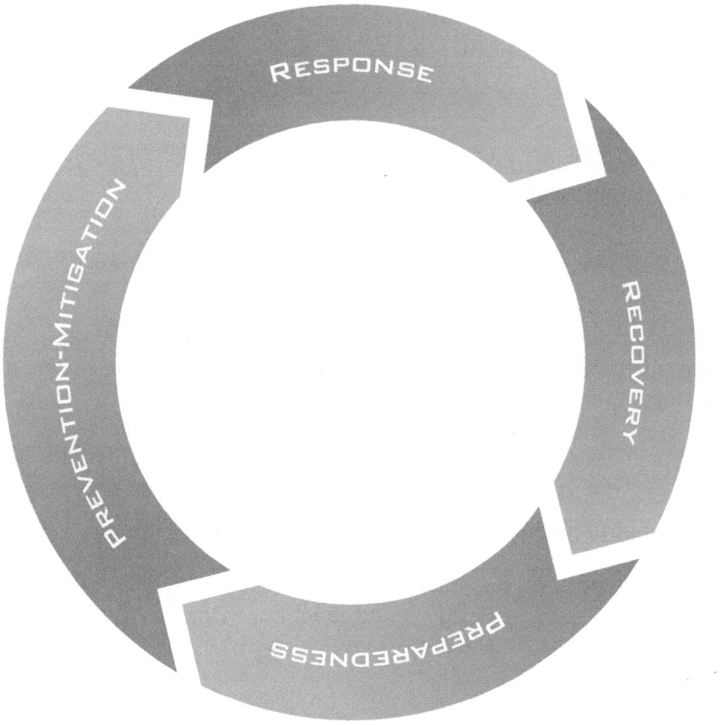

Jones & Bartlett Learning

World Headquarters
Jones & Bartlett Learning
40 Tall Pine Drive
Sudbury, MA 01776
978-443-5000
info@jblearning.com
www.jblearning.com

Jones & Bartlett Learning books and products are available through most bookstores and online booksellers. To contact Jones & Bartlett Learning directly, call 800-832-0034, fax 978-443-8000, or visit our website, www.jblearning.com.

Substantial discounts on bulk quantities of Jones & Bartlett Learning publications are available to corporations, professional associations, and other qualified organizations. For details and specific discount information, contact the special sales department at Jones & Bartlett Learning via the above contact information or send an email to specialsales@jblearning.com.

Production Credits
Chairman, Board of Directors: Clayton Jones
Chief Executive Officer: Ty Field
President: James Homer
Sr. V.P., Chief Operating Officer: Don W. Jones, Jr.
V.P., Design and Production: Anne Spencer
V.P., Manufacturing and Inventory Control: Therese Connell
Executive Publisher: Kimberly Brophy
Executive Acquisitions Editor—Fire: William Larkin
Associate Managing Editor: Robyn Schafer
Associate Editor: Laura Burns
Editorial Assistant: Kara Ebrahim
Associate Production Editor: Jessica deMartin
Marketing Manager: Brian Rooney
Composition: Toppan BestSet
Cover Design: Kristin E. Parker
Assistant Photo Researcher: Elise Gilbert
Printing and Binding: McNaughton & Gunn
Cover Printing: McNaughton & Gunn

Copyright © 2012 by Jones & Bartlett Learning, LLC, an Ascend Learning Company

All rights reserved. No part of the material protected by this copyright may be reproduced or utilized in any form, electronic or mechanical, including photocopying, recording, or by any information storage and retrieval system, without written permission from the copyright owner.

Some images in this book feature models. These models do not necessarily endorse, represent, or participate in the activities represented in the images.

Additional photo and illustration credits appear on page 293, which constitutes a continuation of the copyright page.

Library of Congress Cataloging-in-Publication Data
National incident management system : principles and practices / Donald W. Walsh . . . [et al.].—2nd ed.
        p. cm.
     Includes index.
     ISBN-13: 978-0-7637-8187-3
     ISBN-10: 0-7637-8187-8
  1. Emergency management–United States.   2. Crisis management–United States.   3. Internal security–United States.   I. Walsh, Donald W.
     HV551.3.N375 2012
     363.34068–dc22

                                        2010041569

6048
Printed in the United States of America
24 23 22 21   10

BRIEF CONTENTS

CONTENTS

7   Finance/Administration   71

8   Intelligence/Investigations   79

9   Multiagency Coordination Systems   85

10 Public Information

Chapter Resources

National Incident Management System: Principles and Practice, Section Edition features a variety of case studies, tips, and end-of-chapter materials to facilitate comprehension of critical concepts and help readers synthesize the information learned. These features include:

Rural and Urban Case Studies

Each chapter opens with a rural and urban case study that will capture the reader's attention, stimulate discussion and critical thinking, and provide an overview of the chapter. An additional case study is included at the end of each chapter.

CHAPTER 5

Planning

Rural Case Study

Smith County and Stadtown are completely overwhelmed by the devastation of a flood caused by the breach of several small dams after heavy rainfall. A major part of Stadtown has been flooded by several feet of water. Two hours after the rushing water overwhelmed the town, the Unified Command (UC) group (sheriff's office, fire, and emergency medical services) appoints you as the Planning Section Chief. The scene is chaotic, disorganized, and without direction. Documentation is nonexistent. Your initial discussions with the UC reveal that they have no immediate strategies for managing the incident in a unified manner, and it is clear that the incident is a long-term event.

1. What are your initial actions?
2. As Planning Section Chief, what are your priorities?
3. What personnel do you need immediately to make the Planning Section effective?

Urban Case Study

The Emergency Operations Center (EOC) has been activated, and you are reporting to your assigned position of Planning Section Chief. You find that the Situation Unit is already staffed and working. Information is coming in from the scene regarding additional needs and evacuation issues. The situation is evolving quickly. The incident is in its third hour.

At this juncture, you must set several immediate priorities that will ensure that the EOC is adequately supporting the in-field operations. You also need to plan for several potential operational periods, potentially extending over multiple days or weeks.

1. What situation assessments do you need to make immediately? Why are they important?
2. Besides the Situation Unit, what unit is your next priority?
3. What technical specialists do you immediately want access to? Why?

Introduction

The **Planning Section** is a critical component of the Incident Command System (ICS) and one that is frequently overlooked in local operations, both on the scene and within EOCs. In local environments, this is usually due to a lack of personnel resources

and education. Although not as high profile as the Operations Section, the Planning Section provides unique challenges to individuals who enjoy a more strategic view of incident management while still working in detail-oriented areas. The basis of an effective Planning Section is accurate and timely information acquisition from the Incident Command/

51

Tip

Tips boxes highlight and expand upon important NIMS concepts presented in each chapter.

Tip

Making changes in the command structure of a long-term incident is best done during the normal transfer of command that takes place between defined operational periods. This helps to ensure that all incident personnel are aware of the transition and that the General Staff Section Chiefs are comfortable with their new assignments and are aware of their correct supervisor.

Wrap-Up

End-of-chapter activities reinforce important concepts and improve the readers' comprehension of the text.

Summary

The Summary provides the most important information from the chapter in a bulleted form to help reinforce key concepts.

Glossary

The Glossary provides key terms and definitions from the chapter.

Wrap-Up

Summary

- Disasters and high-impact events result in a logistics-scarce environment.
- The Logistics Section supports all activities needed for efficient incident management.
- The Logistics Section in a fully activated EOC has a Support Branch with a Supply Unit, a Facilities Unit, and a Ground Support Unit, as well as a Service Branch with a Communications Unit, a Food Unit, and a Medical Unit.
- Mass sheltering places high demands on the Logistics Section.
- Logistics functions are based on a push or pull system.
- A communications failure protocol is a critical element in logistics planning.
- Volunteers and donations present management challenges that must be coordinated by the Logistics Section and the Planning Section.

Glossary

Air-to-air nets: Networks for communications among aviation units.

Command net: Network for communications among Command Staff, Section Chiefs, Branch Directors, and Division and Group Supervisors.

Communications failure protocol: Procedures for identifying major communication infrastructures and backup procedures in the case of system failures.

Communications Unit: Plans the effective use of communications equipment and facilities assigned to an incident.

Facilities Unit: Sets up, maintains, and demobilizes all facilities used in support of incident operations.

Food Unit: Plans food operations for facilities and sheltering operations.

Ground Support Unit: Maintains and repairs primary tactical equipment, vehicles, and mobile ground

support equipment, supplies fuel, and provides transportation support.

Ground-to-air net: Network for communications among ground and aviation units.

Incident traffic plan: A plan that specifies traffic routes and procedures for vehicles entering and departing an incident site, command post, or support area.

Logistics Section: Responsible for all support requirements needed to facilitate effective incident management.

Marine nets: Networks for communications among marine units and land-based agencies.

Medical Unit: Develops the Incident Medical Plan and manages medical operations.

Pull logistics: Ordering of personnel, supplies, and equipment from outside local response or support agencies.

Push logistics: Initial response equipment and supplies transported by responding units.

Resources: Personnel, supplies, and equipment needed for incident operations.

Service Branch: Provides communications, food, water, and medical services. Consists of the Communications Unit, the Food Unit, and the Medical Unit.

Supply Unit: Orders, receives, and processes all incident-related resources, personnel, and supplies.

Support Branch: Provides services that assist incident operations by providing supplies, facilities, transport, and equipment maintenance. Consists of the Supply Unit, the Facilities Unit, and the Ground Support Unit.

Support net: Communications network that supports logistics requests, resource status changes, and other nontactical functions.

Tactical net: Communications network that connects operating agencies and functional units.

Unified logistics: Utilization and coordination of two or more agencies or jurisdictions to manage diverse logistics functions.

Wrap-Up Case Study

A severe winter ice storm in upstate New York has caused major power shortages and blocked roads in a 13-county area. Temperatures are close to 0°F and are forecasted to remain low for 10 days. The affected rural population is 250,000 people spread over an area of 6000 square miles.

The nearest urban area is more than 95 miles away. Communications are sparse, at best. Several of the affected counties do not have a dedicated EOC and have not been heard from. Power is not expected to be restored for at least 3 weeks.

1. What pull logistics sources may be available?
   A. Contracted supplies from area local businesses
   B. Supplies from volunteer fire departments
   C. National-level support agencies and state mutual-aid logistics
   D. Supplies from local donations

2. What are the immediate logistics demands?
   A. Additional facilities, food, water, and sanitation
   B. Emergency generators and portable heaters
   C. Coordination with public support agencies, such as the American Red Cross
   D. All of the above

3. What are the key points in a communications failure protocol for this incident?
   A. Modern communications systems rarely fail. A failure protocol is unnecessary.
   B. Additional radio batteries and chargers are needed because dead batteries are the most common type of failure.
   C. Multiple tactical nets need to be established.
   D. Backup systems, storage of backup hardware and software, and a contractual support agreement with private vendors need to be established.

Wrap-Up Case Study

The Wrap-Up Case Study promotes critical thinking and provides additional questions that are answered in Appendix I at the end of the text.

Reporting Relationships

When an Area Command is involved in coordinating multiple incident management activities, the following reporting relationships will apply:

- The Incident Commanders for the incidents under the Area Command's authority report to the Area Commander.
- The Area Commander is accountable to the agency(ies) or to the jurisdictional executive(s) or administrator(s).

- If one or more incidents within the Area Command are multijurisdictional, a unified Area Command should be established. In this instance, Incident Commanders report to the Unified Area Commander for their jurisdiction.

Rural Case Study *Answers*

1. The Smith County EOC has the space (although limited) and communications capabilities that are essential for an effective MACS. The EOC also provides a means for communications with the state EOC and the county's public safety dispatch center.
2. The MACS is organized using the ICS template. Logistics and Planning Sections are required to establish communications and to order, allocate, and track resources. The Finance/Administration Section contracts for and purchases resources.
3. The natural disaster in Smith County is a series of incidents, each having an ICP and an ICS structure. An Area Command is a tool for prioritizing resources and coordinating the various Incident Command Posts. The Area Command becomes unified with the additions of the Sheriff and the Director of Emergency Management, and it is located in the EOC.

Urban Case Study *Answers*

1. The incident has escalated beyond the ICP level. The large-scale evacuations, along with a terrorist attack threat, present interoperability problems and COP requirements that are addressed by a fully activated EOC.
2. This incident requires complex coordination between multiple police, fire, and EMS agencies. State assistance and federal law enforcement support must be interoperable with the local effort. In this incident, the primary functions of the MACS are as follows:
   - Logistics support and resource tracking
   - Coordination of information and interagency issues
   - Implementation of preparedness plans
3. The initial explosion and the threat of another attack classify this as a national security incident. Intelligence information must be protected and effectively utilized for strategic planning. This is accomplished by elevating the Intelligence/Investigations Function to the Section level in the EOC.

Rural and Urban Case Study Answers

Answers to the Rural and Urban Case Study questions featured at the beginning of the chapter are provided in the Wrap-Up, allowing the readers to think about potential responses to the questions as they read the chapter.

Dr. Donald W. Walsh, PhD, EMT-P

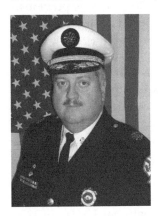

Dr. Donald W. Walsh has a vast array of experience from his 30-year Chicago Fire Department career and continues his involvement at all levels. Between 1976 and 2007, Dr. Walsh worked for the Chicago Fire Department's Bureau of Operations, where he served as a licensed paramedic, EMS manager, educator, instructor, chief officer, and assistant deputy fire commissioner for the EMS Division, where he managed the second-largest EMS system in the United States. His public safety background includes being an adjunct faculty member of the National Fire Academy under the US Department of Homeland Security, president of the Chicago Fire Paramedics Association, and director of the Illinois Paramedics Association. He is on the board of directors and is the currently elected secretary of the National Association of Emergency Medical Technicians.

As a respected international speaker, author, and educator, Dr. Walsh has lectured to public safety and healthcare industry audiences all over the world, addressing various topics in homeland security, EMS, fire rescue operations, law enforcement, and private industry. Dr. Walsh's specialties and expertise include public safety management, strategic planning, incident command, incident management, disaster planning, and antiterrorism responses. Dr. Walsh has lectured and trained throughout the United States, as well as Europe, eastern Europe, Asia, the Middle East, and the former Soviet Union. Dr. Walsh has been a presenter on and has been interviewed by CNN International, Turkish National Television, *20/20*, ABC News Magazine-New York, Discovery Channel, and many local television and radio stations and media outlets throughout the United States, the Middle East, and Europe. Dr. Walsh has published more than 60 national and international articles and scientific abstracts in professional and peer-reviewed journals, and he serves on many professional peer-reviewed journal editorial and advisory boards. Dr. Walsh was elected as a Fellow to the Institute of Medicine of Chicago and also served as a subject matter expert for the US Army and NASA on fire fighter safety issues in coordination with the US Fire Administration.

Throughout his career, Dr. Walsh has been awarded the James O. Page Leadership Award, EMS Fire Chief of the Year from the International Association of Fire Chiefs, Paramedic of the Year from *EMS Magazine*, Paramedic of the Year from the National Association of Emergency Medical Technicians, a City of Chicago Recognition Resolution, and a State of Illinois House of Representatives Recognition Resolution.

Dr. Walsh's extensive background in public safety and private industry has fostered new technologies and programs in the areas of antiterrorism training, incident command, rescue equipment development, and disaster management response programs. His most recent research on fire smoke and cyanide treatments has been published in peer-reviewed and professional publications. Within the fields of fire service, EMS, and organizational planning, Dr. Walsh has assisted with corporate and public safety information technologies and educational programs, as well as global networking and research development programs. In addition to his government and consultant activities, Dr. Walsh is currently working with private-sector businesses and industries to develop corporate educational programs, public safety programs, and information technology systems.

Dr. Walsh is currently working on new fire safety technologies and research on the dangers of fire smoke, cyanide identification and treatment protocols, fire suppression foam systems, and technologies and antiterrorism preparedness programs related to cyanide weapons and disaster management.

Dr. Hank T. Christen, Jr., EdP, MPA

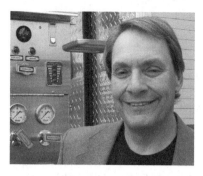

Dr. Hank T. Christen has been a consultant in the fields of emergency response and counterterrorism for US Department of Defense agencies, federal response agencies, and local government public safety agencies since 2000. He was previously a battalion chief for the Atlanta Fire Department and director of Emergency Services for Okaloosa County, Florida. He served as unit commander for the Gulf Coast Disaster Medical Assistance Team (DMAT) and has responded to 12 national disasters, including the attack on the World Trade Center on September 11, 2001.

Dr. Christen is a contributing editor for *Firehouse Magazine* and has published more than 30 articles in technical journals. He is the coauthor of *The EMS Incident Management System, Understanding Terrorism and Managing Its Consequences*, and *Terrorism Response: Field Guide for Law Enforcement*.

Dr. Christen has been a speaker at national conferences for the past 20 years. He was a member of the US Department of Defense, Defense Science Board (Transnational Threats, 1997), and the US Army Interagency Board for Medical Logistics. He was a member of the Executive Session on Domestic Preparedness, a faculty member at the John F. Kennedy School of Government at Harvard University, and he is currently an affiliate faculty member at George Washington University Medical School, Auburn University, and the Gordon Center for Research in Medical Education at the University of Miami.

A Miami native, Dr. Christen completed his undergraduate studies at the University of Florida and his doctoral degree in human performance technology at the University of West Florida.

Christian E. Callsen, Jr., LP

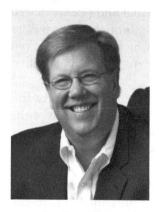

Christian "Chris" E. Callsen, Jr., is an experienced emergency services and homeland security leader and educator with a broad range of professional experience. In his 26-year career in public safety, he has served in volunteer and career organizations nationwide. Recently he retired as the assistant chief of operations for Austin-Travis County Emergency Medical Services in Austin, Texas. Chief Callsen now serves as the chief operating officer for North America at Optima and maintains a consultancy in emergency services and incident management. Credentialed as both an incident commander and planning section chief for Type III IMTs, Chief Callsen has extensive practical experience in major incident response, including Hurricanes Katrina and Rita.

Chief Callsen has been active in several areas of local, regional, and national homeland security planning through participation on the Austin/Travis County Counter Terrorism Planning Group, as the inaugural chair of the Capital Area Planning Council's Homeland Security Task Force, and as a member of the federal Interagency Board for Equipment Standardization. Educated at Georgetown University in Washington, DC, Chief Callsen has had assignments throughout his EMS career as a flight paramedic, a field training officer, and a clinical practice manager, as well as a senior operations chief.

Geoffrey T. Miller, AS, EMT-P

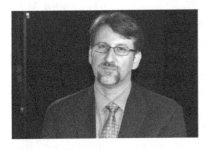

Geoffrey T. Miller is the associate director of Research and Curriculum Development for the Division of Prehospital and Emergency Healthcare at the Michael S. Gordon Center for Research in Medical Education (GCRME) at the University of Miami Miller School of Medicine. Mr. Miller began his career in public safety 20 years ago. Previously, Mr. Miller worked as a paramedic fire fighter with Alachua County Fire Rescue before moving into EMS education. During his time with Alachua County Fire Rescue, he also oversaw projects on system utilization and hospital diversions, and he assisted in the development and implementation of E911 system upgrades, electronic patient tracking, and reporting and medical care protocol refinements. Following his service in fire rescue, Mr. Miller served as associate professor of EMS programs at Santa Fe Community College in Gainesville, Florida. There, he led the school's participation as a field test site in the pilot testing of the US Department of Transportation national standard curriculum for paramedics.

Mr. Miller joined the GCRME more than 9 years ago and has since worked in the areas of patient simulation, interactive multimedia computer learning systems, emergency medical skills training, terrorism response, and disaster medical response and management. He is active in the areas of applied outcomes research in education, with an emphasis on the creation and improvement of methods of clinical competence assessment using advanced educational technology and simulation. Presently Mr. Miller develops, implements, disseminates, and evaluates innovative EMS curricula and assessment systems that are used by prehospital providers, medical schools, and US Army medical teams throughout the United States.

Mr. Miller is actively engaged in scholarly research and publication in EMS practice and education. He has coauthored several books, including *Arrhythmia Recognition: The Art of Interpretation*. Mr. Miller is a frequent author and coauthor in emergency medical services and emergency care journals. He is regularly invited to speak at state, national, and international conferences.

Mr. Miller is a member of numerous local, state, and national EMS professional organizations and committees that advise fire rescue, EMS, law enforcement, public health, and hospitals. Mr. Miller is also an active member of national and Florida state educational organizations and has served twice as the president of the Florida Association of EMS Educators. In 2000, Mr. Miller was recognized as the Paramedic Instructor of the Year by the Florida Association of EMS Educators. In 2003, he was recognized as the EMS Educator of the Year by the State of Florida Department of Health Bureau of EMS. In 2005, he received the Mary Ann Talley award for EMS education from the National Association of Emergency Medical Technicians.

Paul M. Maniscalco, MPA, MS, EMT-P

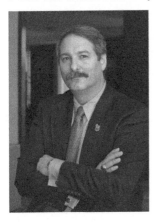

Paul M. Maniscalco is a senior research scientist and principal investigator at George Washington University. He presently serves as the first president of the International Association of EMS Chiefs. Chief Maniscalco is a former president of the National Association of Emergency Medical Technicians (NAEMT), a past chairman of the NAEMT National EMS Chief Officers Division, and a former deputy chief/paramedic for the City of New York. Chief Maniscalco has more than 30 years of public safety response, supervisory, and management experience.

Chief Maniscalco has lectured extensively and is widely published in academic and professional journals on EMS, fire service, public safety, and national security issues. He is the coauthor of *The EMS*

Incident Management System: EMS Operations for Mass Casualty and High Impact Incidents and a contributing author to the following texts: *Hype or Reality? The "New Terrorism" and Mass Casualty Attacks* by the Chemical and Biological Arms Control Institute; *Model Procedures Guide for Emergency Medical Incidents* by the National Fire Service Incident Management System Consortium; and *Understanding Terrorism and Managing the Consequences, Mass Casualty and High Impact Incidents: An Operations Management Guide*, and *Public Health Guide for Emergencies* by the IFRC/RC Society and Johns Hopkins School of Hygiene and Public Health Center for Disaster and Refugee Studies. In collaboration with organizations including the United Nations, Pan American Health Organization, American Health Organization, United States Agency for International Development, World Health Organization, and International Federation of Red Cross and International Committee of the Red Cross, Chief Maniscalco has participated in public safety and emergency and disaster response capacity-building projects in India, St. Maarten, Turkey, Kenya, and Tanzania.

Chief Maniscalco is an appointee to the President's Homeland Security Advisory Council Senior Advisory Committee for Emergency Services, Law Enforcement, and Public Health and Hospitals. He is a member of the US Department of Defense's Defense Science Board (DSB), Transnational Threat Study, and Chemical Weapons Task Force, as well as a member of the Interagency Board for the Departments of Homeland Security, Defense, and Justice. Chief Maniscalco has served as an advisor to the Defense Advanced Research Projects Agency and was appointed to the Centers for Strategic and International Studies Homeland Security Task Force, as well as the Congressionally-mandated National Panel to Assess Domestic Preparedness (Gilmore National Terrorism Commission), where he also served as the chairman of the Threat Reassessment Panel, State, and Local Response Panel and Research Panel. Additionally, he served on the Cyber-Terrorism and Critical Infrastructure Panels during this 5-year commission. Chief Maniscalco also received an appointment to Harvard University's John F. Kennedy School of Government in an Executive Session on Domestic Preparedness fellowship sponsored by the US Department of Justice.

Chief Maniscalco has earned numerous awards and honors for professional achievement and service from government, corporate, and professional organizations. He was awarded more than 100 commendations from the City of New York during his 22-year career, including the Medal of Honor. In 2003, he received the NAEMT's Rocco V. Morando Lifetime Achievement Award for significant sustained professional achievement and contributions of national impact to the profession.

Chief Maniscalco earned a baccalaureate degree in public administration, public health, and safety from the City University of New York and a master's degree in public administration, foreign policy, and national security from the NYU-Wagner Graduate School of Public Service. He is presently pursuing additional graduate studies with a research focus on organizational behavior and emergency response to disasters and terrorism incidents.

Graydon C. Lord, MS, NREMT-P (Retired)

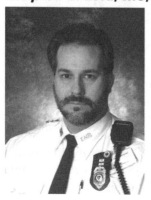

Graydon C. Lord presently serves as associate director of the National EMS Preparedness Initiative at George Washington University's Office of Homeland Security and senior policy analyst on emergency response and homeland security. Chief Lord came to George Washington University after nearly 5 years as division chief of Emergency Medical Services for Cherokee County Fire Department in Cherokee County, Georgia.

In this capacity, Chief Lord evaluated the EMS system and determined that the needs of the community would best be met by creating a fully integrated, dual-role, cross-trained, fire-based EMS system. Chief Lord provided leadership and operational execution to achieve that goal. Cherokee County Fire Department now has 200 EMTs and paramedics who serve 500 square miles in both an urban and rural environment with Advanced Life Support ambulances.

Chief Lord became an EMT and paramedic in 1980 and was promoted through the ranks to become EMS operations chief of the second-largest EMS system in New England at Worcester Emergency Medical Services in Worcester, Massachusetts, until his retirement in 2001.

Chief Lord lectures nationally and internationally on EMS systems development, leadership and operations, disaster response, and homeland security preparedness. He is an adjunct faculty member for various institutions and agencies, including the Institute for International Disaster Emergency Medicine, Group Trauma Services of Portugal, Texas A&M University, US Department of Justice, US Department of Homeland Security, University of Massachusetts Medical Center, Copenhagen Fire Department, Appalachian Technical College, and the Georgia Public Safety Center. He was appointed by former President George W. Bush to serve on the National Commission on Children and Disasters, and he also holds an appointment to the US Department of Defense InterAgency Board.

Chief Lord is a member or officer of several professional organizations, including the International Association of Emergency Medical Services Chiefs (IAEMSC), National Association of Emergency Medical Technicians (NAEMT), National Registry of Emergency Medical Technicians (NREMT), National Association of EMS Physicians (NAEMSP), and Georgia Association of Emergency Medical Services (GAEMS). He is a past member of the board of directors for the NAEMT and the GAEMS.

Neal J. Dolan, BS, MCJ, NREMT-P

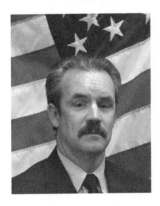

Neal J. Dolan currently serves as deputy director for the South Carolina Law Enforcement Division (SLED), which is the state's designated homeland security agency responsible for planning, budgeting, and distributing grants. In this capacity, Mr. Dolan oversees the statewide operations of approximately 600 employees involved in criminal investigations, homeland security, and statutory regulatory functions.

Prior to his current position at SLED, Mr. Dolan was the special agent in charge for the US Secret Service in the South Carolina District with overall command and managerial responsibility for Secret Service operations and offices in Columbia, Greenville, and Charleston. Mr. Dolan served with the US Secret Service for 25 years. His past assignments include the Miami field office, the Office of Training, the Presidential Protective Division, the Office of the Assistant Director for Investigations, and the Orlando field office.

Mr. Dolan has extensive experience in large event planning, logistics, safety, and security. He was part of the US Department of Homeland Security executive planning board for the G-8 Summit in St. Simons, Georgia. Mr. Dolan is also a nationally registered paramedic who is credited with creating numerous innovative programs in the areas of emergency medicine, tactical medicine, and medical support teams for the US Secret Service. He also served as chairman of the National Association of Emergency Medical Technicians, National Paramedic Division.

In 1993, Mr. Dolan was temporarily assigned as a Secret Service tactical paramedic to the FBI's hostage rescue team to provide medical assistance during the Branch Davidian incident in Waco, Texas. During the 50 days of this siege, more than 200 people were treated for injuries ranging from minor heat-related illnesses to severe burns after the compound was engulfed in flames.

Mr. Dolan has lectured extensively and is widely published in academic and professional journals on EMS, law enforcement, public safety, and national security issues. He is also a contributing author to *Understanding Terrorism and Managing the Consequences*, *Terrorism Response: Field Guide for Law Enforcement*, and *Terrorism Response: Field Guide for Fire and EMS Organizations*.

Prior to his work with the US Secret Service, Mr. Dolan was a police officer in North Attleboro, Massachusetts; a lieutenant with the Lexington County Sheriff Department in Lexington, South Carolina; and director of the Criminal Justice Program at Horry-Georgetown Technical College in Myrtle Beach, South Carolina.

Mr. Dolan has a BS in law enforcement from Bryant University and a master's degree in criminal justice from the University of South Carolina.

> There are no secrets to success. It is the result of preparation,
> hard work and learning from failure.
>
> —*Colin Powell*

> We are what we repeatedly do. Excellence then, is not an act but a habit.
>
> —*Aristotle*

The attacks of September 11, 2001 were the impetus for the federal government to create a comprehensive plan to synchronize the nation's preparedness and response efforts.

On February 28, 2003, President George W. Bush issued a presidential mandate (Homeland Security Presidential Directive/HSPD-5, Management of Domestic Incidents) directly to the secretary of the US Department of Homeland Security to develop a National Response Framework and administer a National Incident Management System (NIMS).

The NIMS Incident Command System (ICS) had its origin in the Fire Ground Command System pioneered by the Phoenix Fire Department in the 1970s. Simultaneously, the ICS was being developed in California to assist in dealing with large-scale events, such as wildfires and earthquakes. Both systems provided a foundation for today's NIMS ICS.

Since its inception in 2004, NIMS has represented the country's first-ever standardized approach to incident management. NIMS has been used as the consistent nationwide template to enable state, federal, tribal, and local governments, nongovernmental organizations (NGOs), and the private sector to effectively work together to prevent, respond, and recover from recent incidents.

In 2006, the NIMS document began revisions in an effort to incorporate best practices and lessons learned from recent incidents. In December 2008, a revised NIMS document emerged, clarifying concepts, principles, and terminology and refining the process used by first responders during incidents.

The revision sought to achieve the following goals:

- Eliminate redundancy
- Emphasize that NIMS is more than the ICS
- Clarify ICS concepts
- Increase emphasis on planning and add guidance on mutual aid
- Clarify roles of the private sector, NGOs, and the chief elected and appointed officials
- Expand the intelligence and investigative function
- Highlight the relationship between the NIMS and the National Response Framework

This book is a primer for emergency responders, organizations, and institutions to respond to emergency events. The examples in the text have been drawn from the experiences of first responders in the field and provide real-life situations where coordinated operations were critical. As emergency responders integrate NIMS ICS into training curricula, this text can act as a guide to the nation's homeland security strategy and provide you with principles and concepts of NIMS ICS.

Neal J. Dolan
Deputy Director, South Carolina Law Enforcement Division
Special Agent in Charge (Retired)
US Secret Service
US Department of Homeland Security

On February 28, 2003, President George W. Bush issued Homeland Security Presidential Directive/HSPD-5, Management of Domestic Incidents (see Appendix A), which directs the secretary of the US Department of Homeland Security (DHS) to develop and administer a National Incident Management System (NIMS).

On March 1, 2004, the first federal publication on NIMS was released by the DHS. Following this publication, the Federal Emergency Management Agency (FEMA) under DHS published a draft revision of NIMS with updates and changes to the original NIMS publication (FEMA 501/Draft August 2007). The second NIMS publication was developed through a collaborative inter-governmental partnership with significant input from the incident management functional disciplines, the private sector, and nongovernmental organizations (NGOs).

In December 2008, DHS published the approved NIMS document. The new, revised NIMS system provides a consistent nationwide template to enable federal, state, tribal, and local governments; NGOs; and the private sector to work together to prevent, protect against, respond to, recover from, and mitigate the effects of incidents, regardless of cause, size, location, or complexity. This consistency provides the foundation for utilization of NIMS for all incidents, ranging from daily occurrences to incidents requiring a coordinated federal response.

This book is based on the new changes and updates published in the December 2008 NIMS document developed by DHS, FEMA, and other federal agencies. The book uses the new NIMS document, along with significant input from the incident management functional disciplines, to update topics including but not limited to public safety agencies, the private sector, NGOs, first responder agencies, institutional groups, and professional associations.

This book further updates the first edition of *National Incident Management System: Principles and Practice* with the latest NIMS updates and information, including the interface of the DHS National Response Framework (NRF). The NRF is a guide to how the nation conducts all-hazards responses. The NRF identifies the key principles as well as the roles and structures that organize national response. In addition, it describes special circumstances where the federal government exercises a larger role, including incidents where federal interests are involved and catastrophic incidents for which a state would require significant support.

NIMS is not an operational incident management or resource allocation plan. NIMS represents a core set of doctrines, concepts, principles, terminology, and organizational processes that enable effective, efficient, and collaborative incident management.

HSPD-5 requires all federal departments and agencies to adopt NIMS and use it in their individual incident management programs and activities, as well as in support of all actions taken to assist state, tribal, and local governments. The directive requires federal departments and agencies to make adoption of NIMS by state, tribal, and local organizations a condition for federal preparedness assistance (through grants, contracts, and other activities). NIMS recognizes the role that NGOs and the private sector have in preparedness and activities to prevent, protect against, respond to, recover from, and mitigate the effects of incidents.

Building on the foundation provided by existing emergency management and incident response systems used by jurisdictions, organizations, and functional disciplines at all levels, NIMS integrates best practices into a comprehensive framework for nationwide use by emergency management and response personnel in an all-hazards context. These best practices lay the groundwork for the components of NIMS and provide the mechanisms for further development and refinement of supporting national standards, guidelines, protocols, systems, and technologies. NIMS fosters the development of specialized technologies that facilitate emergency management and incident response activities and allows for the adoption of new approaches that will enable continuous refinement of the system over time.

The secretary of DHS, through the National Integration Center (NIC), Incident Management Systems Integration Division (formerly known as the NIMS Integration Center), publishes the standards, guidelines, and compliance protocols for determining whether a federal, state, tribal, or local government has implemented NIMS. Additionally, the secretary of DHS, through the NIC, manages publications and collaboratively, with other departments and agencies, develops standards, guidelines, compliance procedures, and protocols for all aspects of NIMS.

National Incident Management System: Principles and Practice, Second Edition was developed to update the significant changes developed by DHS while keeping a variety of case studies, tips, and end-of-chapter materials to facilitate comprehension of critical concepts and help readers understand the information learned in the first edition. This book reflects contributions from emergency management stakeholders, educators, incident management experts, and lessons learned during recent incidents.

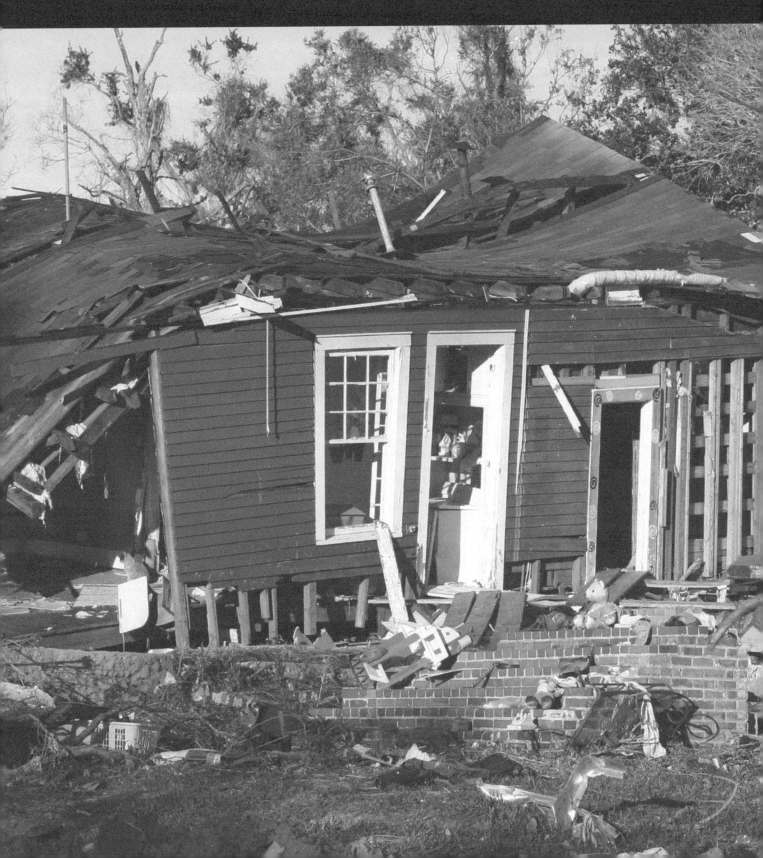

Understanding the National Incident Management System

CHAPTER 1

Introduction to the National Incident Management System

Rural Case Study

Smith County, a rural area located 100 miles from the city of Littletown, has a population of 75,000. In general, Smith County is a quiet and peaceful place for the local fire, emergency medical services (EMS), and police. The greatest challenge occurs early every summer when severe thunderstorms roll through the area.

One day in mid-May, the National Weather Service issues a severe thunderstorm warning for four counties, including Smith County, at about 4:00 P.M. At 6:17 P.M., a funnel cloud is sighted by Deputy Williams of the Smith County Police. The direction of travel places the 900 citizens of Stadtown in the path of the funnel cloud. At 6:21 P.M., Stadtown is struck by an F4 tornado, which completely levels the downtown shopping district and the majority of residential properties. The damage to Stadtown is confirmed by Deputy Williams, who arrives on the scene within 2 minutes.

1. Should an incident management system be used to handle this situation?
2. What response agencies and disciplines will likely be needed to successfully respond to the disaster at Stadtown?

Urban Case Study

Pleasantville is a busy suburb of 25,000 people and is located just 10 miles outside of Metro, a thriving city of 1.6 million people. In Pleasantville, the majority of emergency response calls are for minor motor vehicle accidents that occur on the highway that loops around the suburb. In years past, the fire, EMS, and police have trained together to respond to any potentially major emergency incidents because of Pleasantville's proximity to a major city, the interstate, and the train tracks that run beside the interstate. In recent months, all three departments also have been training together to respond to any potential terrorist incidents.

It is a windy winter day in January at Pleasantville Fire Station 2. The wind is gusting at 16 miles per hour. The dispatcher calls to report a motor vehicle accident between a truck and a freight train on Interstate 101.

1. What agencies will probably respond with the fire department?
2. What agencies or organizations will have a role in the management of this type of incident?

Introduction

Everything changed on September 11, 2001. Organizations from public safety to private industry watched incidents unfold before them with a certainty that things would never be the same again. The Advisory Panel to Assess Domestic Response Capabilities for Terrorism Involving Weapons of Mass Destruction (commonly known as the Gilmore Commission), in its fifth report dated December 15, 2003, to the president of the United States and Congress, referred to this state as the **new normalcy**.

The creation of the National Incident Management System (NIMS) is a key product of this new normalcy. The NIMS represents a fundamental shift in the philosophy of incident management in this country from a discipline-specific incident response and command framework to an all-hazards integrated, multiagency approach to incident management. NIMS defines a comprehensive national approach to incident management that is equally functional for local, state, and federal response agencies, as well as health care, infrastructure, public service, and private industry.

Such an approach improves coordination and cooperation between public and private agencies and organizations in a variety of emergency management and incident response activities, setting the stage for seamless multifunction integration under a single incident command and control system. The NIMS framework sets forth the comprehensive national approach **(Table 1-1)**.

NIMS is appropriate for all jurisdictional levels and across functional disciplines; it improves the effectiveness of emergency response providers and incident management organizations by emphasizing cooperation instead of competition.

Incidents typically begin and end locally and are managed on a daily basis at the lowest possible geographical, organizational, and jurisdictional level. However, there are instances in which successful incident management operations depend on the involvement of multiple jurisdictions, levels of government, functional agencies, and/or emergency responder disciplines. These instances require effec-

tive and efficient coordination across this broad spectrum of organizations and activities.

NIMS uses a systematic approach to integrate the best existing processes and methods into a unified national framework for incident management. Incident management refers to how incidents are managed across all homeland security activities, including prevention and protection, as well as response, mitigation, and recovery.

This framework forms the basis for interoperability and compatibility that will, in turn, enable a diverse set of public and private organizations to conduct well-integrated and effective emergency management and incident response operations. Emergency management is the coordination and integration of all activities necessary to build, sustain, and improve the capability to prepare for, protect against, respond to, recover from, or mitigate against threatened or actual natural disasters, acts of terrorism, or other manmade disasters. It does this through a core set of concepts, principles, procedures, organizational processes, terminology, and standard requirements applicable to a broad community of NIMS users.

Foundations of NIMS

The authorization for the establishment of a national incident management system is found within Homeland Security Presidential Directive/HSPD-5, which was issued on February 28, 2003. This directive establishes that the secretary of the US Department of Homeland Security shall develop and administer a NIMS. Specifically, HSPD-5 states the following:

Table 1-1 Overview of NIMS	
What NIMS Is	What NIMS Is *Not*
■ A comprehensive, nationwide, systematic approach to incident management, including the Incident Command System, Multiagency Coordination Systems, and Public Information	■ A response plan
■ Standardized resource management procedures that enable coordination among different jurisdictions or organizations	■ A communications plan
■ A set of preparedness concepts and principles for all hazards	■ Only used during large-scale incidents
■ Essential principles for a common operating picture and interoperability of communications and information management	■ Only applicable to certain emergency management/incident response personnel
■ Scalable, so it may be used for all incidents (from day-to-day to large-scale)	■ Only the Incident Command System or an organization chart
■ A dynamic system that promotes ongoing management and maintenance	■ A static system

This system will provide a consistent nation-wide approach for Federal, State, and local governments to work effectively and efficiently together to prepare for, respond to, and recover from domestic incidents, regardless of cause, size, or complexity. To provide for interoperability and compatibility among Federal, State, and local capabilities, the NIMS will include a core set of concepts, principles, terminology, and technologies covering the incident command system; multiagency coordination systems; unified command; training; identification and management of resources (including systems for classifying types of resources); qualifications and certification; and the collection, tracking, and reporting of incident information and incident resources.

During the NIMS development process, several other HSPDs were issued that have helped to refine the concepts that were eventually incorporated into the final NIMS document, which was originally issued on March 1, 2004.

HSPD-7 is a comprehensive document that prioritizes critical infrastructures and key resources. In addition to defining specific critical infrastructure components, it also establishes a broad range of specific responsibilities for the **US Department of Homeland Security (DHS)** and other federal agencies with specific authorities. This is critical to the NIMS because it provides for the protection of critical assets that will be employed to successfully implement the NIMS within local, state, and federal organizations.

HSPD-7 requires that command facilities, such as Emergency Operations Centers (EOCs), dispatch centers, and response stations and precincts, must be identified and protected. Efforts are made to enhance key resource protection, or hardening. Organizations are to develop uniform policies, procedures, and guidelines.

According to HSPD-7, communications and information technology are defined as critical infrastructure. Federal agencies are required to assist in the accomplishment of critical infrastructure protection guidelines, and federal agencies must collaborate with the private sector.

HSPD-8 establishes preparedness policies for prevention and response to terrorist attacks and major disasters. This policy specifies a need for "all-hazard preparedness." Preparedness goals for federal agencies are specified, as are requirements for the support of state and local first responders. Several key requirements related to funding and support of planning, preparedness, mitigation, and response activities directly impact local and state response agencies.

Concepts and Principles of NIMS

Every hour of every day thousands of people in the United States call for assistance. The process of living creates emergency incidents that require the response of local agencies to assist citizens, such as robberies, automobile collisions, fires, flooding, medical emergencies, electrical outages, industrial accidents, viruses, or roadways blocked by downed trees. The vast majority of these incidents are successfully resolved with local resources, but some require a larger commitment than a local community can provide. Others, though infrequent, require the involvement of multiple agencies at many levels of government and from a broad range of disciplines. NIMS provides a scalable methodology that can be applied to incidents involving a single local jurisdiction and a single response discipline (such as a bank robbery and associated area search) to incidents as complex and challenging as those experienced on September 11, 2001, in New York, Virginia, and Pennsylvania.

Tip
The most important word in the title of the National Incident Management System is *system*. It is also the most often overlooked word. Many participants in the emergency response community assume that NIMS is simply the new version of the Incident Command System (ICS), but it is much more. NIMS incorporates all of the aspects of preparing for and managing incidents. These include command and management (which includes an ICS), as well as preparedness, resource management, communications and information management, supporting technologies, and ongoing management and maintenance.

NIMS is based on the premise that utilization of a common incident management framework will give emergency management/response personnel a flexible but standardized system for emergency management and incident response activities. NIMS is flexible because the system components can be utilized to develop plans, processes, procedures, agreements, and roles for all types of incidents; it is applicable to any incident regardless of cause, size, location, or complexity. Additionally, NIMS provides an organized set of standardized operational structures, which is critical in allowing disparate organizations and agencies to work together in a predictable, coordinated manner.

Flexibility

The components of NIMS are adaptable for any situation, from routine, local incidents to larger-scale incidents requiring the activation of interstate mutual aid to those requiring a coordinated federal response, whether planned (e.g., a major sporting or community event), notice (e.g., hurricane), or no-notice (e.g., earthquake). This flexibility is essential for NIMS to be applicable across the full spectrum of potential incidents, including those that require multiagency, multijurisdictional (such as incidents that occur along international borders), and/or multidisciplinary coordination. The inherent flexibility provided by the NIMS framework facilitates scalability of emergency management and incident response activities. NIMS also provides the flexibility for unique implementation in specified areas around the nation. When appropriate, the National Integration Center (NIC) will review and support implementation plans, which reflect these individual requirements and organizational structures, to ensure consistency with NIMS concepts and principles.

Standardization

The flexibility to manage incidents of any size requires coordination and standardization among emergency management/response personnel and their affiliated organizations. NIMS provides a set of standardized organizational structures that improve integration and connectivity among jurisdictions and disciplines, starting with a common foundation of preparedness and planning. Personnel and organizations that have adopted the common NIMS framework are able to work together, thereby fostering cohesion among the various organizations involved in all aspects of an incident. NIMS also provides and promotes common terminology, which fosters more effective communication among agencies and organizations responding together to an incident.

Overview of NIMS Components

NIMS integrates existing best practices into a consistent, nationwide, systematic approach to incident management that is applicable at all levels of government, nongovernmental organizations (NGOs), and the private sector, as well as across functional disciplines in an all-hazards context. Five major components make up this systems approach:

- Preparedness
- Communications and information management
- Resource management
- Command and management
- Ongoing management and maintenance

The components of NIMS were not designed to stand alone, but rather to work together in a flexible, systematic manner to provide the national framework for incident management. A more detailed discussion of each component is included in subsequent sections of this chapter.

Preparedness

Effective emergency management and incident response activities begin with a host of preparedness activities conducted on an ongoing basis, in advance of any potential incident. Preparedness involves an integrated combination of the following:

- Assessment
- Planning
- Procedures and protocols
- Training and exercises
- Personnel qualifications
- Licensure and certification
- Equipment certification
- Evaluation and revision

Communications and Information Management

Emergency management and incident response activities rely on communications and information systems that provide a common operating picture to all command and coordination sites. NIMS describes the requirements necessary for a standardized framework for communications and emphasizes the need for a common operating picture. This component is based on the concepts of interoperability, reliability, scalability, and portability, as well as the resiliency and redundancy of communications and information systems.

Resource Management

Resources (such as personnel, equipment, or supplies) are needed to support critical incident objectives. The flow of resources must be fluid and adaptable to the requirements of the incident. NIMS defines standardized mechanisms and establishes the resource management process to identify requirements then order and acquire, mobilize, track and report, recover and demobilize, reimburse, and inventory resources.

Command and Management

The command and management component of NIMS is designed to enable effective and efficient incident management and coordination by providing a flexible, standardized incident management structure **(Figure 1-1)**. The structure is based on three key organizational constructs:

- Incident command system
- Multiagency coordination systems
- Public information

Ongoing Management and Maintenance

Within the auspices of ongoing management and maintenance, there are two components: the NIC and supporting technologies.

National Integration Center

HSPD-5 required the secretary of DHS to establish a mechanism for ensuring the ongoing management and maintenance of NIMS, including regular consultation with other federal departments and agencies; state, tribal, and local stakeholders; NGOs; and the private sector.

The NIC provides strategic direction, oversight, and coordination of NIMS and supports both routine maintenance and the continuous refinement of NIMS and its components. The NIC oversees the program and coordinates with federal, state, tribal, and local partners in the development of compliance criteria and implementation activities. It provides guidance and support to jurisdictions and emergency management/response personnel and their affiliated organizations as they adopt or are encouraged to adopt the system, depending on their status. The NIC also oversees and coordinates the publication of NIMS and its related products. This oversight includes the review and certification of training courses and exercise information.

Supporting Technologies

As NIMS and its related emergency management and incident response systems evolve, emergency management/response personnel will increasingly rely on technology and systems to implement and continuously refine NIMS. The NIC, in partnership with the DHS Science and Technology Directorate, oversees and coordinates the ongoing development of incident management-related technology, including strategic research and development.

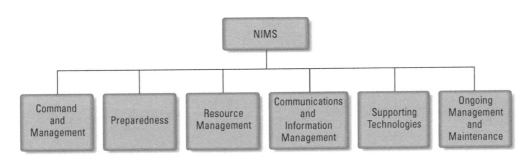

Figure 1-1 Components of NIMS.

Rural Case Study *Answers*

1. Because of the scope of the damage and the potential loss of life, the response to this incident will be large and complex and require the coordination of multiple agencies, jurisdictions, and disciplines. This incident is perfectly suited for the use of an incident management system.

2. The following agencies and disciplines will likely be involved in the response:
   - Fire department
   - Law enforcement
   - EMS
   - Emergency management
   - Public works
   - Utilities
   - Coroner or medical examiner
   - Rescue teams
   - HazMat personnel
   - Human services agencies

Urban Case Study *Answers*

1. Initially the police department would respond. EMS would respond if there is a report of injuries associated with the collision.

2. In addition to fire, police, and EMS services, consider the jurisdiction and responsibility of transportation departments, the railroad, and the trucking company involved in the incident.

Wrap-Up

Summary

- NIMS is the national model for an incident management system that is applicable across jurisdictions and disciplines and is functional for all hazards.
- NIMS was developed after looking at lessons learned from major incident responses, especially those related to the events of September 11, 2001.
- HSPD-5 is the basis for the development of NIMS, and it establishes the DHS as the agency responsible for domestic incident management.
- NIMS consists of five components:
  - Preparedness
  - Communications and information management
  - Resource management
  - Command and management
  - Ongoing management and maintenance

Glossary

New normalcy: Developed by the Advisory Panel to Assess Domestic Response Capabilities for Terrorism Involving Weapons of Mass Destruction (commonly known as the Gilmore Commission), this concept calls upon the United States to develop a new, higher level of preparedness and attentiveness.

US Department of Homeland Security (DHS): The federal agency tasked with all aspects of domestic incident management.

Substantial floods have inundated central Virginia. Dozens of low water crossings are now under high volumes of water moving at extremely high rates of speed. Bridges not previously thought vulnerable to flooding are now under water. People are calling 911 to notify responders of people trapped in low water crossings or surrounded by rising flood waters. Fire, EMS, and police resources are responding to more than 20 swift-water rescue incidents throughout the area, and more than 20 additional incidents are holding with no resources available to respond.

1. Resources have been requested and are arriving from outside the impacted area. Which NIMS concept assists in making sure incident command clearly knows what it is requesting?
    A. Communications and information management
    B. Standardization
    C. Supporting technologies
    D. Flexibility

2. Incidents typically begin and end:
    A. at the federal level.
    B. with state government.
    C. locally.
    D. without a satisfactory solution.

3. What federal organization provides strategic direction, oversight, and coordination of NIMS and supports both routine maintenance and the continuous refinement of NIMS and its components?
    A. National ICS Education Institute
    B. National Integration Center
    C. National Fire Academy
    D. Homeland Security Advisory Council

CHAPTER 2

Integration of the Incident Command System

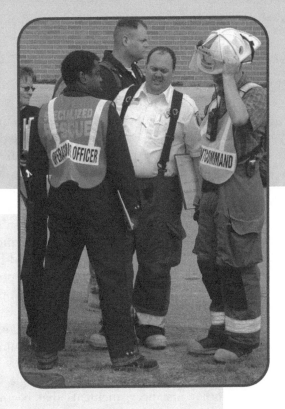

Rural Case Study

The damage caused to Stadtown by the tornado is substantial, and bystanders immediately begin approaching Deputy Williams with reports of injured parties at multiple locations. Several small fires and damage to dozens of buildings have also been reported. Other members of the emergency response forces are still responding or just arriving on the scene.

Remembering his recent Incident Command System (ICS) training, Deputy Williams established a command post at a local elementary school. He is joined there by representatives of Smith County EMS and the Stadtown Fire Department. The damage reports initially received from all sources confirm catastrophic damage to the town center. It is too early to have an accurate estimate of casualties.

1. What form should the initial command structure take? Is Unified Command (UC) appropriate? Why or why not?
2. What are the initial strategic objectives for this incident?
3. What safety issues need to be considered?
4. In addition to the command post, what other incident facilities should be considered?

Urban Case Study

Engine 2 is approaching the scene of the accident on Interstate 101 and has been advised that emergency medical services (EMS) and the police are responding as well. As Engine 2 nears the scene, it is clear that the initial call information is accurate and that the incident involves a freight train and a tractor-trailer. The silhouette of the truck indicates that it is a tanker.

The captain on Engine 2 directs that they stage upwind and uphill. Upon examining the scene with binoculars, a hazardous materials placard is identified on the tanker. The freight train does not have any hazardous materials cars; it was hauling gravel from a local quarry operation. Further examination via binoculars reveals that the driver of the tanker truck is still in the vehicle and does not appear to be moving. The captain of Engine 2 is unable to see any personnel from the train moving around the accident scene.

1. What steps should the captain of Engine 2 immediately take?
2. What are the immediate hazards in this situation?
3. In addition to EMS and police, what additional resources will be required based on this new information?

Introduction

The most familiar component of the National Incident Management System (NIMS) to most members of the public safety community is the **Incident Command System (ICS)**, a system for domestic incident management that is based on an expandable, flexible structure and that uses common terminology, positions, and incident facilities. This chapter will address the various components of ICS in sufficient detail to allow the user to integrate the specific modifications that NIMS has specified or implied by its structure and ongoing development. ICS, in order to be effective, depends on a common framework and common characteristics and definitions.

Most incidents are managed locally and are typically handled by local communications or dispatch centers and emergency management/response personnel within a single jurisdiction. In other instances, incidents that begin with a single response within a single jurisdiction rapidly expand to multidisciplinary, multijurisdictional levels requiring significant additional resources and operational support.

ICS provides a flexible core methodology for coordinated and collaborative incident management, whether an incident requires additional resources provided from different organizations within a single jurisdiction (multidisciplinary) or outside the jurisdiction (multijurisdictional), or for complex incidents with national implications (such as an emerging infectious disease or a bioterrorism attack).

When a single incident covers a large geographical area, multiple local emergency management and incident response agencies may be required. The responding agencies are defined as the governmental agencies, though in certain circumstances nongovernmental organizations (NGOs) and private-sector organizations may be included, such as the American Red Cross, utility companies, the Salvation Army, construction organizations, etc. Effective cross-jurisdictional coordination using processes and systems is absolutely critical in this situation.

ICS is used to organize on-scene operations for a broad spectrum of emergencies from small to complex incidents, both natural and manmade. The field response level is where emergency management/response personnel, under the command of an appropriate authority, carry out tactical decisions and activities in direct response to an incident or threat. Resources from the federal, state, tribal, or local levels, when appropriately deployed, become part of the field ICS as prescribed by the local authority.

As a system, ICS is extremely useful; not only does it provide an organizational structure for incident management, but it also guides the process for planning, building, and adapting that structure. Using ICS for every incident or planned event helps hone and maintain skills needed for the large-scale incidents.

ICS is used by all levels of government—federal, state, tribal, and local—as well as by many NGOs and the private sector. ICS is also applicable across disciplines. It is normally structured to facilitate activities in five major functional areas:

- Command
- Operations
- Planning
- Logistics
- Finance/Administration

Intelligence/Investigations is an optional sixth functional area that is activated on a case-by-case basis.

Acts of biological, chemical, radiological, and nuclear terrorism may present unique challenges for the traditional ICS structure. Incidents that are not site specific, are geographically dispersed, or evolve over longer periods of time will require extraordinary coordination among all participants. The concept of **Area Command** will help organizations begin thinking about how to organize a response of this type and incorporate the various governmental authorities and jurisdictions in a collaborative incident management construct.

Area Command

Area Command is an organization to oversee the management of multiple incidents handled individually by separate ICS organizations or to oversee the management of a very large or evolving incident engaging multiple Incident Management Teams (IMTs). An Agency Administrator/Executive or other public official with jurisdictional responsibility for the incident usually makes the decision to establish an Area Command. An Area Command is activated only if necessary, depending on the complexity of the incident and incident management span-of-control considerations.

Area Commands are particularly relevant to incidents that are typically not site specific, are not immediately identifiable, are geographically dispersed, and evolve over longer periods of time (e.g., public health emergencies, earthquakes, tornadoes, civil disturbances, and any geographic area where several IMTs are being used and these incidents are all requesting similar resources). Incidents such as these, as well as acts of biological, chemical, radiological, and nuclear terrorism, require a coordinated intergovernmental, NGO, and private-sector response, with large-scale coordination typically conducted at a higher jurisdictional level. Area Command is also used when a number of incidents of the same type in the same area are competing for the same resources, such as multiple hazardous material incidents, spills, or fires.

When incidents are of different types and/or do not have similar resource demands, they are usually handled as separate incidents or are coordinated through an Emergency Operations Center (EOC) or Multiagency Coordination Group (MAC Group). If the incidents under the authority of the Area Command span multiple jurisdictions, a Unified Area Command should be established **(Figure 2-1)**. This allows each jurisdiction to have appropriate representation in the Area Command.

Area Command should not be confused with the functions performed by Multiagency Coordination System(s) (MACS): Area Command oversees management coordination of the incident(s), while a MACS element, such as a communications/dispatch center, EOC, or MAC Group, coordinates support.

Management Characteristics of ICS

ICS bases its well-proven structure on a series of common management characteristics. These charac-

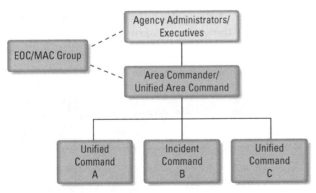

The dotted line connecting EOC/MAC Group with the Agency Administrators/Executives and Area Commander/Unified Area Command represents the coordination and communication link between an EOC/MAC Group and the Command structure.

Figure 2-1 Chain of command and reporting relationships.

teristics enable ICS to function in a consistent manner across geographic areas, disciplines, and incident sizes. Clearly, this aspect of ICS is critical to the effective function of NIMS from a truly nationwide perspective.

Common Terminology

Like any system or profession, the effective use of ICS depends on clear communication. This communication is facilitated by common terminology that has long been a key aspect of ICS. NIMS incorporates the vocabulary of ICS, allowing those familiar with it to function comfortably. Those unfamiliar with ICS prior to being introduced to NIMS need to learn and use this terminology in order to operate with other organizations involved in the management of an incident. Like any language, the routine use of terminology during normal operations will make it much easier to incorporate the language during a stressful incident response.

> ### Tip
>
> The use of clear language during all radio communications is critical. Many organizations continue to use various code systems for communications, which can be very problematic during multiagency and multidisciplinary incidents. Although many of these code systems are well established, organizations should adopt a clear-text standard and eliminate the use of code systems as part of implementing NIMS.
>
> Common terminology also serves to alleviate the impact of geographic differences as well as language and cultural issues that often adversely impact communication, particularly in high-stress situations. The use of a common set of terms and definitions also helps to ensure that diverse incident management and support entities are able to work together in a wide variety of incident management functions and hazard scenarios.

Organizational Functions

Major functions and functional units with domestic incident management responsibilities are named and defined by NIMS. Terminology for the organizational elements involved is standard and consistent. Examples of such functions and functional units include the following:

- Command
- Operations
- Logistics

- Groups
- Divisions
- Leaders
- Supervisors

Resource Descriptions

Major resources—including personnel and teams; facilities; special capability assets, such as Urban Search and Rescue Teams (USAR); and major equipment and supply items (e.g., fire engines, ambulances, law enforcement units, electric utility restoration equipment, and personnel specializing in managing donations)—used to support incident management activities are given common names and are typed or classified with respect to their capabilities to help avoid confusion and to enhance interoperability. The process for accomplishing this task is specified in Chapter 12.

The most current list of federally recognized resource-typing definitions is available from DHS/FEMA on the National Integration Center Web site. Eventually, all types of potential public safety and public works resources will be included in this system to allow incident management personnel to order exactly what they require. The detail of the system is well illustrated in the classification/typing system for ground ambulances (Table 2-1).

Incident Facilities

Common terminology is used to designate the facilities in the vicinity of the incident area that will be used in the course of incident management activities. These can include the **Incident Command Post**, the location where the Incident Command or Unified Command manages an incident; a **staging area**, the location in which resources assigned to an incident but not yet deployed are held ready; or a **treatment area**, a fixed location arranged for the collection and treatment of patients at a mass casualty incident.

Modular Organization

The ICS organizational structure typically develops in a top–down modular fashion that is based on the size and complexity of the incident, as well as the specifics of the hazard environment created by the incident. When needed, separate functional elements can be established, each of which may further be subdivided to enhance internal organizational management and external coordination. Responsibility for the establishment and expansion of the ICS modular organization ultimately rests with **Incident Command (IC)**.

IC deploys specific structures based on the nature of the incident. As incident complexity increases, and therefore as the incident management organization complexity increases, the organization expands from the top down as functional responsibilities are delegated. Although this expansion is characterized as top down, it is important to remember that ICS expands both horizontally and vertically during the course of the incident. Concurrently with structural expansion, the number of management positions expands to adequately address the requirements of the incident. NIMS has not modified this approach, but it does require incident command personnel to broaden their concept of what the ICS organizational structure might incorporate, especially in terms of new types of response functions across a far broader realm of disciplines and specialties (e.g., public works professionals, utilities management organizations, responsible parties, and transportation organizations).

Figure 2-2 illustrates a **Unified Command (UC)** for a structure fire with significant patients, and the fire is creating substantial traffic issues. UC is established with fire suppression, EMS, and law enforcement branches that manage both the strategic and tactical objectives of the incident. This branching structure

Table 2-1 Classification System for Ground Ambulances

Resource Type	Ambulance (Ground)	Minimum Staff	Minimum HazMat Status
Type I	Advanced Life Support (ALS)	1 EMT, 1 Paramedic	HazMat Level B capable
Type II	ALS	1 EMT, 1 Paramedic	Non-HazMat response
Type III	Basic Life Support (BLS)	2 EMTs	HazMat Level B capable
Type IV	BLS	2 EMTs	Non-HazMat response
Other	Nontransporting (EMS response resources)	1 BLS or ALS responder	Non-HazMat response

Note: Ambulances may be categorized as health and medical. They may be designated team, equipment, personnel, supplies, or vehicle.

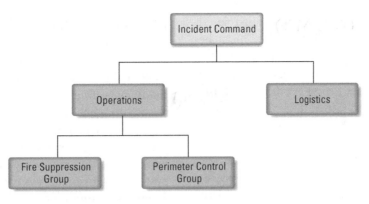

Figure 2-2 Simple ICS structure.

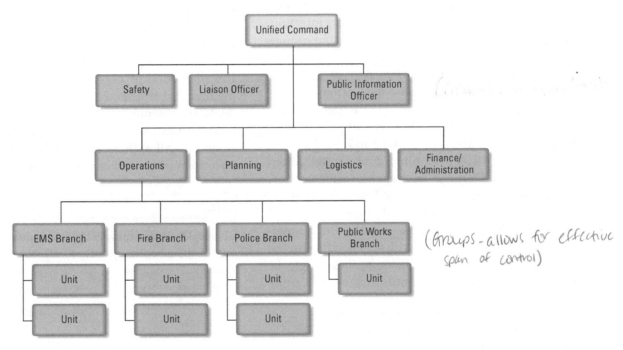

(Groups - allows for effective span of control)

Figure 2-3 Complex ICS structure. *Note:* Sectors are usually called groups or divisions in the wildland-fire model.

is a common use of ICS with UC and is frequently used by organizations during routine operations. In this example, the responsibility for operations is assigned to a single Operations Section Chief (Fire) who is appointed by the UC group, and the specific tactical issues are handled by the Branch Directors in the fire suppression, EMS, and law enforcement branches. This ability to customize the ICS system, while maintaining the consistent use of appropriate terminology, demonstrates the flexibility inherent in the ICS system.

Figure 2-3 illustrates a complex UC structure for a major incident. All **General Staff** positions are filled, and the organization has expanded both vertically (the introduction of operations and logistics) and horizontally (the use of groups to maintain an effec-

tive span of control). This type of structure would typically be used for a large, long-term incident, such as the response to the Pentagon or the World Trade Center incidents on September 11, 2001, or a large wildfire response operation. The full deployment of ICS helps to ensure that all incident needs are met in an organized manner, and the structure allows the incident objectives to be met consistently between operational periods.

Management by Objectives

Management by objectives represents an approach to defining actions related to managing an incident that is communicated throughout the entire ICS organization. IC begins the process by establishing overarching or strategic incident objectives (e.g., evacuate, triage, treat, and transport all incident-related victims). When these are established, they must be communicated to the General Staff, which includes the Operations Section Chief, the Logistics Section Chief, the Finance/Administration Section Chief, the Planning Section Chief, and the Intelligence/Investigations Section Chief in a major law enforcement incident.

Operations has the task of translating strategic objectives into specific, measurable tactical objectives (e.g., evacuate all casualties from the incident scene to the triage area in 15 minutes using evacuation teams). Tactical objectives are then further developed into specific assignments and plans. This can be done at any level of the ICS organization, depending on specific assignments, roles, and responsibilities. An example is directing police officers to secure a specific intersection as part of a specific tactical objective to secure an outer perimeter.

The last component of the management-by-objectives approach is documenting results to measure performance and making indicated corrective actions. This is most often done through after-action reports. During a longer-term incident, these specific actions may be translated into the strategic and tactical objectives during the next operational period, or sooner if activities are judged to be ineffective in achieving the objectives. Depending on the size and complexity of the incident, these might be completed internally or by an outside organization.

Reliance on an Incident Action Plan

Incident Action Plans (IAPs) are oral or written plans containing general objectives reflecting the overall strategy for managing an incident. Drafted by the Planning Section Chief, the IAP provides a coherent means of communicating the overall incident objectives in the contexts of both operational and support activities (see Appendix D: ICS Form 202 Incident Objectives).

Generally, the IAP includes a summary of the incident details (usually including a simple incident map) and current actions. The IAP also includes established incident objectives, a communications plan (how various aspects of the incident command organization will communicate with one another), specific ICS organizational/position assignments (e.g., who is assigned as the Operations Section Chief), incident safety information, and an incident medical plan, if appropriate. A detailed description of the IAP, including its specific components, is included in Chapter 5.

Manageable Span of Control

Span of control is a key concept within the structure of the ICS system. Span of control recognizes that each ICS supervisor or manager has a limit to how many personnel he or she can effectively manage. Based on general business management concepts, this number has been set at between five and seven direct reports. A span of control of three or four is appropriate for emergency operations. The use of ICS system expansion allows the IC/UC to maintain these numbers throughout the organization. Although this number is generally accepted, each situation is unique, and a specific supervisor may be responsible for a greater number of individuals when similar resources perform similar functions (e.g., police officers managing the perimeter of a large crime scene). It is important to remember that like all of ICS, this concept needs to be applied in a flexible manner that is sensitive to the specific type of incident, the nature of the task, hazards and safety factors, and the distance between personnel and resources. All of these factors can substantially influence span-of-control considerations.

Tip

Examples of Manageable Span of Control
In ICS, the span of control of any individual with incident management supervisory responsibility should range from 3 to 7 subordinates, with 5 being optimal. During a large-scale law enforcement operation, 8 to 10 subordinates may be optimal.

Predesignated Incident Locations and Facilities

Various types of operational locations and support facilities are established in the vicinity of an incident to accomplish a variety of purposes, such as decontamination, donated goods processing, mass care, and evacuation. The IC/UC will direct the identification and location of facilities based on the requirements of the situation at hand. Typical predesignated facilities include Incident Command Posts, staging areas, mass casualty triage areas, and others, as required.

Comprehensive Resource Management

Successful incident management depends on ensuring that the status and availability of resources is constantly updated and accurate. For example: Is a needed Type I Fire Engine Strike Team (defined as five Type I Fire Engines) located in staging, or is it out of service? When did it arrive at the incident location? When was the team assigned a task? When was the task completed? All of these questions are important to understanding the status of your incident management resources, and the answers are provided through an effective, comprehensive resource management system.

Recognizing the importance of this function, the ICS has developed comprehensive systems for managing resources (defined as personnel, teams, equipment, supplies, and facilities) that are available or potentially available for assignment or allocation in support of incident management and emergency response activities. Resource management also includes processes specific to how resources are requested, staged, deployed, demobilized, and accounted for in terms of reimbursement and incident recordkeeping. To make this system work, each resource that arrives on an incident should be required to report its status to the supervisor to which it is assigned. It is then the responsibility of the specific supervisors to provide updated status information on all assigned resources to the ICS management structure. This process allows for the development of a comprehensive and complete picture of incident resources.

Integrated Communications

Incident communications is one of the most difficult aspects of successful incident management. It requires organizations, jurisdictions, and personnel to integrate and invest in new communications infrastructures and to develop communications policies and plans that enable integrated information exchange among operational and support units. Preparedness planning must address the equipment, systems, and protocols necessary to achieve integrated voice and data incident management communications.

Tip

The development of an incident communications plan should be a high priority as the ICS structure is expanded. The needs of command and supervisory personnel to communicate effectively while allowing the units performing the specific tasks to have tactical communications channels requires the careful delegation of communications infrastructure. In some cases, too much communication can be as problematic as too little.

The effective use of ICS also requires that organizations think about the development of effective communications plans for both routine and major incidents. This area is frequently overlooked when developing IAPs and can substantially impact the success of the incident management effort.

Establishment and Transfer of Command

To be effective, the Command function (the individual or individuals who have the leadership responsibility for managing an incident) needs to be clearly established from the initiation of incident operations. Failure to do so can substantially affect an incident in a negative manner. The agency or agencies with jurisdictional authority over an incident designate the individual(s) at the scene who are responsible for establishing command. It is critical for local jurisdictions to clearly define this expectation and the processes associated with it so that all ICS participants clearly understand their responsibilities.

When command is transferred, the process must include a briefing that captures all essential information for continuing safe and effective operations. The effective use of IAPs can substantially ease the difficulties associated with the transfer of command, especially during extended incidents with multiple operational periods. During the response to the World Trade Center attacks, the use of IAPs ensured that ongoing search and rescue operations were coordinated from one shift of search personnel to the next. This helped eliminate the problem of searching the same area several times, especially as the appearance of the site changed due to removal of debris layers.

Effective IAPs are key planning and operational tools for long-term incidents and allow for continuity between IC/UC personnel from one shift to the next and for the maintenance of an overall incident management strategic plan.

Chain of Command and Unity of Command

Chain of command simply means that there is a clear line of authority within the structure of the ICS organization. Operations reports to Command, the triage group reports to the medical branch, and each supervisory member of the ICS organization clearly understands to whom they report and who provides them with their tactical objectives. Unity of command means that every individual has one, and only one, supervisor at the scene of the incident.

Unified Command

As implied earlier, many incidents involve the overlap of jurisdictional authority due to functional areas, legal authority, geography, or other factors. This realization, probably the most important in the evolution of ICS, has resulted in the development of the UC concept.

Unless otherwise defined by local protocol or agreement, UC should be used in incidents involving multiple jurisdictions, a single jurisdiction with multiagency involvement, or multiple jurisdictions with multiagency involvement. In many jurisdictions, the majority of incidents meet one of these criteria.

The strength of UC is that it allows agencies with different legal, geographic, and functional authorities and responsibilities to work together effectively without affecting individual agency authority, responsibility, or accountability. Like the rest of the ICS, the effective use of UC depends on its routine use and a strong relationship among personnel who are likely to assume command roles.

Tip

Integrating UC into local operations can be a challenge. Consider setting up a regular opportunity for command personnel from different organizations to meet and get to know one another in a setting without a specific agenda or purpose (such as a routine lunch or breakfast meeting). When personnel become familiar with one another, the concept of working together in a UC environment becomes much easier to understand and accept.

Accountability

Incident safety depends on the use of an effective personnel and resource accountability system. To achieve and implement an accountability system, several key components and processes must be incorporated into the system. First, resources must be checked in when they arrive in the staging area or with their supervisor when they are assigned a specific function. Second, resources should be deployed in coordination with specific tactical objectives or tasks associated with the IAP. To ensure unity of command, each resource must know to which supervisor he or she is accountable. In addition, resources must be deployed within a span of control that allows supervisory personnel to maintain knowledge of resource location and operations. The development of new systems to ease and automate this process is an area of ongoing development and is a substantial portion of the supporting technologies initiatives within NIMS.

Deployment

Personnel and equipment should respond only when requested or when dispatched by an appropriate authority. Unfortunately, public safety personnel and others continue to respond to incidents without being requested. Although in many cases the intent of these individuals is admirable, they can create substantial challenges for the ICS structure and may compromise the safety of incident victims, other responders, or themselves.

Information and Intelligence/Investigations Management

NIMS has added a new focus to this area of the ICS structure. Though information management has always been a part of ICS, the addition of new technologies and the ability to display information in real time has made information management and display an evolving specialty within ICS. The integration of a comprehensive intelligence function, though common in law enforcement ICS operations, is now recognized as critically important to all response disciplines, especially during incidents potentially linked to terrorism. Not only does this function support the effective conduct of incident operations, it also can directly impact personnel safety.

INCIDENT OBJECTIVES	1. INCIDENT NAME	2. DATE	3. TIME
Determine immediate resource needs to save lives and prevent further harm	Stadtown Flood	9-15-2009	1630 hours

4. OPERATIONAL PERIOD (DATE/TIME)
9-15-2009/1630 to 2230 hours

5. GENERAL CONTROL OBJECTIVES FOR THE INCIDENT (INCLUDE ALTERNATIVES)

Determine resource availability for rescue and life saving. Assign resources currently available for immediate operations and deploy under the ICS structure. Determine resource requirements not available and make requests through mutual aid system via the EOC.

6. WEATHER FORECAST FOR OPERATIONAL PERIOD
Light rain subsiding into the evening and night with temps in the low 60s and mild winds from the west.

7. GENERAL SAFETY MESSAGE
All personnel working in the rescue zone must wear life preservers and work in teams of four.

8. ATTACHMENTS (☑ if attached)

☐ Organization List (ICS 203)　　☐ Medical Plan (ICS 206)　　☐　Weather Forecast

☐ Assignment List (ICS 204)　　☐ Incident Map　　☐ _____

☐ Communications Plan (ICS 205)　　☐ Traffic Plan　　☐ _____

9. PREPARED BY (PLANNING SECTION CHIEF)	10. APPROVED BY (INCIDENT COMMANDER)
Assistant Chief Jones	

Figure 2-4 ICS form 202: sample incident objectives.

Rural Case Study *Answers*

1. UC is appropriate because the strategic incident objectives involve multiple agencies **(Figure 2-4)**. Additionally, the care of casualties, the conduct of search and rescue operations, and the securing of perimeters and access and egress routes is the responsibility of different agencies.
2. The initial strategic objectives include the following: perform search and rescue operations, identify and evacuate casualties, treat and transport casualties, secure an incident perimeter, secure hazardous materials and threats, and ensure responder safety.
3. Safety considerations may include ongoing weather threats, debris, normal biohazard issues, traffic safety issues, building collapses, fall hazards, and loose animals.
4. In addition to the command post, incident facilities such as staging, casualty collection points, transport areas, treatment areas, logistics, and morgues need to be considered in this scenario.

Urban Case Study *Answers*

1. The captain should assume the Fire Command, advise other incoming response agencies and units of the hazards, and suggest a safe staging location.
2. The immediate hazards include the following: hazardous materials leakage, the potential for fire/explosion, and the impact of the hazardous materials on victims downwind and downhill. Additionally, the train poses specific hazards that need to be addressed.
3. The following additional resources should be considered: a hazardous materials team, environmental protection personnel, emergency management if evacuation is being considered, and health personnel due to the possible effects of hazardous materials on victims.

Wrap-Up

Summary

- NIMS incorporates the previously established components of the ICS, making them a cornerstone of domestic incident management.
- The components of the ICS have not been substantially altered by NIMS. Instead, a focus on integrated incident management (illustrated by the UC concept) has been added.
- The ICS is based on specific, well-defined management characteristics. These characteristics include such things as common terminology, a modular organization structure, management by objectives, integrated communications, and unity of command, among others.

Glossary

Area Command: An organization established to oversee the management of either multiple incidents that are each being handled by an Incident Command System organization or one large incident that has multiple Incident Management Teams assigned to it.

General Staff: Consists of the following Incident Command System positions: the Operations Section Chief, the Logistics Section Chief, the Planning Section Chief, the Finance/Administration Section Chief, and possibly an Intelligence/Investigations Section Chief.

Incident Action Plan (IAP): A formal document that includes several components and provides a coherent means of communicating overall incident objectives in the contexts of both operational and support activities. The most important section is the incident objectives. An IAP is often verbal during fast-moving tactical events.

Incident Command (IC): The Incident Command System position responsible for overall incident management. This person establishes all strategic incident objectives and ensures that those objectives are carried out effectively.

Incident Command Post: The location from which Incident Command manages the incident. The command post should be easily identified and its location known to all responding resources.

Incident Command System (ICS): A system for domestic incident management that is based on an expandable, flexible structure and that uses common terminology, positions, and incident facilities.

Staging area: The location at which resources assigned to an incident are held until they are assigned to a specific function.

Treatment area: An incident facility that is used as a location for the collection and treatment of patients prior to transport; typically organized according to patient status.

Unified Command (UC): The command structure in which multiple individuals are cooperatively responsible for all the strategic objectives of the incident; typically used when an incident is within multiple jurisdictions or is managed by multiple disciplines.

Wrap-Up Case Study

A large river-barge convoy has struck the support structure of a main highway bridge over the Mississippi River. The initial emergency response to the incident has been completed, and the scene has been turned over to the State Department of Transportation. A substantial amount of work needs to be done to eventually return the freeway to full operation.

The District Manager is responsible for the restoration of function after the impact. This is the largest emergency project she has ever encountered, and she is getting substantial pressure from the State Transportation Board. She has already received phone calls from the governor's office, among others, requesting her estimate of when the bridge will reopen.

1. Which components of the ICS General Staff will be most helpful in organizing this project?
    A. Finance/Administration
    B. Logistics
    C. Safety
    D. Both A and B
2. Based on the situation presented, in which section of ICS would you place a Damage Assessment Unit?
    A. Planning
    B. Liaison
    C. Operations
    D. Logistics
3. The decision is made to operate the reconstruction project around the clock using an 8-hour operational period. Who is responsible for developing the IAP?
    A. Command
    B. Operations
    C. Planning
    D. A, B, and C

CHAPTER 3

Command

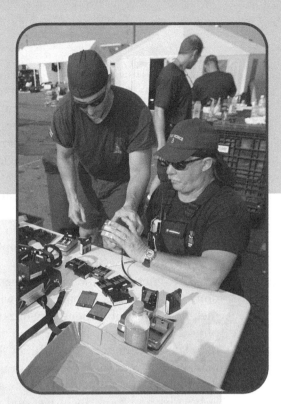

Rural Case Study

Deputy Williams, along with representatives from emergency medical services (EMS) and the Stadtown Fire Department, establishes a Unified Command (UC) structure and announces the location of the command post to all responding units. To provide some order to the ongoing operations, each member of the UC group gives a brief summary of what he or she knows and what activities are underway. After each organization completes its initial report, the three UC Agency Representatives take a deep breath and realize they are dealing with an incident far larger than any of them have ever encountered. They realize that they need to craft an informal initial Incident Action Plan (IAP).

1. At this point in the incident, what are the specific responsibilities of each organization?
2. Now that the UC has been established, what Incident Command System (ICS) position should be filled? Why?
3. Why is UC the most appropriate command structure for this incident?

Urban Case Study

Battalion 1, Ladder Truck-10 (Pleasantville Fire Department), and EMS unit 200 (Pleasantville EMS) have arrived on the scene of the accident. At this point in the incident, one victim is visible, and the presence of a highly lethal hazardous material is indicated. The captain of Engine 2 provides the Command Staff with an initial briefing.

The command group analyzes the initial information and begins discussions related to incident organization and structure. The incident takes place completely within the jurisdiction of the City of Pleasantville, although a chemical plume could potentially involve territory in the unincorporated areas of the county as well as the city of Metro.

1. Based on your knowledge of the incident, what command structure would you choose? Why?
2. What are the strategic incident objectives at this point?
3. When does this incident evolve from a single-jurisdiction to a multijurisdiction event?

Introduction

In 2003, the National Incident Management System (NIMS) signaled the need for a change in the culture of command. Organizations throughout the public safety community began to realize that a silo-based approach to incident management and, particularly, how the structure of the Command function was managed required a substantial shift in organizational culture. With the 2008 revision of the NIMS, the US Department of Homeland Security (DHS) has continued to ask all response agencies to take an inclusive approach to the deployment and use of ICS. The days of a singular dedication to a lone Incident Commander, especially in complex multijurisdictional and/or multidisciplinary incidents, are long past. This singular focus, often represented by different agencies at the same scene that are using ICS but are not operating in a unified manner, is an incident management approach that can no longer be sustained due to the diverse and complex threats that face the response community.

The intent of NIMS is to open the doors to domestic incident management wide enough to include a range of response organizations and disciplines that is much broader than previously contemplated. Although the core of initial incident management most often consists of the public safety disciplines—law enforcement, EMS, and fire—NIMS is broader and more inclusive, and the use of ICS must be as well. Although public safety often thinks that incidents end when their role is complete, members of the emergency management community, as well as public works, public health, and utilities, know that incidents frequently are measured not in hours or days, but in weeks or months.

This new culture of domestic incident management must be characterized by an approach that contemplates the use of NIMS and the incident command function from an end-to-end perspective. This includes the more consistent use of a UC approach in any incident that includes either multiple jurisdictions or multiple disciplines. In today's environment, it is clear that this constitutes the vast majority of responses and indicates that all response disciplines need to consider a UC methodology as the common response configuration. Incident Command (IC) personnel from all response organizations must operate from the perspective that UC is indicated until it is clearly defined that an incident is singular in both jurisdiction and discipline **(Table 3-1)**.

Command and General Staff Overview

To effectively manage incidents, the ICS organization depends on five major functions: Command, Operations, Planning, Logistics, and Finance/ Administration. A sixth function—Intelligence/ Investigations—may be added at the direction of Command **(Figure 3-1)**. Detailed information about Command, including the associated Command Staff positions, is included in this chapter. The remaining General Staff positions are discussed in their own chapters later in the text.

In brief terms, Operations is responsible for the actual activities directly related to the management of the tactical incident objectives. Planning, as the name implies, is responsible for developing IAPs, maintaining an accurate situation status, and coordinating resource and technical support activities. Logistics is responsible for food, water, supplies, lodging, and equipment; this function is often the most underappreciated aspect of the General Staff. Finance/Administration manages the business aspects of ICS and is absolutely critical, especially

Table 3-1 Advantages of Using UC
■ A single set of objectives is developed for the entire incident.
■ A collective approach is used to develop strategies to achieve incident objectives.
■ Information flow and coordination are improved among all jurisdictions and agencies involved in the incident.
■ All agencies with responsibility for the incident have an understanding of joint priorities and restrictions.
■ No agency's legal authorities will be compromised or neglected.
■ The combined efforts of all agencies are optimized as they perform their respective assignments under a single IAP.

Source: National Incident Management System. US Department of Homeland Security. December 2008.

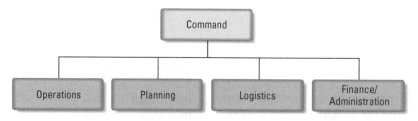

Figure 3-1 Command, Command Staff, and General Staff positions.

when organizations attempt to get reimbursement from state or federal disaster funds. The last component of the General Staff—Intelligence/Investigations—is new and is used in specific situations during which the collection and analysis of intelligence is of such importance that it drives substantial components of the incident management strategy and/or tactics.

Command

Structurally, Command comprises IC and the Command Staff. Command Staff is responsible for overall management of the incident. Command, although it is the chosen term of the ICS system, is perhaps misleading. It is important to remember that incidents are managed; personnel are commanded. IC, whether conducted by an individual or through UC, is a management and leadership position. IC is responsible for setting strategic objectives and maintaining a comprehensive understanding of the impact of an incident as well as identifying the strategies required to manage it effectively. The Command function is structured in one of two ways: single or unified **(Table 3-2)**.

Single Command

Single command is the most traditional representation of the command function and is the genesis of the term Incident Commander. When an incident occurs within a single jurisdiction, and when there is no jurisdictional or functional agency overlap, a single Incident Commander should be identified and designated with overall incident management responsibility. This designation is done by the appropriate jurisdictional authority. This does not mean that other agencies do not respond or do not have a role in supporting the management of the incident.

Single command is best used when a single discipline in a single jurisdiction is responsible for the strategic objectives associated with managing the incident. As an example, if a local EMS organization provides tactical paramedics to support the police special missions team, single command (e.g., the police department) is indicated during a tactical incident because EMS is not responsible for any of the strategic objectives. Single command also is appropriate in the later stages of an incident that was initially managed through UC. Over time, as many incidents stabilize, the strategic objectives become increasingly focused in a single jurisdiction or discipline. In this situation, it is appropriate to transition from UC to single command. This is best done during a transfer of command at a routine operational period transition, but it may be done anytime that the Command Staff feels it is appropriate.

> **Tip**
>
> Making changes in the command structure of a long-term incident is best done during the normal transfer of command that takes place between defined operational periods. This helps to ensure that all incident personnel are aware of the transition and that the General Staff Section Chiefs are comfortable with their new assignments and are aware of their correct supervisor.

It also is acceptable, if all agencies and jurisdictions agree, to designate a single Incident Commander in multiagency or multijurisdictional incidents. In this situation, however, Command personnel should be carefully chosen or predesignated to ensure that they understand the strategic issues important to each discipline or jurisdiction. A frequent and successful example of this approach is the use of defined Incident Management Teams (IMTs) that have highly skilled, experienced, credentialed Incident Commanders.

The Incident Commander is responsible for developing the strategic incident objectives on which the IAP will be based. The Incident Commander is responsible for approving the IAP and all requests pertaining to the ordering and release of incident resources.

Table 3-2 Single and Unified Command

Single Command

- A single Incident Commander has sole responsibility for establishing incident objectives and strategies.
- The single Incident Commander is directly responsible for ensuring that all functional areas and activities are focused on accomplishing the management strategy.

Unified Command

- There is a joint determination of incident objectives, strategies, plans, resource allocations, and priorities.
- Agencies/jurisdictions work together to execute integrated incident operations and maximize the use of assigned resources.
- Joint determinations are made by Section Chiefs (as indicated by incident scope).

Unified Command

Unified Command (UC) is a critical evolution of the ICS system that recognizes an important reality of incident management. The response to a multiagency or multijurisdictional incident is a routine occurrence. UC provides a framework that allows agencies with different legal, geographic, and functional responsibilities to coordinate, plan, and interact effectively. UC, through a consensus-based approach, addresses the challenges encountered nationwide when multiple organizations responding to the same incident establish separate, but concurrent, incident management structures. This approach leads to inefficiency and a duplication of effort that results in ineffective incident management, on-scene conflict, and substantial safety issues. UC is crafted specifically to address these issues.

The concept of UC is a clear departure from the traditional view of IC. Unfortunately, it is frequently misunderstood and difficult for some organizations to implement. To be effective in implementing UC, agencies and individuals need to worry less about the structural change and more about the changes required in organizational culture and interagency relationships. As incidents become increasingly complex, the probability of any one individual having the knowledge and expertise required to effectively develop, implement, and evaluate strategic objectives for a major incident decreases rapidly.

UC is effective in the early stages of incidents because it addresses a routine challenge. During the initial management of many incidents, the various strategic objectives (e.g., scene security, rescue, patient treatment, safety, etc.) are all critical and are all happening concurrently. Although several organizations have attempted to introduce the concept of *lead agency* into UC, it can prove ineffective, especially during the early phases. The concurrent nature of the strategic objectives would essentially require that the lead agency change from moment to moment. In truth, this results in no lead agency and a true unified approach. The lesson is to be concerned less with who is in charge and more with what is required to safely and effectively manage the incident.

The agencies or jurisdictions represented in the UC group, for the most part, depends on the nature of the incident and the geographic location. The incident nature not only indicates the types of disciplines involved, but it also may dictate the involvement of various levels of government agencies. For example, terrorism-related incidents would require the involvement of the Federal Bureau of Investigation (FBI),

and air transport incidents would involve the Federal Aviation Administration (FAA). Effective incident managers will use the flexibility inherent in the UC model to develop innovative, but effective, UC groups. For UC to be effective, the management of the incident depends on a collaborative process to establish incident objectives and designate priorities that accommodate those objectives.

NIMS states that UC functions as a single integrated management organization that involves the following:

- Colocated Command at the IC post
- One Operations Section Chief to direct tactical efforts
- Coordinated process for resource ordering
- Shared Planning, Logistics, and Finance/Administration functions wherever possible
- Coordinated approval of information releases

NIMS also states that all agencies in the UC structure contribute to the following processes:

- Selecting objectives
- Determining overall incident strategies
- Ensuring that joint planning for tactical activities is accomplished in accordance with approved incident objectives
- Ensuring the integration of tactical operations
- Approving, committing, and making optimum use of all assigned resources

UC, therefore, results in the development of a single set of integrated and prioritized incident objectives that form the basis of a single IAP. In many incidents (especially those that are multidisciplinary), the specific roles and responsibilities may be clear (e.g., investigation and security are the responsibility of law enforcement), but in multijurisdictional incidents, it may be much more complex. Consider, for example, an incident that results in a hazardous materials component in both a city and a county, both of which have hazardous materials response capabilities. Which HazMat team will manage that component of the incident?

Tip

Making UC work often depends on the relationships among agency Command Staffs. Although it is not always possible to know other agency commanders, consider organizing a routine lunch or breakfast that allows Command Staff to get to know one another in a nonstressful environment.

Other components of the system must be unified as well. Resource availability and capabilities have to be tracked and understood by all incident participants through the appropriate components of ICS. Limitations and safety issues also are critically important to all ICS components and must be clearly defined in the IAP. A unique component of the IAP in the UC environment is a clear statement of specific areas of agreement and, more importantly, disagreement among agency officials/representatives and the methods used to address the disagreements. The IAP should include an explanation of the strategy that will be used to resolve disagreements.

The use of UC also reinforces those other aspects of ICS that make it effective for managing incidents. Because Command utilizes the UC model, the incident is managed using a single organizational structure (limiting duplication and freeing more resources for overall incident management duties). This enhances the effectiveness and efficiency of incident management activities, especially in large-scale incidents with limited resources. UC also ensures that the incident will be managed from a single Incident Command Post (ICP). This helps to ensure that critical information, especially involving responder safety, is distributed quickly and effectively to all incident personnel. The lack of a UC post has been cited as a contributing factor in public safety deaths at disaster incidents. UC also allows for a single Planning section, which helps prevent multiple, redundant requests for similar items and the inefficient use of limited supplies and resources. A single Planning section also enhances the development of a comprehensive, unified IAP. When complete, the IAP is submitted to the UC for approval. UC also will appoint a single Operations Section Chief, typically with deputies representing key functional disciplines for the operational period.

The effective use of UC requires that responding organizations make a commitment to this concept. Although it is possible for UC to be effective when the Command personnel are unfamiliar with one another, it is substantially enhanced when organizations, particularly senior personnel, have taken the time to establish relationships prior to having to manage a large incident. The ability to combine the experience of multiple Command personnel and bring it to bear on complex problems is the most powerful tool organizations have to manage difficult, complex incidents.

Command Staff

Complementing and supporting the Command function (whether single or unified) are the members of the Command Staff. The filling of these positions is at the discretion of Command, and their responsibilities fall to Command if the positions are not filled. When filled, these positions report directly to IC and are assigned responsibility for key activities that are not a part of the ICS General Staff (i.e., Operations, Planning, Logistics, Finance/Administration, and Intelligence/Investigations) functional elements. Three Command Staff positions are routinely identified in the ICS: Public Information Officer, Safety Officer, and Liaison Officer. Additional positions may be required, depending on the nature, scope, complexity, and location(s) of the incident(s), or according to specific requirements established by the IC **(Figure 3-2)**. **Figure 3-3** provides a sample assignment list.

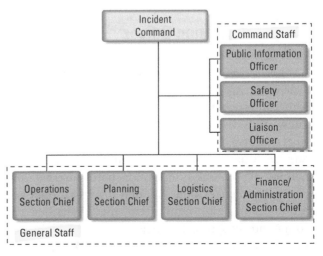

Figure 3-2 Command Staff and General Staff.

1. BRANCH Rescue	2. DIVISION/GROUP North	**ASSIGNMENT LIST**			

3. INCIDENT NAME Stadtown Flood	4. OPERATIONAL PERIOD DATE 9-15-2009 TIME 1630 to 2230 hours

5. OPERATIONAL PERSONNEL

OPERATIONS CHIEF Fallsvie   DIVISION/GROUP SUPERVISOR Connelly

BRANCH DIRECTOR Carver   AIR TACTICAL GROUP SUPERVISOR

6. RESOURCES ASSIGNED TO THIS PERIOD

STRIKE TEAM/TASK FORCE/ RESOURCE DESIGNATOR	EMT	LEADER	NUMBER PERSONS	TRANS. NEEDED	PICKUP PT./TIME	DROP OFF PT./TIME
Rescue North	N	Nollan	4	N		

7. CONTROL OPERATIONS

8. SPECIAL INSTRUCTIONS

Search the north part of town via boat to collect trapped persons. Deliver to Main Street-north at Chandler for processing by Red Cross.

9. DIVISION/GROUP COMMUNICATIONS SUMMARY

FUNCTION		FREQ.	SYSTEM	CHAN.	FUNCTION		FREQ.	SYSTEM	CHAN.
COMMAND	LOCAL	155.750	Citywide	4	SUPPORT	LOCAL			
	REPEAT					REPEAT			
DIV./GROUP TACTICAL		155.95	Tack	6	GROUND TO AIR				

PREPARED BY (RESOURCE UNIT LEADER) Lorry	APPROVED BY (PLANNING SECT. CH.) Marker	DATE 9-15-2009	TIME 1630 to 2230 hours

Figure 3-3 ICS form 204: sample assignment list.

Public Information Officer

The **Public Information Officer (PIO)** is responsible for interfacing with the public, the media, and/or with other agencies with incident-related information requirements. The PIO gathers, verifies, coordinates, and disseminates accurate, accessible, and timely information on the incident's cause, size, and current situation; resources committed; and other matters of general interest for both internal and external audiences. The PIO may also perform a key public information-monitoring role. Whether the Command structure is single or unified, only one PIO should be designated per incident. Assistants may be assigned from other involved agencies, departments, or organizations. The IC/UC must approve the release of all incident-related information. In large-scale incidents or where multiple command posts are established, the PIO should participate in or lead the Joint Information Center (JIC) to ensure consistency in the provision of information to the public. (A more complete discussion of JICs can be found in Chapter 10.)

In addition to providing information, the PIO also serves as a valuable resource for monitoring the media's coverage of an incident. In today's age of immediate access to satellite imagery, it is not unusual for local and national news sources to have information that is not available to the IMT. This function requires the on-scene or incident PIO to stay in close contact with personnel who have access to media information.

Safety Officer

The **Safety Officer (SO)** monitors incident operations and advises Command on all matters relating to operational safety, including the health and safety of emergency responder personnel. It is important to remember that responsibility for incident safety is clearly assigned to IC/UC and supervisors at all levels of incident management. The SO is responsible for establishing a method to ensure the ongoing assessment of hazardous environments. This can be done in cooperation with environmental management agencies and hazardous materials specialists. The SO also is responsible for coordinating multiagency safety efforts, most often through the use of Deputy SOs who are better qualified to assess specific activities in various disciplines. The responsibilities of the SO encompass not only responders, but also victims and bystanders in the incident area.

The SO, Deputy SOs, and Command Staff all have emergency authority to stop and/or prevent unsafe acts during incident operations. In a UC structure, a single SO should be designated and supplemented (as needed) with assistants from other UC agencies or jurisdictions **(Figure 3-4)**. Additionally, specific, high-risk operations may require Deputy

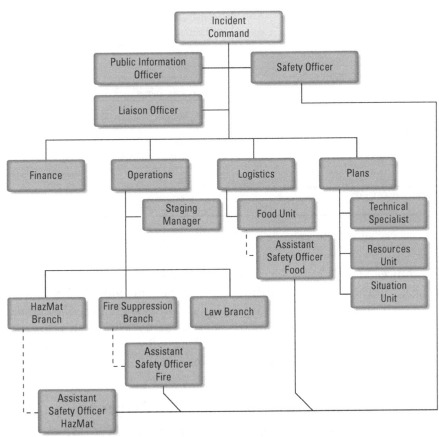

The dotted-line connections represent coordination and communication between the two points, not necessarily a direct link within the chain of command.

Figure 3-4 Example of the role of Safety Officer and Assistant Safety Officers in ICS in a multibranch incident.

ORGANIZATION ASSIGMENT LIST	1. INCIDENT NAME	2. DATE PREPARED	3. TIME PREPARED
	Stadtown Flood	9-15-2009	1630 hours

POSITION: Fire Chief   NAME: Mickelson

4. OPERATIONAL PERIOD (DATE/TIME)
9-15-2009/1630 to 2230 hours

5. INCIDENT COMMAND AND STAFF

INCIDENT COMMANDER	Mickelson
DEPUTY	
SAFETY OFFICER	Carlson
INFORMATION OFFICER	N/A
LIAISON OFFICER	N/A

6. AGENCY REPRESENTATIVES

AGENCY	NAME
SPD	Skirmanki
SEMS	Claredon
EOC	Donaldson

7. PLANNING SECTION

CHIEF	Marker
DEPUTY	
RESOURCES UNIT	Lorry
SITUATION UNIT	
DOCUMENTATION UNIT	
DEMOBILIZATION UNIT	
TECHNICAL SPECIALISTS	

8. LOGISTICS SECTION

CHIEF	O'Neil
DEPUTY	

a. SUPPORT BRANCH

DIRECTOR	
SUPPLY UNIT	
FACILITIES UNIT	
GROUND SUPPORT UNIT	

b. SERVICE BRANCH

DIRECTOR	
COMMUNICATIONS UNIT	
MEDICAL UNIT	
FOOD UNIT	

9. OPERATIONS SECTION

CHIEF		Fallsview
DEPUTY		

a. BRANCH I- Rescue

BRANCH DIRECTOR		Carver
DEPUTY		
DIVISION/GROUP	North	Connelly
DIVISION/ GROUP	South	Wilson
DIVISION/ GROUP		
DIVISION/GROUP		
DIVISION /GROUP		

b. BRANCH II- EMS

BRANCH DIRECTOR		Paterson
DEPUTY		
DIVISION/GROUP	North	Sampson
DIVISION/GROUP	South	Dillon
DIVISION/GROUP		
DIVISION/GROUP		

c. BRANCH III- DIVISIONS/GROUPS

BRANCH DIRECTOR	
DEPUTY	
DIVISION/GROUP	
DIVISION/GROUP	
DIVISION/GROUP	

d. AIR OPERATIONS BRANCH

AIR OPERATIONS BR. DIR.	
AIR TACTICAL GROUP SUP.	
AIR SUPPORT GROUP SUP.	
HELICOPTER COORDINATOR	
AIR TANKER/FIXED WING CRD.	

10. FINANCE/ADMINISTRATION SECTION

CHIEF	
DEPUTY	
TIME UNIT	
PROCUREMENT UNIT	
COMPENSATION/CLAIMS UNIT	
COST UNIT	

PREPARED BY (RESOURCES UNIT)

Figure 3-5 ICS form 203: sample organization assignment list.

SOs with detailed technical knowledge associated with the operation (e.g., heavy equipment operations, law enforcement tactical operations, etc.).

To ensure that safety is a key component of incident operations, the SO, Operations Section Chief, and Planning Section Chief must coordinate closely regarding operational safety and emergency responder health and safety issues. The SO also must ensure the coordination of safety management functions and issues across jurisdictions, across functional agencies, and with private-sector and nongovernmental organizations (NGOs). It is important to note that the agencies, organizations, or jurisdictions that contribute to joint safety management efforts do not lose their individual identities or responsibility for their own programs, policies, and personnel. Rather, each entity contributes to the overall effort to protect all responder personnel involved in incident operations.

Liaison Officer

The **Liaison Officer (LNO)** is the point of contact for representatives of other governmental agencies, NGOs, or private entities. In either a single or UC structure, representatives from assisting or cooperating agencies and organizations (defined as those not represented in the UC group) coordinate through the LNO. The LNO provides a conduit to the IC/UC from these supporting organizations without the additional confusion that would be inherent if all of these representatives were in the command post. In the simplest terms, if an organization is not represented in Command, then they access Command through the LNO. **Figure 3-5** provides a sample organization assignment list.

A key functional component of the LNO concept is that agency and/or organizational representatives assigned to an incident must have the authority to speak for their parent agencies and/or organizations on all matters, following appropriate consultations with their agency leadership. Assistants and personnel from other agencies or organizations (public or private) involved in incident management activities may be assigned to the LNO to facilitate coordination.

Assistants

In the context of large or complex incidents, Command Staff members may need one or more assistants to help manage their workloads. Commonly, these personnel can monitor communications, keep track of incoming information, and generally support the personnel filling the Command Staff positions. Personnel who anticipate being assigned to Command Staff positions at incidents should consider, in advance, how to effectively use assistants and when to request them. Like most aspects of incident management, being proactive and requesting resources early substantially enhances incident management effectiveness.

Additional Command Staff

Additional Command Staff positions may also be necessary, depending on the nature and location of the incident and/or specific requirements established by the IC/UC. A Legal Counsel may be assigned directly to the Command Staff to advise the IC/UC on legal matters, such as emergency proclamations, the legality of evacuation orders, and the legal rights and restrictions pertaining to media access. Similarly, a Medical Advisor may be designated and assigned directly to the Command Staff to provide advice and recommendations to the IC/UC in the context of incidents involving medical and mental health services, mass casualty, acute care, and so on.

Rural Case Study *Answers*

1. The Sheriff's Office is responsible for security and assisting in search and rescue operations. The Fire Department is responsible for search and rescue, assisting with patient management, hazardous materials and utilities management, and fire suppression. EMS is responsible for patient care, assisting in search and rescue, casualty transport, and responder rehabilitation.

2. Several options exist:

- Operations due to the complex, ongoing nature of rescue, fire suppression, and patient care
- Logistics due to the heavy supplies needs this incident will require, especially in the long term
- Planning due to the complex long-term components of the incident
- Alternately, establish EMS, fire, search and rescue, and law enforcement branches

The best option is the latter because the limited personnel available allows for UC to initially manage both the strategic and tactical issues.

3. UC is the most appropriate because the incident crosses disciplinary boundaries, and all the agencies have specific strategic objectives related to the incident.

Urban Case Study *Answers*

1. A single command structure should be implemented under the Fire Department. At this point, there are no strategic objectives for the police or EMS, although both organizations have supporting roles in managing a HazMat incident. Although potential victims exist in the vehicle and the train, they are not currently accessible, and rescue operations are not indicated.

2. The strategic management objectives include the following: manage the identification and impact analysis of the hazardous materials release, specifically addressing the potential for expansion based on weather conditions and chemical properties.

3. It becomes a multijurisdiction event when incident analysis indicates, through modeling, that the chemical plume will encompass or threaten the unincorporated area of the county and the city of Metro.

Wrap-Up

Summary

- Command is either single or unified in structure. Single command is a structure in which a single individual is responsible for all of the strategic objectives of the incident, and it is typically used when an incident is within a single jurisdiction and is managed by a single discipline. UC is a structure in which multiple individuals are cooperatively responsible for all the strategic objectives of the incident. UC is indicated in incidents that involve multiple jurisdictions or multiple agencies with overlapping responsibilities and authorities.

- Effective UC depends on a collaborative approach to incident management and requires a single IAP and a single command post. UC also depends on effective relationships and mutual respect among members of the UC group.

- The Command Staff consists of Command, the PIO, the SO, and the LNO. Additionally, assistants and special advisors may be appointed as needed based on the type of incident and its complexity.

- The General Staff consists of the Section Chiefs for Operations, Planning, Logistics, and Finance/Administration. Additionally, NIMS has added Intelligence/Investigations as a new, optional member of the General Staff.

Glossary

Joint Information Center (JIC): The office within NIMS responsible for ensuring that all public information released about an incident is consistent; also responsible for screening any inappropriate facts that may damage an investigation.

Liaison Officer (LNO): The Command Staff position responsible for providing a method of communication between the Incident Command/Unified Command and other supporting organizations.

Public Information Officer (PIO): The position within NIMS responsible for gathering and releasing incident information to the media and other appropriate agencies.

Safety Officer (SO): The Command Staff position responsible for the management of the incident safety plan. This person has the authority to immediately stop any on-scene activity that is deemed to be unsafe.

Single command: The Command structure in which a single individual is responsible for all of the strategic objectives of the incident. Typically used when an incident is within a single jurisdiction and is managed by a single discipline.

A tour bus with 55 passengers has left a roadway and overturned, striking a major bridge support during the collision. The bridge has been substantially damaged and is unstable, but it is not a direct threat to the bus. No other vehicles were involved in the collision. Local public safety (fire, police, EMS), public works, and transportation organizations are on the scene, and morning rush hour is just beginning. The affected highway is a major inbound artery for the city.

The various organizations begin to manage their specific aspects of the incident, but conflicts immediately develop among the law enforcement personnel (who are trying to investigate the collision) and fire and EMS personnel (who are still managing patients). It is clear that ICS would help the situation and assist in managing conflicting objectives. Answer the following questions based on what you know about the incident.

1. What is the most appropriate initial configuration of IC?
   A. Single command (police)
   B. Single command (fire)
   C. UC (fire, police, EMS)
   D. UC (fire, police, EMS, local transportation official)

2. After all casualties have been evacuated from the scene, it is appropriate for EMS to withdraw from ongoing representation in the UC group.
   A. True
   B. False

3. As Command transitions during this incident, what would be an appropriate final configuration for a UC group?
   A. EMS, transportation, public works
   B. Police, transportation, public works
   C. Fire, police, EMS
   D. A, B, or C

CHAPTER 4

Operations

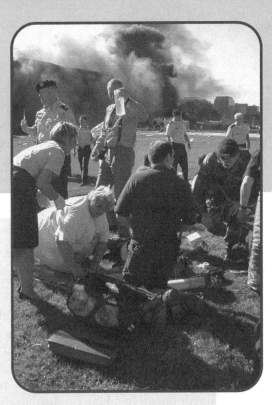

Rural Case Study

As additional fire, law enforcement, and emergency medical services (EMS) units begin to arrive on scene to support the first incident unit and its Incident Commander, the span of control is quickly exceeded. The Incident Commander decides to create an Operations Section and assigns a lieutenant from Engine 4 as the Operations Section Chief. He is briefed by the Incident Commander and tasked with rescuing individuals from damaged residential and commercial properties, fire control, emergency medical treatment, evacuation of causalities, and security of the scene.

Within minutes, the Operations Section Chief organizes his available personnel to perform these tasks. Using a map of the downtown area, he designates two geographic areas (divisions), identified as East and West, and begins to assign his limited personnel to each of these. He assigns a supervisor to each division. He communicates his plan to the Incident Commander and requests additional resources.

The Operations Section Chief has a serious challenge ahead of him. Additional personnel, rescue equipment, and on-scene resources, such as medical equipment and mobile treatment areas, are needed. As these resources arrive, however, a structured deployment plan must be in place to ensure the most effective and efficient use of these resources. Furthering the complexity of this event is the loss of the public safety communications system due to storm damage.

1. What additional resources does this Operations Section Chief require?
2. What are the primary responsibilities of the Operations Section Chief?

Urban Case Study

Responders are now massing on the scene of the train accident. The initial focus is on stabilizing the incident site and awaiting technical resources. However, with the detonation of the chemical trailer, the incident takes a new direction that requires a change in scene tactics, additional resources, and enlargement of the incident site to include everyone downwind of the plume.

Incident Command assigns a fire officer as Operations Section Chief for the initial incident site at the train tracks. A request is made to the Emergency Operations Center (EOC) in nearby Pleasantville to activate its resources and begin the evacuation of the potential downwind area. At this point, there are multiple command sites: one at the initial incident site and one in the neighboring town. In effect, an Area Command is established to accommodate the unique needs of the two primary affected areas.

1. What additional operational resources are required at the scene of the explosion?
2. How should the Operations Section be divided when the number of resources exceeds the Operations Section Chief's span of control?
3. How should the EOC develop its operational strategy to begin the evacuation?

Introduction

As indicated in both of the opening scenarios, a large number of personnel will be responding to these incidents. Responding personnel need to be assigned to perform specific functions at these scenes, and a systematic method of assigning these resources by discipline, function, or geographic need must be utilized for an efficient, coordinated, and safe effort.

Operations Section

The **Operations Section** is responsible for managing all tactical operations at the incident site. These objectives are typically directed toward reducing the immediate hazard, saving lives and property, establishing situational control, and restoring normal conditions. The Operations Section functions at the direction of Incident Command (IC), whether the incident requires simple, single-unit responses or involves many jurisdictions and responding agen-cies. Oftentimes, the Operations Section is employed and utilized by public safety and health entities during day-to-day operations.

The Operations Section is a component of the Incident Command System (ICS) and generally has the greatest number of assigned personnel, and hence the greatest number of functions. Most public safety and health professions, such as law enforcement **(Figure 4-1)**, fire **(Figure 4-2)**, EMS **(Figure 4-3)**, and hospitals **(Figure 4-4)**, have developed organizational charts for their ICS structure.

Because of its functional unit-management structure, ICS is applicable across a spectrum of incidents of differing size, scope, and complexity. The types of agencies included in the Operations Section are defined by the incident objectives and typically include fire, law enforcement, EMS, hospitals, public health, and public works. Additionally, many incidents may involve private individuals, companies, or nongovernmental organizations (NGOs), which may be trained and qualified to participate in the Operations Section.

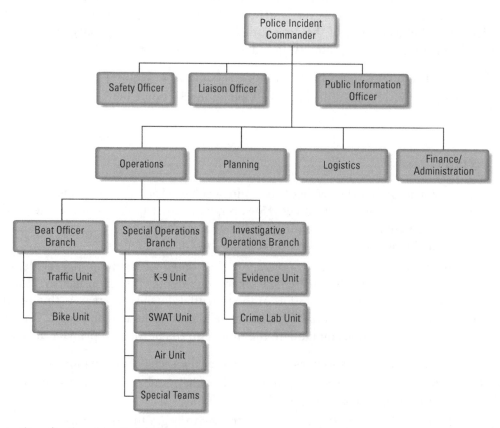

Figure 4-1 Operations Section: Law Enforcement.

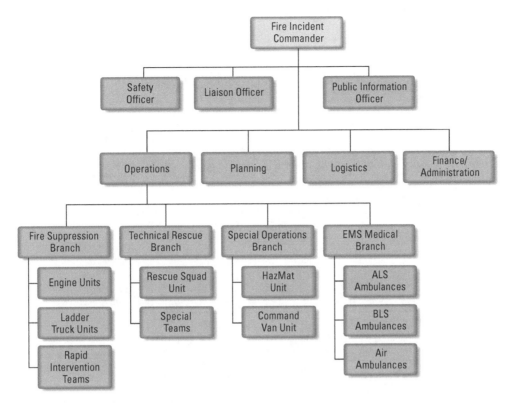

Figure 4-2 Operations Section: Fire.

Tip

The Operations Section Chief and the primary leadership should be well informed regarding Logistics Section resources. Without a well-organized flow of ground support, personnel, supplies, and specialized equipment, the Operations Section will quickly come to a standstill.

Incident operations can be organized and executed in many ways. The specific method selected will depend on the type and magnitude of the incident, the agencies needed to complete the objectives, and the strategies of the particular incident management effort. The following discussion presents several different methods of organizing incident tactical operations. In some cases, a method will be selected to accommodate jurisdictional boundaries. In other cases, the approach will be strictly functional. In still others, a mix of functional and geographic approaches is appropriate.

ICS offers extensive flexibility in determining the appropriate approach. **Figure 4-5** shows the primary organizational structure of the Operations Section. Everyone within the Operations Section, as well as all personnel on the scene, is responsible for a common set of responsibilities at any incident. These are essential to the successful response to and performance of on-scene activities and demobilization following the incident. **Table 4-1** outlines the common responsibilities for all ICS personnel.

Tip

Communication among the many different agencies and resources at the scene of a large-scale incident can become complicated. Use common terminology rather than jargon, codes, or agency-specific terminology. This facilitates effective communication.

Operations Section Chief

The **Operations Section Chief** (OPS), who is a member of the General Staff, directly manages all incident tactical activities and implements the Incident Action Plan (IAP). The OPS will develop and manage the Operations Section to accomplish the incident objectives set by the Incident Commander. The OPS is normally the person with the greatest technical and tactical expertise in dealing with the problem at hand.

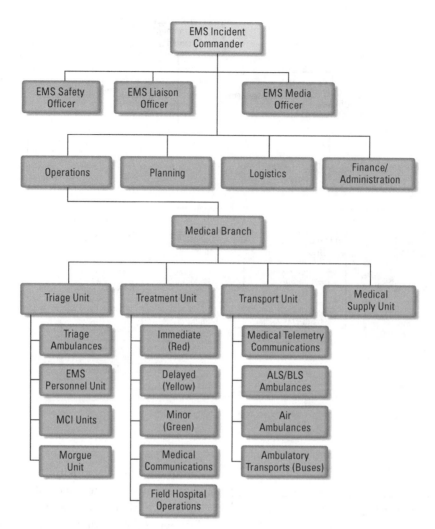

Figure 4-3 Operations Section: EMS.

The Operations Section Chief may have one or more deputies (preferably from other agencies or jurisdictions in multijurisdictional or multidisciplinary incidents). Deputies will be qualified to a similar level as the OPS (and should be capable of seamlessly filling the OPS position if needed). The OPS should be designated for each operational period and have direct involvement in the preparation of the IAP for the period of responsibility.

The OPS has designated responsibilities beyond the common responsibilities of all responders at the incident site. The OPS also must assist in developing the IAP, brief the appropriate personnel, supervise the Operations Section, and determine the need for additional resources. The OPS also may assemble Strike Teams; report special activities, events, or occurrences; and provide a constant review of active resources. The OPS also is responsible for maintaining a unit/activity log. **Table 4-2** lists the responsibilities of the OPS. The ICS medical plan form identifies

the incident medical station, ambulance services, incident ambulances, hospitals, and medical emergency procedures coordinated by the OPS **(Figure 4-6)**.

Tip
As you prepare and train with other responders in your community, include and identify qualified individuals, from all respective agencies, who can perform the functions of the OPS. This will help in implementing the Operations Section in the event of a real incident. It will also ease operations and enhance communication among the different agencies at the scene.

Because of the complexity of the tactical fieldwork that is typically performed at the scene, most operational resources are assigned to the Operations Section. The number of resources can rapidly exceed the OPS's manageable span of control. Additionally,

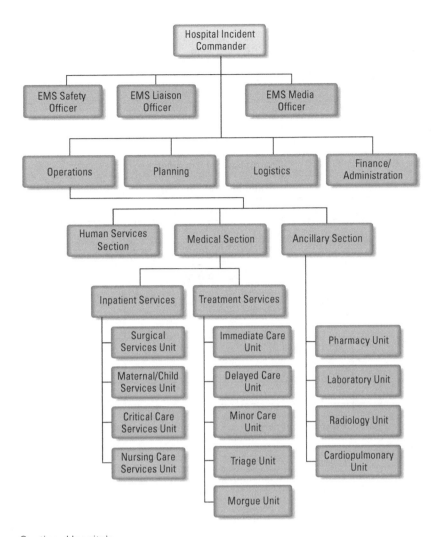

Figure 4-4 Operations Section: Hospitals.

the most hazardous activities are frequently carried out in the operational area. This loss of control can compromise the effectiveness of the OPS and cause an unsafe working environment at the incident scene.

With this in mind, it is necessary to carefully monitor the number of resources that report to any

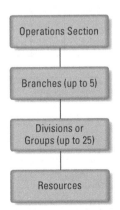

Figure 4-5 The primary organizational structure of the Operations Section.

one supervisor. A ratio of 1:3 to 1:7 is considered the ideal number of subordinates to a leader. When the ratio exceeds 1:7, there is a potential for loss of control and coordination. The following supervisory levels can be added to the Operations Section to help maintain and manage the span of control:

- Branch Director(s)
- Division or Group Supervisor(s)
- Strike Team and Task Force Leader(s)
- Single Resource Leader

Table 4-3 provides an easy way to determine the degree of subdivision that may be needed in the Operations Section.

Divisions, Groups, Resources, and Branches

In order for operations to keep control and maintain optimal staffing and ratios at an incident, resources are assigned into divisions, groups, and branches.

MEDICAL PLAN

	1. Incident Name	2. Date Prepared	3. Time Prepared	4. Operational Period
MEDICAL PLAN	Stadtown Flood	09-15-2009	1630 hours	9-15-2009/ 1630 to 2230 hours

5. Incident Medical Aid Station

Medical Aid Stations	Location	Paramedics Yes	No
North Div	North Main at Chandler	X	
South Div	South Main at Demsey	X	

6. Transportation

A. Ambulance Services

Name	Address	Phone	Paramedics Yes	No
SEMS	911 City Hall	555-555-1212	X	

B. Incident Ambulances

Name	Location	Paramedics Yes	No
SEMS	North Main at Chandler	X	
SEMS	South Main at Demsey	X	

7. Hospitals

Name	Address	Travel Time Air	Ground	Phone	Helipad Yes	No	Burn Center Yes	No
Stadtown C. H.	123 Chandler	4	6	555-555-1111	X			X

8. Medical Emergency Procedures

None

9. Prepared by (Medical Unit Leader)	10. Reviewed by (Safety Officer)
Planning	Carlson

Figure 4-6 ICS form 206: sample medical plan.

Table 4-1 Common Responsibilities for All Personnel in an ICS Organization

Receive your assignment from your agency, including the following:

- Job assignment (e.g., Strike Team designation, position, etc.)
- Resource order number and request number
- Reporting location
- Reporting time
- Travel instructions
- Any special communications instructions (e.g., travel, radio frequency)

Upon arrival at the incident, check in at the designated check-in location.

Note: If you are instructed to report directly to a line assignment, check in with the Division or Group Supervisor. Check-in locations may be found at any of the following locations:

- The Incident Command Post (ICP)
- Bases or camps
- Staging areas
- Helibases

Receive a briefing from an immediate supervisor.

Agency representatives from assisting or cooperating agencies report to the Liaison Officer (LNO) at the ICP after checking in.

Acquire work materials.

Supervisors shall maintain accountability for their assigned personnel with regard to where their personnel are located and the personal safety and welfare of their personnel at all times, especially when working in or around incident operations.

Organize and brief subordinates.

Know the assigned radio frequency for your area of responsibility, and ensure that communications equipment is operating properly.

Use clear text and ICS terminology (no codes) in all radio communications. All radio communications to the incident communications center will be addressed as follows: "(Incident Name) Communications" (e.g., "Pleasantville Communications").

Complete forms and reports required of the assigned position, and send them through the supervisor to the Documentation Unit.

Respond to demobilization orders, and brief subordinates regarding demobilization.

Table 4-2 Responsibilities of the OPS

A single Incident Commander has sole responsibility for establishing incident objectives and strategies.

Review common responsibilities.

Develop the Operations Section tasks for the IAP.

Brief and assign Operations Section personnel in accordance with the IAP.

Supervise the Operations Section.

Determine needs, and request additional resources.

Review the suggested list of resources to be released, and initiate recommendations for release of resources.

Assemble and disassemble Strike Teams assigned to the Operations Section.

Report information about special activities, events, and occurrences to the Incident Commander.

Maintain a unit/activity log.

Divisions

Divisions are used to divide an incident geographically. The person in charge of each Division is designated as a Supervisor. The geographical division of the incident scene is usually determined by the needs of the incident, natural geographic barriers (e.g., rivers, mountains, lakes, shorelines, and valleys), or manmade obstacles (e.g., buildings, roadways, and walls). When geographic features are used to determine boundaries, the size of the Division should correspond to appropriate span-of-control guidelines **(Figure 4-7)**.

The most common method for identifying or labeling Divisions is by using letters (A, B, C, etc.). Other identifiers ("city park," "west city," etc.) may be used as long as the Division identifier is known to all assigned responders. The important thing to remember about the ICS Divisions is that they are established to divide the incident into geographic areas of operation.

Groups

Groups are used to describe functional areas of an operation. Like Divisions, the individual assigned to be in charge of each Group is designated as a Supervisor. The type of Groups established will be determined by the needs of the incident. Groups

Table 4-3 Decision Table for the Implementation of Branches, Divisions, and Groups	
Current span of control chief	**Action by OPS**
Three to five individuals working under a single leader (three is optimal)	Maintain current staffing.
More than five individuals working under a single leader	Create Branches, Divisions, or Groups as needed and assign the appropriate number of personnel to maintain optimal ratios.

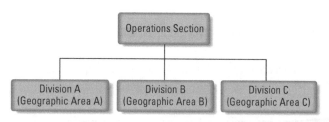

Figure 4-7 Geographic division of an incident.

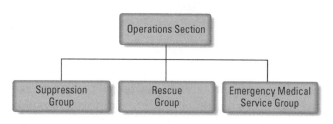

Figure 4-8 Functional division of an incident.

are usually labeled according to the job that they are assigned (e.g., Decontamination Group, Traffic Control Group, etc.). Groups work within the incident wherever their assigned task is needed and are not limited by geographic boundaries **(Figure 4-8)**.

Combined Geographic Divisions and Functional Groups

Divisions and Groups can be utilized together at an incident. Divisions and Groups are at an equal level in the organization. One does not supervise the other. When a Group is working within a Division on a special assignment, the Division and Group Supervisors must closely work together to coordinate their activities.

Division and Group Supervisors also have unique responsibilities beyond their common responsibili-

Table 4-4 Responsibilities of the Division and/or Group Supervisor(s)
Review common responsibilities.
Implement the IAP for the Division/Group.
Provide the IAP to Strike Team Leaders, when present.
Identify increments assigned to the Division/Group.
Review Division/Group assignments and incident activities with subordinates and assign tasks.
Ensure that the Incident Commander and/or Resources Unit is advised of all changes in the status of resources assigned to the Division/Group.
Coordinate activities with adjacent Divisions/Groups.
Determine need for assistance on assigned tasks.
Submit situation and resources status information to the Branch Director or the OPS.
Report hazardous situations, special occurrences, or significant events (e.g., accidents, sicknesses, and discovery of unanticipated sensitive resources) to the immediate supervisor.
Ensure that assigned personnel and equipment get to and from assignments in a timely and orderly manner.
Resolve logistics problems within the Division/Group.
Participate in the development of Branch plans for the next operational period.
Maintain a unit/activity log.

ties during an incident. These include implementing and assigning the IAP to appropriate resources, reviewing activities and assignments, coordinating with adjacent Groups and Divisions, and determining the need for additional resources. Division and Group Supervisors also are responsible for reporting to the OPS regarding Division/Group status, hazardous situations, special occurrences, and significant events. A complete list of responsibilities is provided in **Table 4-4**.

It also is possible to have both Divisions and Groups within the Operations Section. For example, Divisions A, B, and C (based on jurisdictional boundaries) might each have Groups 1 and 2 to provide a management structure for different types of resources within each Division.

Resources

Initially, in any incident, individual resources that are assigned will report directly to the Incident Commander. As the incident grows in size or complexity, individual resources may be organized and employed in a number of ways to facilitate incident management:

- Single resources
- Task Forces
- Strike Teams

Single Resources

Single resources are employed on an individual basis. This is typical in an initial response to an incident. During sustained operations, situations typically arise that call for the use of a single helicopter, vehicle, piece of mobile equipment, and so on. Single resources share the same common incident responsibilities when activated. Beyond these responsibilities, single resources are focused on a specific mission. These resources review the assignment, obtain necessary equipment, review safety concerns, perform the mission, report to their supervisor (the Single Resource Leader), and are responsible for completing and submitting appropriate paperwork. A detailed list of the Single Resource Leader's responsibilities is provided in **Table 4-5.**

Task Forces

Task Forces are any combination of resources assembled to accomplish a specific mission. Task Forces have a designated leader and operate with common communications. Combining resources into Task Forces allows several key resource elements to be managed under one individual's supervision, thus aiding in span of control. One example of a Task Force would be two police units, a rescue unit, and two EMS units working as an assigned team with a leader.

Tip

Because Task Forces are made of different types of resources from a combination of agencies, it is critical to communicate in a common manner. Law enforcement, fire, and EMS personnel may be assigned to the same Task Force to complete a unique mission. Avoid using radio- or agency-specific codes and jargon so that everyone will understand the messages being communicated.

Strike Teams

A **Strike Team** consists of a set number of resources of the same kind and type that operate under a designated leader with common communications among them. Strike Teams represent known capabilities and are highly effective management units. One example of a Strike Team is five engine companies or four police units with a team leader.

Responsibilities for Task Forces and Strike Teams

Task Forces and Strike Teams have a common set of responsibilities during an incident **(Table 4-6)**. When activated, they review their assignments, ensure coordination among adjacent teams and resources, complete the mission assignment, and submit all appropriate paperwork and situation and resource status information.

Table 4-5 Responsibilities of a Single Resource Leader
Review common responsibilities.
Review assignments.
Obtain necessary equipment and supplies.
Review weather/environmental conditions for assignment area.
Brief subordinates on safety measures.
Monitor work progress.
Ensure adequate communications with supervisor and subordinates.
Keep supervisor informed of progress and any changes.
Inform supervisor of problems with assigned resources.
Brief relief personnel, and advise them of any change in conditions.
Return equipment and supplies to appropriate unit.
Complete and turn in all time and use records on personnel and equipment.
Maintain a unit/activity log.

Table 4-6 Responsibilities of Task Force and Strike Team Leaders
Review common responsibilities.
Review common Unit Leader responsibilities.
Review assignments with subordinates, and assign tasks.
Monitor work progress, and make changes when necessary.
Coordinate activities with adjacent Strike Teams, Task Forces, and single resources.
Travel to and from the active assignment area with assigned resources.
Retain control of assigned resources while in available or out-of-service status.
Submit situation and resource status information to Division/Group Supervisor.
Maintain a unit/activity log.

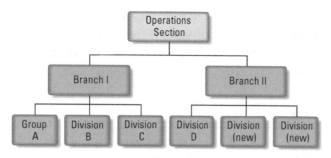

Figure 4-9 Two-Branch organization.

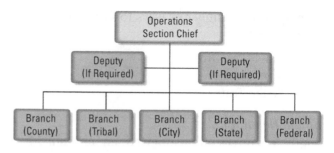

Figure 4-10 Multijurisdictional incident.

Branches

As an incident escalates in size or complexity, it is necessary to create larger subdivisions of the Operations Section. This is accomplished through the formation of **Branches**. In a situation in which the OPS has too many personnel under his or her supervision in Groups, Divisions, or resources, Branches are established to delegate a more appropriate span of control **(Figure 4-9)**. Branches are established to serve several purposes.

The Number of Divisions and/or Groups Exceeds the Recommended Span of Control

The recommended span of control for the OPS is 1:5. (A ratio of 1:3 is best in fast-moving tactical operations.) The span of control can be higher for large-scale law enforcement operations. When the span is exceeded, the OPS should set up two or more Branches and allocate Divisions and Groups among them. For example, if one Group and four Divisions are reporting to the OPS, and two Divisions and one Group are to be added, a two-Branch organization should be formed.

The Nature of the Incident Calls for a Functional Branch Structure

In some cases, the nature of the incident may call for a functional Branch structure. For example, if a large aircraft crashes within a city, various departments within the city (including police, fire, EMS, and public health services) would each have a functional Branch operating under the direction of a single OPS. In this example, the OPS is from the fire department, with deputies from police and public health services. Other alignments could be made, depending on the city plan and type of emergency. Note that in this situation the IC could be either a single command or a Unified Command (UC), depending on the jurisdiction.

Multijurisdictional Incidents

Large incidents that cross city, township, county, or state lines are multijurisdictional. In multijurisdictional incidents, resources are best managed under the agencies that normally control them. For example, the response to a major flood might require combining federal, state, county, city, and tribal resources. Along the floodplain of the river, many communities will be affected by the same problem. The flood is not a series of incidents, but rather a singular incident with multiple management areas. Each town will deploy its resources, as will county, state, and federal agencies. All of these groups work together in a multiagency command structure **(Figure 4-10)**.

Branch Directors have a great deal of responsibility because they supervise a large number of personnel and resources. Branch Directors attend Operations Section planning meetings, continuously review Division and Group assignments, assign and modify work tasks to Divisions and Groups, and supervise the overall operations of the Branch. The Branch Director is responsible for resolving logistic problems; tracking, modifying, and reporting the IAP; and ensuring that all appropriate paperwork is completed and submitted from each area within the Branch **(Table 4-7)**.

Air Operations Branch

The OPS may establish an **Air Operations Branch** to meet mission requirements in certain situations. For example, a large vehicle accident in a remote area may require helicopter transport of victims to specialized medical centers. Military transport also has been utilized to evacuate hospital patients from areas threatened by an incoming hurricane (e.g., the Florida Keys). **Figure 4-11** shows a typical organizational structure for an Air Operations Branch. Many law enforcement agencies also have helicopter units for surveillance and rescue.

When an air operation is requested at an incident, the OPS may designate an Air Operations

Table 4-7 Responsibilities of the Branch Director

Review common responsibilities.

Develop alternatives for Branch operations with subordinates.

Attend planning meetings at the request of the OPS.

Review Division/Group assignment lists for Divisions/Groups within the Branch.

Modify lists based on the effectiveness of current operations.

Assign specific work tasks to Division/Group Supervisors.

Supervise Branch operations.

Resolve logistic problems reported by subordinates.

Report to the OPS when the IAP is to be modified, additional resources are needed, surplus resources are available, or hazardous situations or significant events occur.

Approve accident and medical reports (home agency forms) originating within the Branch.

Maintain a unit/activity log.

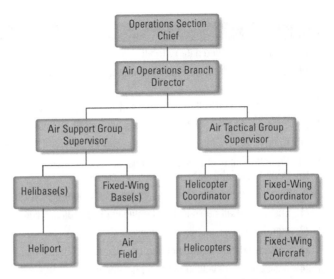

Figure 4-11 Air Operations Branch organizational structure.

Branch Director. Air operations at major incidents are complicated. Flight safety is a paramount concern in complex operations and supports the requirement for a designated Air Operations Branch. The Air Operations Branch Director may have to mix tactical and logistical utilization of helicopters and other aircraft to support operational planning and mission execution.

Whenever both helicopters and fixed-wing aircraft must operate simultaneously within the incident air space, an **Air Tactical Group Supervisor** should be designated. This individual coordinates all airborne activity with the assistance of a Helicopter Coordinator and a Fixed-Wing Coordinator. The **Air Support Group** is responsible for all appropriate recordkeeping for aviation assets assigned to the incident.

Managing the Operations Section

Table 4-8 provides a comprehensive set of instructions for managing the Operations Section, from implementation to demobilization.

Figure 4-12 depicts the entire operational period planning cycle.

Table 4-8 Managing the Operations Section

1. Obtain and assemble information and materials necessary to perform the job upon initial activation.
2. Provide for the safety and welfare of the assigned personnel during the entire period of supervision.
3. Establish and maintain positive interpersonal and interagency working relationships.
4. Gather information necessary to assess incident assignments and determine immediate needs and actions.
5. Obtain a briefing from the Incident Commander, either one-on-one or at an Incident Management Team (IMT) briefing.
6. Collect information from the outgoing OPS, Incident Commander, or other personnel responsible for the incident prior to your arrival.
7. Evaluate and share all information on the Operations Section, and determine what is anticipated for incident operations based on the expected size, type, and duration of the incident.
8. Evaluate and monitor the current situation.
9. Observe and review current operations to prepare tactics for the next operational period planning meeting.
10. Periodically evaluate resource status and tactical needs to determine if resource assignments are appropriate.
11. Participate in preparation of the IAP.
12. Participate in the operational period briefing and emphasize any changes from the written IAP.

(Continues)

Table 4-8 Managing the Operations Section *(Continued)*

13. Interact and coordinate with all Command and General Staff.

14. Supervise and adjust operations organization and tactics as needed, based on changes in the incident situation and resource status.

15. Evaluate the overall effectiveness of the IAP and adjust as necessary for the next operational period.

16. Ensure that the Logistics Section is advised of all changes in the status of assigned resources.

17. Update the Incident Commander on current accomplishments and/or problems.

18. Complete all operational period paperwork as prescribed for each operational period.
19. Report special events, incidents, or accidents.

20. Brief the replacement OPS as to the operational period situation and resource status.

21. Ensure that all personnel and equipment records are complete and have been submitted at the end of each operational period.

22. Identify excess section resources.

23. Consider demobilization during the incident so that an adequate plan is implemented prior to releasing resources.

24. Assist in the development and implementation of the incident demobilization plan.

25. Ensure that demobilization procedures are followed and all resources are accounted for.

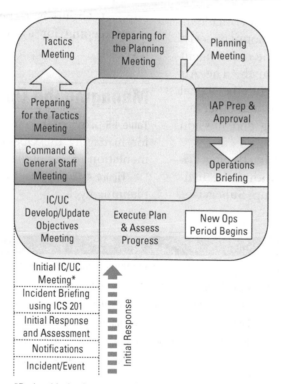

*During this timeframe a meeting with the Agency Administrator/Executive can occur.

Figure 4-12 Operational planning period cycle.

Rural Case Study *Answers*

1. The OPS requires the following resources:
   - Specialized teams, such as search and rescue, extrication, and disaster medical assistance teams
   - Disaster relief groups, such as the American Red Cross and the Salvation Army
   - Public health officials and staff
   - Public works officials and staff (water, electrical, etc.)
   - Civilian communications organizations, such as ham radio operators
2. The primary responsibilities of the OPS include the following:
   - Review common responsibilities.
   - Develop the Operations portion of the IAP.
   - Brief and assign Operations Section personnel in accordance with the IAP.
   - Supervise the Operations Section.
   - Determine needs and request additional resources.
   - Review the suggested list of resources to be released and initiate recommendations for the release of resources.
   - Assemble and disassemble Strike Teams assigned to the Operations Section.
   - Report information about special activities, events, and occurrences to the Incident Commander.
   - Maintain a unit/activity log.

Urban Case Study *Answers*

1. Additional resources include, but are not limited to the following:
   - Additional fire, EMS, and law enforcement personnel
   - Specialized terrorism response units and additional HazMat technicians
   - Public health personnel
   - Municipal and state administration
   - Public transportation
   - Metropolitan Medical Response System (MMRS) teams and Disaster Medical Assistance Teams (DMATs)
   - State and federal terrorism investigation teams
   - Disaster relief groups (American Red Cross, Salvation Army, etc.)
2. The OPS should implement and assign Branches, Divisions, Groups, and specialized resources (Strike Teams, Task Forces) to ensure appropriate span of control (at a ratio of 1:5); lines of reporting; and responder safety.
3. The EOC should implement its Emergency Operations Plan (EOP) and work with the Incident Commander to create a more specific IAP.

Wrap-Up

Summary

- The Operations Section is the most recognized area of incident management. It is involved in tactical operations for reducing immediate hazards, saving lives and property, and establishing situational control. This section involves a broad cross-section of the entire response community on large-scale incidents, which works together as a unit or in combinations of disciplines, depending on the nature of the incident.
- The National Incident Management System (NIMS) provides the critical framework and guidance to implement the Operations Section at the scene of any incident, regardless of its size, scope, or complexity.
- The organization of the Operations Section depends on the specific incident mission requirements and the IAP. It may be organized based on jurisdictional areas, geographic boundaries, functional needs, or a combination of any of the three.
- NIMS and ICS offer the flexibility to apply the appropriate approach to developing an Operations Section with lines of authority and reporting, span of control, and common and specific responsibilities at each level.

Glossary

Air Operations Branch: The component of the ICS responsible for all air resources. This includes both fixed- and rotor-wing aircraft, their support personnel, and landing areas.

Air Support Group: Component of the Air Operations Branch that is responsible for all recordkeeping related to the aviation assets at an incident site.

Air Tactical Group Supervisor: The individual responsible for the coordination of all airborne activity at an incident site.

Branches: Areas of incident management established to delegate an appropriate span of control under the Operations Section Chief.

Division: A geographic area of an incident. Divisions are created to maintain span of control at large incident sites.

Groups: Functional areas of an incident. Groups are usually labeled according to their assigned job (e.g., law enforcement or intelligence). Groups are not limited by geographic boundaries.

Operations Section: Component of the ICS responsible for tactical operations at the incident site. The goal of the Operations Section is to reduce the immediate hazard, save lives and property, establish situational control, and restore normal conditions.

Operations Section Chief (OPS): The member of the general staff who directly manages all incident tactical activities and implements the IAP. This individual usually has the greatest technical and tactical expertise with the incident problem.

Single resource: An individual response unit that is employed at or during an incident (e.g., a helicopter, water tanker, police vehicle, etc.).

Strike Team: A set number of the same type of resources operating under one leader.

Task Force: A combination of resources that work together to complete a specific mission.

Wrap-Up Case Study

Heavy rains and localized flooding have caused a levee outside of Lewiston, a city of 90,000 residents, to breach. Within hours, most of the downtown areas are submerged under 5 feet of water, forcing an emergency evacuation of most of the city, including the local hospital. The floodwaters have essentially split the city into two sections. The OPS begins to assign resources to both sides of the city and develops an Operations IAP.

The flooded area is completely evacuated, and displaced residents are sheltered in predesignated schools. Three hours into the incident, the Incident Commander is notified by the EOC that the drinking water supply for Lewiston has become contaminated, including the water supplying the emergency shelters. Specialized resources have been requested from the State to assist with this new problem.

1. Recall that the floodwaters have split the city of Lewiston into two different geographical areas, creating different needs in each area. What functional element in an Operations Section is based on a geographic area?

    A. Group

    B. Branch

    C. Division

    D. Section

2. When the additional water treatment specialists from public works arrive at the scene, they report to staging. The OPS assembles them into a _____, designates a leader, and assigns it to the shelters to provide potable water.

    A. strike Team

    B. task Force

    C. division

    D. none of the above

3. The East Lewiston Division Supervisor is now supervising 18 people and has requested three law enforcement units, two fire rescue units, and a helicopter to evacuate a near-drowning victim. Which ICS principle has this Supervisor overlooked?

    A. Delegation of authority

    B. Span of control

    C. Unity of command

    D. Common communications

4. Which general staff position develops tactical objectives and directs all tactical resources?

    A. Incident Operations Officer

    B. Planning Section Chief

    C. Logistics Section Chief

    D. Operations Section Chief

CHAPTER 5

Planning

Rural Case Study

Smith County and Stadtown are completely overwhelmed by the devastation of a flood caused by the breach of several small dams after heavy rainfall. A major part of Stadtown has been flooded by several feet of water. Two hours after the rushing water overwhelmed the town, the Unified Command (UC) group (sheriff's office, fire, and emergency medical services) appoints you as the Planning Section Chief. The scene is chaotic, disorganized, and without direction. Documentation is nonexistent. Your initial discussions with the UC reveal that they have no immediate strategies for managing the incident in a unified manner, and it is clear that the incident is a long-term event.

1. What are your initial actions?
2. As Planning Section Chief, what are your priorities?
3. What personnel do you need immediately to make the Planning Section effective?

Urban Case Study

The Emergency Operations Center (EOC) has been activated, and you are reporting to your assigned position of Planning Section Chief. You find that the Situation Unit is already staffed and working. Information is coming in from the scene regarding additional needs and evacuation issues. The situation is evolving quickly. The incident is in its third hour.

At this juncture, you must set several immediate priorities that will ensure that the EOC is adequately supporting the in-field operations. You also need to plan for several potential operational periods, potentially extending over multiple days or weeks.

1. What situation assessments do you need to make immediately? Why are they important?
2. Besides the Situation Unit, what unit is your next priority?
3. What technical specialists do you immediately want access to? Why?

Introduction

The **Planning Section** is a critical component of the Incident Command System (ICS) and one that is frequently overlooked in local operations, both on the scene and within EOCs. In local environments, this is usually due to a lack of personnel resources and education. Although not as high profile as the Operations Section, the Planning Section provides unique challenges to individuals who enjoy a more strategic view of incident management while still working in detail-oriented areas. The basis of an effective Planning Section is accurate and timely information acquisition from the Incident Command/

Unified Command (IC/UC). An effective Planning Section is a combination of "fortune-tellers," intelligence analysts, and technical experts in every conceivable specialty combined with an exceptional understanding of incident management in the field and in the EOC.

Planning Section

The Planning Section comprises four primary units:

- Resources
- Situation
- Documentation
- Demobilization

Figure 5-1 illustrates these primary units, as well as the concept of technical specialists. **Intelligence/Investigations** is a special situation that will be discussed later in the chapter.

Officially, the Planning Section collects, evaluates, and disseminates incident situation information and intelligence to the IC/UC and incident management personnel; prepares status reports; displays situation information; maintains the status of resources assigned to the incident; and develops and documents the Incident Action Plan (IAP) based on guidance from the IC/UC. The Planning Section is critically important to the conduct of incident management operations.

The concept of UC also applies to the Planning Section. **Unified Planning (UP)** is the utilization of two or more planners from different agencies or jurisdictions functioning in a coordinated planning environment. It is highly unlikely that a single indi-

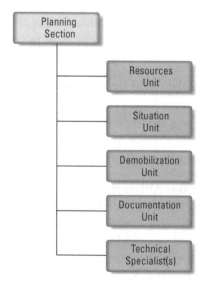

Figure 5-1 Planning Section organization.

vidual has the skills to develop an effective plan when multiple disciplines are functioning in a complex event. An example is an emergency medical services (EMS) professional, a law enforcement officer, and a fire planner managing a Unified Planning Section in the event of a terrorist attack. Other major incidents may require planning expertise from public works, utility, transportation, or public health agencies.

Planning Section Chief

The **Planning Section Chief (PSC)** oversees all incident-related data gathering and analysis regarding incident operations and assigned resources, develops alternatives for tactical operations, conducts planning meetings, and prepares the IAP for each operational period. This individual will normally come from the jurisdiction with primary incident responsibility (or be specifically qualified in this position) and may have one or more deputies from other participating jurisdictions.

It is critical for the PSC to stay in constant contact with the IC/UC and the Operations Section. Incident Commanders should consider the appointment of the PSC to be a critical priority, along with the appointment of an Operations Section Chief (OPS). A PSC can utilize deputies from key response organizations. The complexities inherent in crafting strategic and tactical objectives as part of an IAP for events involving multiple agencies and/or jurisdictions can quickly overwhelm a single PSC.

The technical complexities of many of the tasks assigned to the Planning Section make the effective formation of the team critical. This is especially true when making extensive use of technical specialists who may not be comfortable working in a hierarchical structure. The PSC must act as a coach and a supervisor.

The successful PSC develops a unified IAP with the assistance of personnel from organizations represented in UC as well as other personnel whose skills and/or knowledge are utilized in achieving the tactical objectives of the incident during the next operational period. This unified approach also extends into key units within the Planning Section, especially the Resources Unit and the Situation Unit. The Intelligence/Investigations Function is an optional component (see Chapter 8). It can be established within the Planning Section if it has not been established previously as a separate Intelligence/Investigations Section.

Resources Unit

The Resources Unit ensures that all assigned personnel and other resources have checked in at the incident. **Physical resources** consist of personnel, teams, facilities, supplies, and major items of equipment available for assignment to or employment during incidents. The Resources Unit should have a system for keeping track of the incident location and status of all assigned resources, and it should maintain a master list of all resources committed to incident operations.

In the ICS structure, units are typically subsets sections, especially in the Logistics, Planning, and Finance/Administration Sections. For the Resources Unit to effectively manage and deploy resources, each resource must be categorized by capability and capacity across disciplines and tracked continuously as to status. Following the status condition of each resource is essential for maintaining an up-to-date and accurate picture of resource utilization:

- **Assigned resources** are personnel or teams that have checked in or, in the case of equipment and facilities, have been received and are supporting incident operations.
- **Available resources** are personnel, teams, equipment, or facilities that have been assigned to an incident and are ready for a specific work detail or function.
- **Out-of-service resources** are personnel, teams, equipment, or facilities that have been assigned to an incident but are unable to function for mechanical, rest, or personal reasons or because their condition makes them unusable.

Normally, the individual who changes the status of a resource, such as equipment location, is responsible for promptly informing the Resources Unit.

Situation Unit

The **Situation Unit** collects, processes, and organizes ongoing situation information; prepares situation summaries; and develops projections and forecasts of future events related to the incident. This unit is responsible for forming the current operational picture for the PSC. The Situation Unit must be capable of receiving the real-time information being conveyed throughout the incident management process. The Situation Unit also prepares maps and gathers and disseminates information and intelligence for use in the IAP. This unit may also require the expertise of technical specialists and operations and information security specialists.

Documentation Unit

The **Documentation Unit** maintains accurate and complete incident files, including a complete record of the major steps taken to resolve the incident; provides duplication services to incident personnel; and files, maintains, and stores incident files for legal, analytical, and historical purposes. Documentation is part of the Planning Section primarily because this unit prepares the IAP and maintains many of the files and records that are developed as part of the overall IAP and Planning Function.

Demobilization Unit

The **Demobilization Unit** develops an Incident Demobilization Plan that includes specific instructions for all personnel and resources that will require demobilization. This unit should begin its work early in the incident, creating rosters of personnel and resources and obtaining any missing information as check-in proceeds.

Technical Specialists

Because the ICS is designed to function effectively for any situation that may occur, it is anticipated that **technical specialists** will be used extensively within the Planning Section. Although technical specialists can be attached or serve anywhere within the ICS organization, they are critical to the Planning Section, especially during the development of the tactical objectives in the IAP.

> **Tip**
>
> The ongoing health problems experienced by personnel who responded to the World Trade Center collapse illustrate the importance of quickly deploying technical specialists to assess the threat to response personnel from environmental factors.

Typically, technical specialists contribute specialized skills to the incident management effort. These personnel are frequently maintained on resources lists by response organizations and are activated when needed to address specific situations.

Technical specialists assigned to the Planning Section may report directly to the PSC or to any function in an existing unit, or they may form a separate unit within the Planning Section, depending on the requirements of the incident and the needs of the Section Chief. Technical specialists also may be assigned to other parts of the organization (e.g., to the Operations Section to assist with tactical matters or to the Finance/Administration Section to assist with fiscal matters). Generally, if the expertise is needed for only a short period and involves only one individual, that individual should be assigned to the Situation Unit. If the expertise will be required on a long-term basis and requires several personnel, it may prove more effective to establish a separate **Technical Unit** in the Planning Section. Technical Units are frequently used in hazardous materials incidents, disease epidemics, or hostage situations. In routine incidents, a Technical Unit frequently provides comprehensive weather data specific to the incident location.

The incident dictates the need for technical specialists. Examples of the types of specialists who may be required include the following:

- Meteorologists
- Environmental impact specialists
- Resource use and cost specialists
- Explosives specialists
- Structural engineering specialists
- Medical intelligence specialists
- Pharmaceutical specialists
- Veterinarians
- Agricultural specialists
- Toxic substance specialists
- Radiation health physicists
- Intelligence specialists
- Infectious disease specialists
- Chemical or radiological decontamination specialists
- Attorneys or legal counsel
- Industrial hygienists
- Transportation specialists
- Scientific support coordinators
- Epidemiologists

A specific example of the need to establish a distinct Technical Unit within the General Staff is the requirement to coordinate and manage large volumes of environmental sampling and/or analytical data from multiple sources in certain complex incidents, particularly those involving biological, chemical, and radiation hazards. To meet this requirement, an Environmental Unit is established within the Planning Section to facilitate interagency environmental data management, monitoring, sampling, analysis, and assessment. The Environmental Unit prepares environmental data for the Situation Unit and works in close coordination with other units and sections within the ICS structure to enable effective decision support to Command technical specialists. The Environmental Unit might include a scientific support coordinator. It might also include sampling, response technologies, weather forecast, resources at risk, cleanup assessment, and disposal technical specialists. Example tasks that might be accomplished by the Environmental Unit include the following:

- Identifying sensitive areas and recommending response priorities
- Developing a plan for collecting, transporting, and analyzing samples
- Providing input on wildlife protection strategies
- Determining the extent and effects of site contamination
- Developing site cleanup and hazardous material disposal plans
- Identifying the need for and obtaining permits and other authorizations

The Planning Process and the IAP

An effective and timely planning process is critical because it provides the foundation for effective domestic incident management. The National Incident Management System (NIMS) planning process described in the following discussion represents a template for strategic, operational, and tactical planning that includes all steps the IC/UC and other members of the Command and General Staffs should take to develop and disseminate an IAP. The planning process may begin with the scheduling of a planned event, the identification of a credible threat, or with the initial response to an actual or impending event. The process continues with the implementation of the formalized steps and staffing required to develop a written IAP.

A clear, concise IAP template is essential in guiding the initial incident management decision process and in continuing collective planning activities. The planning process should provide a snapshot of current information that accurately describes the incident situation and resource status (how many tactical objectives have been achieved, the status of strategic incident objectives, and assigned and available resources); predictions of the probable course of events (based on the experience of the Planning, Operations, and Command Staffs); alternative strategies to achieve critical incident objectives; and a realistic IAP for the next operational period. It is imperative that the PSC integrates the experience of the previous operational periods so that the IC/UC may change strategies and tactics based upon the lessons learned in the previous operational period.

Creating a comprehensive IAP involves five phases (described in the next section), which are designed to enable the accomplishment of incident objectives within a specified time. The IAP must provide clear strategic direction and include a comprehensive listing of the tactical objectives, resources, reserves, and support required to accomplish each strategic incident objective. The comprehensive IAP states the sequence of events in a coordinated way for achieving multiple incident objectives.

The phases of the planning process are essentially the same for the IC/UC who develops the initial plan, for the IC/UC and OPS who revises the initial plan for extended operations, and for the incident management team that develops the formal IAP. During the initial stages of incident management, planners must develop a simple plan that is communicated through concise oral briefings. Frequently, this plan is developed very quickly, often with incomplete situation information. As the incident management effort evolves, additional lead time, staff, information systems, and technologies enable more detailed planning and cataloging of events and lessons learned.

Frequently used components of an IAP and the person/unit that normally prepares them are shown in **Table 5-1**.

Table 5-1 Preparation of Frequently Used Components of an IAP

Component	ICS Form	Prepared by
Incident objectives	202	Incident Commander
Organization assignment list or chart	203	Resources Unit
Assignment list	204	Resources Unit
Incident radio communications plan	205	Communications Unit
Medical plan	206	Medical Unit

Note: The ICS forms are included in Appendix D.

Planning Process Phases

The five phases of the planning process are as follows:

1. Understand the situation.
2. Establish incident objectives and strategy.
3. Develop the plan.
4. Prepare and disseminate the plan.
5. Evaluate and revise the plan.

Understand the Situation

The first phase of the planning process includes gathering, recording, analyzing, and displaying situation and resource information in a manner that will ensure a clear picture of the magnitude, complexity, and potential impact of the incident and the ability to determine the resources required to develop and implement an effective IAP.

Establish Incident Objectives and Strategy

The second phase of the planning process involves formulating and prioritizing incident objectives and identifying an appropriate strategy. The incident objectives and strategy must conform with the legal obligations and management objectives of all affected agencies.

Reasonable alternative strategies that will accomplish overall incident objectives are identified, analyzed, and evaluated to determine the most appropriate strategy for the situation at hand. Evaluation criteria include public health and safety factors, estimated costs, and various environmental, legal, and political considerations.

Develop the Plan

The third phase of the planning process involves determining the tactical direction and the specific resources, reserves, and support requirements for implementing the selected strategy for one operational period. This phase is usually the responsibility of the IC/UC. The direction taken is based on resources allocated to enable a sustained response. After determining the availability of resources, the IC/UC develops a plan that makes the best use of these resources.

Prior to the formal planning meetings, each member of the Command Staff and each functional Section Chief is responsible for gathering information to support the decisions being made. During the planning meeting, the Section Chiefs develop the plan collectively.

Prepare and Disseminate the Plan

The fourth phase involves preparing the plan in a format that is appropriate for the level of complexity of the incident. For the initial response, the format is a well-prepared outline suitable for an oral briefing. For incidents that span multiple operational periods, the plan is developed in writing according to ICS procedures.

Evaluate and Revise the Plan

The planning process includes the requirement to evaluate planned events and check the accuracy of information used in planning for subsequent operational periods. The General Staff should regularly compare planned progress with actual progress. When deviations occur and when new information emerges, that information is included in the first step of the process used for modifying the current plan or developing the plan for the subsequent operational period.

Rural Case Study *Answers*

1. You should attempt to obtain situational awareness by quickly questioning the existing Command group. Their answers will help you to determine your next priorities.

2. Assist the UC in developing an initial IAP in outline format. Estimate the time line for the incident. Determine what resources are en route, assigned, available, and out of service.

3. Additional personnel are needed to staff a Situation Unit and a Resources Unit. Technical specialists are required for consultation on structural integrity and utility issues.

Urban Case Study *Answers*

1. A report is needed from the Situation Unit as well as a summary of current requests. Additionally, a consultation with the on-scene Planning Section Chief is indicated to develop a common operational picture (COP) to allow personnel in multiple locations to access common incident-related information. The report and consultation are important because they provide you with information on issues addressed in the current operational period and allow you to plan for the next operational period.

2. The Technical Unit is the next unit you should be concerned with. This unit can provide substantial information on hazardous materials, evacuations, health problems caused by exposure to toxic materials, and infrastructure/environmental issues. Additionally, local meteorological information is critical for this incident.

3. Experts in the following areas would be of immediate assistance: hazardous materials, meteorology, utilities management, water quality/environmental cleanup, medical/public health, transportation, and toxicology. These experts could address the issues identified in the previous answer.

Wrap-Up

Summary

- The Planning Section consists of four primary units: the Resources Unit, the Situation Unit, the Documentation Unit, and the Demobilization Unit.
- Technical specialists may play a critical role in effective incident management. They may be assigned to any component of the ICS structure. Consider forming a Technical Unit if long-term use of technical expertise is expected or if the expertise is needed by multiple components of the ICS structure.
- An effective planning process is critical to domestic incident management.
- The NIMS-approved planning process consists of five phases:
    1. Understand the situation.
    2. Establish incident objectives and strategy.
    3. Develop the plan.
    4. Prepare and disseminate the plan.
    5. Evaluate and revise the plan.

Glossary

Assigned resources: Resources that are engaged in supporting an incident.

Available resources: Resources that are immediately capable of being assigned to a mission to support incident management operations.

Demobilization Unit: The unit in the Planning Section that develops the specific plan related to the release and return of resources to their original status.

Documentation Unit: The unit in the Planning Section that is responsible for all event documentation and administrative functions (copying, filing, etc.).

Intelligence/Investigations: Responsible for the collection and analysis of information related to the incident. Usually exists as part of the Command Staff, a section, a unit within the Planning Section, or as part of the Situation Unit, depending upon the scope and nature of the incident and the need for intelligence.

Out-of-service resources: Resources that are unavailable.

Physical resources: Personnel, teams, facilities, supplies, and major items of equipment available for assignment or employment during incidents.

Planning Section: One of the major components of the ICS. This section collects, evaluates, and disseminates incident situation information and intelligence to the IC/UC and incident management personnel, prepares status reports, displays situation information, maintains the status of resources assigned to the incident, and develops and documents the IAP based on guidance from the IC/UC.

Planning Section Chief (PSC): The supervisor of the Planning Section.

Situation Unit: This unit collects, processes, and organizes ongoing situation information; prepares situation summaries; and develops projections and forecasts of future events related to the incident. The Situation Unit also prepares maps and gathers and disseminates information and intelligence for use in the IAP.

Technical specialists: Personnel activated on an as-needed basis who bring specific skills or knowledge to the incident management effort.

Technical Unit: A unit within the Planning Section that can be set up to house technical specialists who will have long-term commitments to the incident and who will provide ongoing information to the incident management effort.

Unified Planning (UP): The utilization of two or more planners from different agencies, disciplines, or jurisdictions who function as a coordinated Planning Section (similar to the UC concept).

Unit: A component of the ICS that is subordinate to a section.

Wrap-Up Case Study

You are serving as the PSC for the local EOC, which has been activated to assist with the management of a severe influenza event that is impacting the entire region. The primary issues being managed are shortages of hospital beds, medical supplies, and medical personnel due to secondary illnesses (approximately 30 percent of the medical practitioners are too sick to work).

The impact on hospitals is also affecting local EMS organizations, which are having trouble finding open hospital beds for patients suffering from flulike symptoms as well as those resulting from normal EMS system activity. The local and regional medical infrastructure is challenged and nearing a point of collapse.

1. What technical specialists are needed at the EOC?
   A. Medical specialists
   B. Infectious disease specialists
   C. Epidemiologists
   D. All of the above

2. What is the first priority of the Resources Unit?
   A. Implement a tracking mechanism for local medical provider status.
   B. Identify and inventory medical equipment.
   C. Obtain a physical count of available hospital beds.
   D. The Resources Unit is not involved in the crisis at this point.

3. What information should the Planning Section make available to Command on a continuing basis during this incident?
   A. The number of available hospital beds
   B. The weather
   C. EMS system incident activity and volume
   D. Both A and C

CHAPTER 6

Logistics

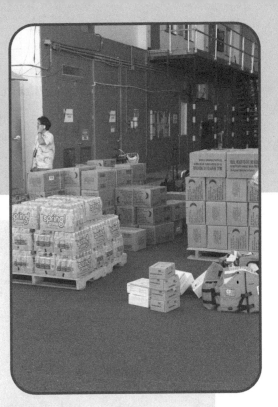

Rural Case Study

Multiple tornado touchdowns in rural Smith County have created critical logistics shortages. The Stadtown Volunteer Fire Department and Rescue Squad are immediately overwhelmed. The Smith County Sheriff's Office is understaffed and is requesting assistance from State Patrol units.

The Stadtown Fire Chief has established limited communications with the state Emergency Operations Center (EOC) via ham radio operators; all other communications networks have failed. The Fire Chief has requested mutual-aid resources. The immediate logistics concerns are as follows:

- *Communications:* Satellite communications and a mobile cellular system
- *Facilities:* Immediate sheltering for most of Stadtown's residents
- *Food:* Food and water support for public shelters
- *Ground support:* Emergency lighting, fuel, and transport vehicles
- *Equipment:* Debris-clearing Strike Teams and cranes
- *Medical:* Emergency medical services (EMS) units, trauma supplies, and supplies for patients and children as well as the special needs population
- *Supplies:* Batteries, clothing, building materials, and comfort items
- *Personnel:* Shelter managers, nurses, urban search and rescue teams, and fire fighters

1. Is Stadtown operating in a push or pull logistics mode? Justify your answer.
2. Prioritize the three most significant issues in this scenario.
3. What communications networks are required in this incident?

Urban Case Study

The Pleasantville incident has rapidly escalated into a major incident. An Incident Command Post (ICP) was established with a Logistics Section Chief. Logistics needs were initially met by supplies and equipment from responding units (i.e., push logistics). The EOC activation generates a full Logistics Section with a Service and Support Branch. Logistics functions are outlined as follows:

- *Logistics Section Chief:* The Logistics Section Chief coordinates with the Multiagency Coordination System (MACS), the Planning Section Chief, and the state EOC.
- *Supply Unit:* The Supply Unit develops a supply order list based on the needs identified by the Incident Commander and orders and processes supplies.

(Continues)

- *Facilities Unit:* The Facilities Unit initially assisted in setting up the EOC, and it now must transition into a mass-sheltering mode with the American Red Cross. Evacuations generate needs for food, water, shelter, and sanitation.
- *Ground Support Unit:* The Ground Support Unit anticipates needs for generators, vehicle maintenance, and fuel. Evacuation actions require buses supplied by the Pleasantville School Board and the Metro Transit Authority.
- *Communications Unit:* The Communications Unit must cope with an immediate overload of the cellular telephone system. The Pleasantville dispatch center is in the evacuation zone and must be relocated to a console at the Metro Communications Center. A command net, support net, and multiple tactical nets are established to ensure fire service, EMS, and law enforcement interoperability.
- *Food Unit:* The Food Unit initiates plans for a food/water schedule at the incident command post, evacuation control points, and the EOC. The unit begins coordination with the American Red Cross and private vendors to support mass-sheltering operations.
- *Medical Unit:* Incident requirements dictate that an EMS Operations Branch be established in the Operations Section. The EMS Commander is assigned to the EOC Operations Section to coordinate medical operations, develop an Incident Medical Plan, transport patients from the evacuation zone, and provide medical support to public shelters.

1. Why is the Medical Unit transitioned to an EMS Branch in the Operations Section?
2. What are the logistical complications when an incident requires mass sheltering?
3. List at least four key implementation steps to plan and establish an effective system.

Introduction

The difference between a routine response and a disaster or high-impact event is often an issue of logistics. In the routine incident, response agencies arrive with enough supplies and equipment to meet on-scene demands. In a disaster or high-impact incident, supply and equipment requirements exceed normal capacity. In essence, a disaster is a logistics-scarce environment. In operating a Logistics Section, it is important to remember that supplies, services, and facilities that are normally scarce or difficult to acquire (e.g., baby supplies, day care resources, and specialized medical care items) will require additional effort and foresight if they are to be available when requested.

Operations agencies, when operating at peak capacity, consume resources at a fast rate. In the Incident Command System (ICS) template, the Logistics Section exists to ensure that operations functions maintain an operational tempo by keeping everyone supplied.

Logistics activities require a special skill set that is not always present in traditional response agencies. Activities such as supply ordering and tracking, equipment support, and feeding and sheltering are not hot topics. However, without logistics support, law enforcement, fire, EMS, and sheltering operations quickly lose momentum **(Table 6-1)**.

> **Tip**
>
> Logistics supports operations functions, such as law enforcement, fire, EMS, and food and sheltering operations.

Logistics Section

The **Logistics Section** is responsible for all support requirements needed to facilitate effective and efficient incident management, including ordering resources from off-incident locations. It also provides facilities, transportation, supplies, equipment maintenance and fuel, food services, communications and information technology support, and emergency responder medical services, including inoculations.

The Logistics Section meets all support needs for the incident, including ordering resources through appropriate procurement authorities from outside locations. For example, equipment and supplies are ordered through prearranged agreements with national or regional vendors or via local government

Table 6-1 Keys to Successful Logistics Implementation

1. Follow logistics procedures in the Emergency Operations Plan (EOP).
2. Conduct logistics officer training.
3. Establish a local cache system.
4. Coordinate state/federal caches.
5. Set up a system of supply management at the command post and EOC, including order processing and storing, distributing, and tracking of supplies.
6. Develop procedures for major facility operations, including public sheltering and coordination protocols, to support agencies such as the Salvation Army and the American Red Cross.
7. Coordinate with the school transportation system and transit agencies for mass civilian evacuation or movement of emergency personnel.
8. Develop procedures for refueling large numbers of vehicles, including aircraft and marine units.
9. Develop and implement a local regional communications plan to ensure interoperability among diverse agencies.
10. Develop and implement a state and federal communications plan, including data transmission.
11. Develop and implement procedures for communications interoperability among local Department Operations Centers (DOCs), EOCs, the command post, and area commands.
12. Develop and implement plans for mass feeding, including coordination with volunteer organizations and contracting with private-sector companies.
13. Coordinate disaster cache procedures for response and support agencies.

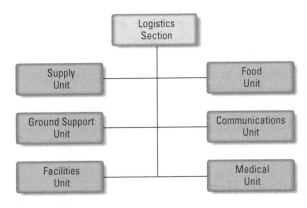

Figure 6-1 Logistics Section organization (high-impact incident)

purchasing agents. Damage to local stores or vendors does not threaten the logistics effort. The Logistics Section also provides facilities, transportation, supplies, equipment maintenance and fueling, food service, communications, and medical services for incident personnel **(Figure 6-1)**.

The Logistics Section is led by a Section Chief, who may also have a deputy. Having a deputy is encouraged when all designated units are established at an incident site. When the incident is very large or requires several facilities with large numbers of equipment, the Logistics Section is divided into Support and Service Branches to maintain a narrow span of control.

Unified Logistics

The concept of **unified logistics** is similar to Unified Command. Unified logistics is the utilization and coordination of two or more agencies or jurisdictions in the Logistics Section.

Unified logistics applies to high-impact, long-duration incidents where several diverse agencies have specialized logistics requirements. A single Logistics Section Chief may not have the skills and proficiency to support multiple agencies with differing support needs. Consider incidents such as the Loma Prieta earthquake (California), the Pentagon attack, or Hurricane Charley (Florida). In each case, fire, law enforcement, and medical agencies had enormous but diverse logistics requirements. Fire fighters needed air cylinders, chemical suits, and respirators. EMS needed medications, oxygen, and cardiac monitors. Law enforcement agencies needed barricades, body armor, and evidence-collection kits. It is unlikely that a single Logistics Chief exists who could have adequately responded to such a diverse shopping list.

Tip

Unified logistics is the coordination of multiple agencies or jurisdictions in the Logistics Section.

Unified logistics is implemented by assigning two or more Logistics Section Chiefs from different agencies or jurisdictions to a unified Logistics Section. Private-sector logistics managers also may be assigned. For example, fire, law enforcement, and private-provider EMS logistics officers are assigned to manage a unified Logistics Section in a terrorist attack.

Unified logistics also is accomplished by assigning appropriate specialists to the units within the Logistics Section. For example, an EMS specialist is assigned to the Supply Unit to manage orders for medications and specialized medical devices or equipment. Fire maintenance personnel and public works maintenance personnel are assigned to the Ground Support Unit.

Because of the flexibility of the ICS, a unified Logistics Section can be implemented in several different ways. The desired end state is a Logistics Section that supports a wide range of supplies, tools, vehicles, equipment, and personnel needs.

Support Branch

The **Support Branch** provides services that assist incident operations by providing supplies, facilities, transport, and equipment maintenance. The Support Branch consists of the following units:

- Supply Unit
- Facilities Unit
- Ground Support Unit

Supply Unit

The **Supply Unit** orders, receives, stores, and processes all resources. **Resources** are personnel, supplies, and equipment needed for incident operations. When established, the Supply Unit also has the basic responsibility for ordering all resources, including the following:

- All tactical and support resources (including personnel)
- All expendable and nonexpendable supplies required for incident support

Tactical resources include tools, helicopters, fire units, ambulances, and equipment such as chain saws or generators. Support resources include fuel, tents, and food. Personnel resources include fire fighters, police officers, special teams, and medical teams.

Expendable supplies are materials that are consumed and cannot be reused. Such supplies include oxygen, medications, bandages, and water. Nonexpendable supplies can be reused. They include backboards, fire hoses, and body armor.

The Supply Unit provides the support required to receive, process, store, and distribute all supply orders. The Supply Unit also handles tool operations, which includes storing, disbursing, and servicing all tools and portable, nonexpendable equipment.

Facilities Unit

The **Facilities Unit** establishes, maintains, and demobilizes all facilities used in support of incident opera-

tions. The unit also provides facility maintenance and security services required to support incident operations.

The Facilities Unit sets up the EOC, area commands, the command post, incident base, and camps, as well as trailers and/or other forms of shelter for use in and around the incident area. The incident base and camps often may be established in areas that have existing structures, which may be used in their entirety or in part. The Facilities Unit also provides and sets up necessary personnel support facilities, including areas for the following:

- Food and water services
- Sleeping
- Sanitation and showers
- Staging

This unit also orders, through the Supply Unit, additional support items, such as portable toilets, shower facilities, and lighting units.

Providing shelter for victims is a critical operational activity. Sheltering for victims is normally conducted by appropriate nongovernmental organization (NGO) staff, such as the American Red Cross or similar entities. Sheltering functions should be moved from the Logistics Section Facilities Unit to the Operations Section when a disaster or attack escalates into a mass-sheltering incident. When thousands of people are displaced, sheltering demands escalate exponentially. The entire ICS structure has to redirect operations and support efforts to respond effectively to public needs for housing, food, water, sanitary facilities, and clothing.

Ground Support Unit

The **Ground Support Unit** maintains and repairs primary tactical equipment, vehicles, and mobile ground support equipment; records usage time for all ground equipment (including contract equipment) assigned to the incident; supplies fuel for all mobile equipment; provides transportation in support of incident operations (except aircraft); and develops and implements the **incident traffic plan**. This plan specifies traffic routes and procedures for vehicles entering and departing an incident site, command post, or support area.

In addition to its primary functions of maintaining and servicing vehicles and mobile equipment, the Ground Support Unit also maintains a transportation pool for major incidents. This pool consists of vehicles (e.g., staff cars, buses, and pickups) that are suitable for transporting personnel. A vehicle pool may require coordination with mass transit authorities, school transportation services, or contracted transportation companies. The Ground Support Unit also provides up-to-date information on the location and status of transportation vehicles to the Resources Unit.

Service Branch

The **Service Branch** provides communications, food, water, and medical services. The Service Branch consists of the following:

- Communications Unit
- Food Unit
- Medical Unit

Communications Unit

The **Communications Unit** develops the communications plan (ICS form 205) to make the most effective use of the communications equipment and facilities assigned to the incident, installs and tests all communications equipment, supervises and operates the incident communications center, distributes and recovers communications equipment assigned to incident personnel, and maintains and repairs communications equipment on site. The Communications Unit must coordinate with dispatch centers, DOCs, and the EOC during major incidents.

Tip

The Communications Unit must coordinate with dispatch centers, DOCs, and the EOC during major incidents or events.

The Communications Unit's major responsibility is effective communications planning for the ICS, especially in the context of a multiagency incident. This is critical for determining required radio nets, establishing interagency frequency assignments, and ensuring the interoperability and optimal use of all assigned communications capabilities. A radio net is a network of like functions or units assigned to a specific radio frequency for coordination purposes. For example, all units in the EMS transport sector are assigned to communicate on the Med 8 frequency.

The Communications Unit Leader should attend all incident planning meetings to ensure that the communications systems available for the incident can support the tactical operations planned for the next operational period.

Incident communications are managed through the use of a common communications plan and an incident-based communications center established solely for the use of tactical and support resources assigned to the incident. Advance planning is required to ensure that an appropriate communications system is available to support incident operations requirements. This element is critical for interoperability and is often lacking in many communities. This planning includes the development of frequency inventories, frequency-use agreements, and interagency radio caches.

Most complex incidents will require an incident communications plan. The Communications Unit is responsible for planning the use of radio frequencies; establishing networks for command, tactical, support, and air units; setting up on-site telephone and public address equipment; and providing any required off-incident communication links. Codes should not be used for radio communication; a clear spoken message—based on common terminology that avoids misunderstanding in complex and noisy situations—reduces the chances for error. Radio networks for large incidents will normally be organized as follows:

- Command net
- Tactical nets
- Support net
- Ground-to-air net
- Air-to-air nets
- Marine nets

Command Net

The **command net** links together Command Staff, Section Chiefs, Branch Directors, and Division and Group Supervisors. The command net must be interoperable with US Department of Defense and other federal agencies. Presently, Federal Communications Commission (FCC) requirements prohibit local and state agencies from installing and using federal radio frequencies.

Tactical Nets

Several **tactical nets** may be established to connect agencies, departments, geographical areas, or specific functional units. The determination of how nets are set up should be a joint Planning, Operations, and Logistics function. The Communications Unit Leader will develop the overall plan.

Support Net

A **support net** may be established primarily to handle changes in resource status, but it may also handle logistical requests and other nontactical functions. This net is a key coordination element between the Supply Unit and the Resources Unit (Planning Section).

Ground-to-Air Net

The **ground-to-air net** is utilized for communications and coordination among ground and aviation units. To coordinate ground-to-air traffic, either a specific tactical frequency may be designated or regular tactical nets may be used.

Air-to-Air Nets

Air-to-air nets will normally be planned and assigned for use at the incident. These units use approved Federal Aviation Administration (FAA) frequencies. These nets become more complex when coordinating civilian and military aviation assets due to incompatible military and civilian frequencies.

Marine Nets

Many incidents occur in coastal areas where federal and local marine units are involved with operational assignments. **Marine nets** are used for communications between marine patrol/rescue boats and land-based agencies. Land-based command posts should have marine frequencies to ensure coordination among marine and land units.

Tip

Failure of communications systems and networks is a common factor in disasters and terrorist attacks.

Communications Failure Protocol

A realistic and effective incident communication plan must include a **communications failure protocol**. This protocol is a plan and operational procedure that identifies major communications networks and backup systems in the case of infrastructure failures (Table 6-2).

Major disasters or terrorism attacks often severely disable or damage seemingly dependable communications systems. Telephone systems (landlines and cellular) often fail. Dispatch center antennas and network repeaters are destroyed or malfunction.

Table 6-2 Communications Failure Protocol

- Identify all major communications networks and systems.
- Analyze potential weaknesses and failure points in each network.
- Identify secondary and tertiary backup systems for critical networks.
- Develop a contractual relationship with communications system vendors for 24/7 emergency support.
- Invest in backup hardware, software, and infrastructure.

Partial or total failures of the public 911 system are common. Information and data networks such as e-mail and Web-based systems may fail.

A communications failure protocol is a collaborative effort among agency communications officers, the National Incident Management System (NIMS) preparedness committee, and private vendors/suppliers. Effective planning dictates that response agencies anticipate communications failure and develop appropriate procedures.

Food Unit

The **Food Unit** determines food and water requirements, plans menus, orders food, provides cooking facilities, cooks and serves food, maintains food-service areas, and manages food security and safety concerns.

Efficient food service is important, especially for any extended incident. The Food Unit must be able to anticipate incident needs, both in terms of the number of people who will need to be fed and whether the type, location, or complexity of the incident indicates that there may be special food requirements. The unit must supply food needs for the entire incident, including all remote locations (i.e., camps and staging areas) and operations personnel who are unable leave their operational assignments. The Food Unit must interact closely with the following elements:

- Planning Section (to determine the number of personnel that must be fed)
- Facilities Unit (to arrange food-service areas)
- Supply Unit (to order food)
- Ground Support Unit (to obtain ground transportation)
- Air Operations Branch Director (to obtain air transportation)
- Mass-sheltering agencies (to obtain shelter)

- Contracted food purveyors (to obtain food services)
- Organizations donating food/water (to ensure adequate amounts of food/water are available)

Careful planning and monitoring are required to ensure food safety before and during food service operations. This includes the assignment, as indicated, of public health professionals with expertise in environmental health and food safety.

Note that feeding victims is a critical operational activity that will be incorporated into the Incident Action Plan (IAP). Feeding activities will normally be conducted by members of an appropriate NGO, such as the American Red Cross or similar entities.

Medical Unit

A **Medical Unit** in the Logistics Section should not be confused with EMS operations. The NIMS template is based on the wildland-fire ICS model where a Medical Unit (usually an individual with basic life support skills) is assigned to a base camp. In non-wildland-fire incidents, medical services are operational in nature and assigned to the Operations Section. The medical agency is usually a local/regional EMS agency or a federal disaster medical assistance team (DMAT) (see Chapter 4).

The assignment of a Medical Unit in the Logistics Section versus EMS in the Operational Section demonstrates the flexibility of the NIMS. If the medical mission is limited in scope, it is practical to utilize a Medical Unit as a support function under the Logistics Section Chief. In incidents that demand operational medical services, EMS units (ground, water, or air) are assigned to the Operations Section Chief.

The primary responsibilities of the Medical Unit or the EMS Commander include the following:

- Develop the Incident Medical Plan (for incident personnel).
- Develop procedures for handling any major medical emergency involving incident personnel.
- Provide continuity of medical care by coordinating with public health agencies.
- Provide transportation for injured incident personnel.
- Ensure that incident personnel patients are tracked as they move from origin, to care facility, to final disposition.

- Assist in processing all paperwork related to injuries or deaths of incident personnel.
- Coordinate personnel and mortuary affairs for personnel fatalities.

The Medical Unit or the EMS Commander is responsible for the effective and efficient provision of medical services to incident personnel. The Medical Unit Leader will develop an Incident Medical Plan, which will, in turn, form part of the IAP. The Incident Medical Plan should provide specific information on medical assistance capabilities at incident locations, potential hazardous areas or conditions, and off-incident medical assistance facilities and procedures for handling complex medical emergencies. The Medical Unit or the EMS Commander also will assist the Finance/Administration Section with the administrative requirements related to injury compensation, including obtaining written authorizations, billing forms, witness statements, administrative medical documents, and reimbursement, as required. The Medical Unit or the EMS Commander will ensure patient privacy and protect confidential medical information to the fullest extent possible.

Note that patient care and medical services for those who are not incident personnel (victims of a bioterror attack, hurricane victims, etc.) are critical operational activities associated with a host of potential incident scenarios. As such, these activities are incorporated into the IAP as key considerations of the Planning and Operations Sections. These sections should be staffed accordingly with appropriately qualified EMS, public health, and medical personnel; technical experts; and other professional personnel, as required.

Push and Pull Logistics

Logistics functions are either *push* or *pull* in nature. In a **push logistics** system, response agencies carry equipment and supplies to emergency scenes. The predetermined list of equipment and supplies is based on years of experience. On routine responses, fire, law enforcement, and EMS units bring their logistics with them.

In disasters and high-impact events, push logistics is no longer effective. Operations units quickly consume their resources. These incidents quickly transition into a pull logistics scenario. **Pull logistics** is when vehicles, personnel, and support equipment have to be ordered from sources outside of local response or support agencies. When an incident transitions to a pull logistics model, the logistics function becomes infinitely more complicated.

Tip

Pull logistics functions require complicated interagency and private-sector coordination.

In a pull system, the supply chain gets longer. It takes time to identify, allocate, and transport resources. Resource requests begin to take days to complete instead of hours.

Ordering and tracking problems also emerge. In a pull system, the chance that items will be lost or misrouted or that the wrong resources will be sent becomes greater. The critical element in a pull logistics system is planning.

Tip

Planning is required to effectively pull logistics from outside sources. The NIMS preparedness organization must develop an effective pull logistics system.

Supply shopping in the middle of a disaster or attack is doomed to failure. An effective logistics plan is a priority for local and state preparedness organizations. The essence of the plan is the identification of anticipated resources and ordering procedures. Information on the following pull logistics sources must be included in the logistics plan:

- *Mutual aid:* The plan should list mutual-aid agencies and their contact information and identify the resources available from each.
- *Contracting:* The plan should list private contractors and businesses and their 24-hour contact information. This requires coordination with Administration/Finance for purchasing agreements.

- *Donations:* The plan should describe the system for managing donations, including allocation, storage, tracking, and distribution.

Tip

Resource management procedures (see Chapter 12) are essential for an effective pull logistics system.

Volunteers and Donations

Volunteers and donations are coordinated at the EOC level. Americans donate generously to disaster causes, especially those receiving widespread media coverage. Such donations are a mixed blessing. On the positive side, donations and volunteers provide much-needed services. On the negative side, donations can overwhelm a logistics system. Clothing must be sorted and stored. Food, especially perishable items, must be inspected and distributed. Equipment and supplies must be categorized and stored.

All donated materials, regardless of type, must be distributed to the proper location in a timely manner. Effective distribution must be coordinated with the Ground Support Unit to ensure transportation. Coordination with the Resources Unit (Planning Section) for resource tracking and status also is important.

Volunteers are the core of support in any major incident. However, unsolicited volunteers who are not affiliated with a formal volunteer organization present special problems. Volunteers often do not bring a support infrastructure with them. If they do not bring equipment, food, and shelter, they drain an overtaxed Logistics Section. Volunteers must be formally credentialed and logged into the system. This is especially important for medical volunteers who must be properly credentialed or licensed to perform medical care. Volunteer processing should be assigned to the Resources Unit and coordinated with the Logistics Section.

Rural Case Study *Answers*

1. Stadtown is operating with a pull logistics system. Normal response systems have been overwhelmed; logistics must be ordered over long distances from mutual-aid agencies, state agencies, volunteer organizations, and private contractors.
2. The three primary logistics issues are as follows:
   - Medical issues are of importance because mass casualties have been reported and the local EMS and treatment facilities are nonfunctional.
   - Heavy lifting equipment is needed to clear roads and to assist in search and rescue operations.
   - Mass-sheltering operations require emergency power, facilities, transportation, and food.
3. A communications infrastructure must be reestablished. A command net is needed to coordinate agency managers. A tactical net is needed for interoperability between operations units. A support net is needed to coordinate pull logistics efforts and sheltering.

Urban Case Study *Answers*

1. A single Medical Unit in the Logistics Section is not practical when an incident demands an aggressive EMS response. In this case, an EMS Operations Branch is established. If the EMS demands escalate even further, an EMS Chief should be assigned to the Unified Command (UC) group.
2. Mass sheltering places a very high demand on all units in the Logistics Section. Facilities and water requirements are immediate. Sheltering also consumes supplies and requires medical, communications, and ground support.
3. Key implementation steps for establishing a logistics system are:
   - Develop a logistics plan.
   - Train and certify at least one Logistics Section Chief.
   - Plan and implement a local regional communications plan that includes a communications failure protocol.
   - Coordinate with a preparedness organization, emergency management agencies, and volunteer agencies to implement a mass-sheltering support plan.

Wrap-Up

Summary

- Disasters and high-impact events result in a logistics-scarce environment.
- The Logistics Section supports all activities needed for efficient incident management.
- The Logistics Section in a fully activated EOC has a Support Branch with a Supply Unit, a Facilities Unit, and a Ground Support Unit, as well as a Service Branch with a Communications Unit, a Food Unit, and a Medical Unit.
- Mass sheltering places high demands on the Logistics Section.
- Logistics functions are based on a push or pull system.
- A communications failure protocol is a critical element in logistics planning.
- Volunteers and donations present management challenges that must be coordinated by the Logistics Section and the Planning Section.

Glossary

Air-to-air nets: Networks for communications among aviation units.

Command net: Network for communications among Command Staff, Section Chiefs, Branch Directors, and Division and Group Supervisors.

Communications failure protocol: Procedures for identifying major communication infrastructures and backup procedures in the case of system failures.

Communications Unit: Plans the effective use of communications equipment and facilities assigned to an incident.

Facilities Unit: Sets up, maintains, and demobilizes all facilities used in support of incident operations.

Food Unit: Plans food operations for facilities and sheltering operations.

Ground Support Unit: Maintains and repairs primary tactical equipment, vehicles, and mobile ground support equipment, supplies fuel, and provides transportation support.

Ground-to-air net: Network for communications among ground and aviation units.

Incident traffic plan: A plan that specifies traffic routes and procedures for vehicles entering and departing an incident site, command post, or support area.

Logistics Section: Responsible for all support requirements needed to facilitate effective incident management.

Marine nets: Networks for communications among marine units and land-based agencies.

Medical Unit: Develops the Incident Medical Plan and manages medical operations.

Pull logistics: Ordering of personnel, supplies, and equipment from outside local response or support agencies.

Push logistics: Initial response equipment and supplies transported by responding units.

Resources: Personnel, supplies, and equipment needed for incident operations.

Service Branch: Provides communications, food, water, and medical services. Consists of the Communications Unit, the Food Unit, and the Medical Unit.

Supply Unit: Orders, receives, and processes all incident-related resources, personnel, and supplies.

Support Branch: Provides services that assist incident operations by providing supplies, facilities, transport, and equipment maintenance. Consists of the Supply Unit, the Facilities Unit, and the Ground Support Unit.

Support net: Communications network that supports logistics requests, resource status changes, and other nontactical functions.

Tactical net: Communications network that connects operating agencies and functional units.

Unified logistics: Utilization and coordination of two or more agencies or jurisdictions to manage diverse logistics functions.

Wrap-Up Case Study

A severe winter ice storm in upstate New York has caused major power shortages and blocked roads in a 13-county area. Temperatures are close to 0°F and are forecasted to remain low for 10 days. The affected rural population is 250,000 people spread over an area of 6000 square miles.

The nearest urban area is more than 95 miles away. Communications are sparse, at best. Several of the affected counties do not have a dedicated EOC and have not been heard from. Power is not expected to be restored for at least 3 weeks.

1. What pull logistics sources may be available?
   A. Contracted supplies from area local businesses
   B. Supplies from volunteer fire departments
   C. National-level support agencies and state mutual-aid logistics
   D. Supplies from local donations

2. What are the immediate logistics demands?
   A. Additional facilities, food, water, and sanitation
   B. Emergency generators and portable heaters
   C. Coordination with public support agencies, such as the American Red Cross
   D. All of the above

3. What are the key points in a communications failure protocol for this incident?
   A. Modern communications systems rarely fail. A failure protocol is unnecessary.
   B. Additional radio batteries and chargers are needed because dead batteries are the most common type of failure.
   C. Multiple tactical nets need to be established.
   D. Backup systems, storage of backup hardware and software, and a contractual support agreement with private vendors need to be established.

CHAPTER 7

Finance/Administration

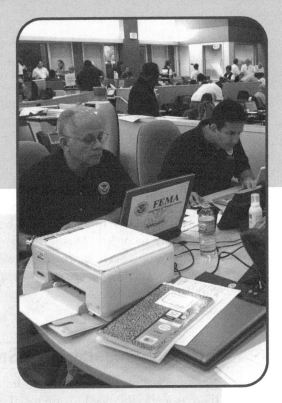

Rural Case Study

Following the Stadtown F4 tornado, you are assigned by the Incident Commander to establish a Finance/Administration Section. Working with the Logistics and Planning Sections, you determine that your top priorities are to establish a Time Unit for on-scene personnel usage documentation and a Procurement Unit to coordinate purchase orders for shelters, water, food, and medical supplies needed at the incident site.

As the Time and Procurement Units begin to put their plans into action, you are notified by the Incident Commander that the Medical Unit has several responders who are injured and will be transported to a hospital emergency department for care. You are requested to document the injury claims and report back to the Incident Commander.

1. Which unit of the Finance/Administration Section will be tasked with the purchase of shelter, food, and medical supplies?
2. Personnel injury claims are one role of the Finance/Administration Section. What other type(s) of claims may be handled by the Finance/Administration Section?

Urban Case Study

As the incident escalates in complexity and size, the Incident Commander recognizes the potential for a long, complex operational period and assigns a Finance/Administration Section Chief. The first priority for the Section Chief is to work with the Logistics Section to procure transit and school buses to begin the evacuation of residents from the predicted downwind plume area.

The Finance/Administration Section Chief contacts the local school district and makes a request for school buses. He directs them to be delivered to the incident staging area for deployment. The Section Chief also works with the Metro Emergency Operations Center (EOC) to arrange buses for resident evacuation in their jurisdiction.

When these arrangements have been made, the Section Chief develops units to take on the responsibility of recording personnel time and gathering information on the cost of the assigned resources at the incident.

1. What costs should be tracked and documented by the Finance/Administration Section?
2. What additional responsibilities is the Finance/Administration Section responsible for?

Introduction

Without funding and reimbursements, the ability to respond and recover from incidents would be limited. It is easy to see in the aftermath of recent manmade and natural disasters the enormous and far-reaching financial impact that is created. Because incident response is a very expensive business—whether it is a small, local response or a response to a larger event—costs and finances must be carefully and thoroughly recorded. This task falls to the Finance/Administration Section. This Section will manage all activities related to cost summaries and contracts for supplies and services as well as reimbursement issues at all levels of government.

Finance/Administration Section

Nearly every major incident will incur costs. When there is a specific need for financial and/or administrative services to support incident management activities, a **Finance/Administration Section** should be established. Under the Incident Command System (ICS), not all agencies will require such assistance. However, in large, complex scenarios involving significant funding originating from multiple sources, the Finance/Administrative Section is an essential part of the ICS. The basic organizational structure for a Finance/Administration Section is shown in **Figure 7-1.**

Tip

Although the functions of Finance/Administration are critical components of effective command and management, components of the Finance/Administration Section are not necessarily staffed at the incident scene. Wireless communications systems enable some of the Finance/Administration functions to be performed away from the incident scene, typically in the workstations where these functions would customarily be performed.

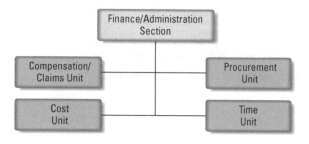

Figure 7-1 Finance/Administration Section organization.

In addition to monitoring multiple sources of funds, the Finance/Administration Section must track and report projected and actual cost totals, current available funds, and potential funds as the incident progresses to the Incident Commander. This enables the Incident Commander to forecast incident needs before operations are affected negatively. This is particularly important if significant operational assets are under contract from the private sector.

The Finance/Administration Section Chief also must monitor cost expenditures to ensure that the local, regional, state, and federal statutory rules that apply are met. For example, spending by a local government may be limited by statute. In response to an incident, as resources are purchased above and beyond the normal day-to-day approved spending, the local government's budget may be exceeded. Some local governments require council approval on items that exceed or do not match the approved annual budget. Close coordination with the Planning and Logistics Sections also is essential so that operational records can be reconciled with financial documents.

It is important to understand that not every incident will require a separate Finance/Administration Section. Some incidents may require only one specific function of the Finance/Administration Section (e.g., cost analysis). In these cases, the service may be provided by a technical specialist in the Planning Section. A Procurement Unit is needed to facilitate vendor contracts. This unit would be responsible for coordinating and securing the rental of buses, as identified in the Urban Case Study. A second example is the management and monitoring of purchase orders for anticipated shelters, water, food, and medical supplies, as identified in the Rural Case Study.

The Finance/Administration Section is overseen and managed by a **Finance/Administration Section Chief**. The Section Chief has the overall responsibility for monitoring the financial and administrative activities of the incident **(Table 7-1)**. The Finance/Administration Section Chief reports to the Incident Commander and is a member of the General Staff. The Section Chief will determine, given current and anticipated requirements, the need for establishing specific subordinate units. In cases of extremely large incidents, a Deputy Section Chief may be appointed.

The subordinate units of the Finance/Administration Section include the Time Unit, the Procurement Unit, the Compensation/Claims Unit, and the Cost Unit. Each of these subgroups is managed by a Unit Leader.

Table 7-1 Responsibilities of the Finance/Administration Section Chief

Review and understand the common National Incident Management System (NIMS) and Section Chief responsibilities.

Attend planning meetings of the General Staff.

Manage all financial aspects of the incident.

Provide financial and cost-analysis information.

Develop an operating plan for the Finance/Administration Section.

Ensure that all personnel time records are accurately completed and transferred according to policy.

Provide financial information for the demobilization plan.

Ensure that all "obligation" documents are prepared and completed.

Brief section personnel on all incident-related financial issues.

Maintain appropriate NIMS/ICS forms.

Table 7-2 Responsibilities of the Time Unit Leader

Review and understand the common NIMS and Unit Leader responsibilities.

Ensure daily personnel time recording documents are prepared and compliant.

Maintain overtime logs.

Submit cost estimates for personnel and equipment needs.

Brief the Finance/Administration Section Chief on Time Unit activities.

Release reports to assisting agencies regarding their personnel.

Maintain ICS activity logs.

Table 7-3 Responsibilities of the Procurement Unit Leader

Review and understand the common NIMS and Unit Leader responsibilities.

Coordinate with local jurisdiction(s) regarding plans and supply sources.

Prepare, establish, and authorize contracts and agreements with vendors.

Draft memoranda of understanding (MOU) as needed.

Ensure proper accounting for all new property and assets.

Coordinate with the Compensation/Claims Unit for processing claims.

Brief the Finance/Administration Section Chief on Procurement Unit activities.

Maintain ICS activity logs.

Finance/Administration Section Organizational Areas

Time Unit

The **Time Unit** is primarily responsible for ensuring daily recording of personnel time, equipment usage, and commissary management in accordance with the policies and procedures of the relevant agencies (Table 7-2). During large incidents, it may be more efficient and manageable to subdivide the Time Unit into specific functional areas. These positions include the Personnel Time Recorder, the Equipment Time Recorder, and the Commissary Manager.

The Time Unit is responsible for personnel time records, which should be collected and processed for each operational period. The Time Unit Leader may require the assistance of personnel familiar with the relevant policies and procedures of any assisting agencies. Examples of these expert assistants include agency timekeepers, claims adjusters, bookkeepers, and private payroll service contractors. These records must be verified, checked for accuracy, and posted according to existing policies. Excess hours worked (overtime) also must be determined, and separate overtime logs must be maintained. This documentation becomes critical in the reimbursement process when federal funds or grants become available to agencies and organizations after the incident.

The Time Unit works with the Logistics Section to ensure that records regarding equipment usage time are maintained. This function may be tasked to the Ground Support Unit for ground equipment and the Air Support Group for aircraft.

The final role of the Time Unit is to establish, staff, supply, and maintain a commissary at large, prolonged incident sites. This role includes providing adequate commissary operations to meet the needs of the incident, security for the commissary stock (via the Supply Unit Leader), and maintenance of appropriate forms and ICS documents related to the operation of the commissary.

Procurement Unit

The **Procurement Unit** administers all financial matters pertaining to vendor contracts. This unit coordinates with local jurisdictions to identify sources for equipment, prepares and signs equipment rental agreements, and processes all administrative requirements associated with equipment rental and supply contracts (Table 7-3). In some agencies, the

Supply Unit in the Logistics Section is responsible for procurement activities. The Procurement Unit also works closely with local governmental authorities responsible for issuing purchase orders for supplies and equipment.

> **Tip**
>
> It is a good idea to have disaster resource contracts or ongoing working agreements with local supply vendors (e.g., home improvement centers, food caterers, heavy equipment transportation and vehicle rental services, etc.) in place before an incident ever takes place. Such agreements reduce complex purchasing during the incident.

Compensation/Claims Unit

The **Compensation/Claims Unit** is responsible for two primary areas: injury compensation and claims related to incident activities other than injuries. The specific activities of the unit are varied and may not always be accomplished by the same person **(Table 7-4)**. During large incidents, the Compensation/Claims Unit may be further divided into the Compensation for Injury and Claims Groups. The individual or group responsible for handling injury compensation ensures that all forms required by workers' compensation programs and local agencies are completed. This individual or group maintains files on reported injuries and illnesses associated with the incident. This includes specific and thorough documentation that may include witness statements. Because the Medical Unit may perform some of the same tasks, close coordination between the Medical Unit and the Compensation/Claims Unit is essential.

The second function of the Compensation/Claims Unit is to coordinate investigations of all civil tort claims involving property associated with or involved in the incident. The Compensation/Claims Unit maintains logs on the claims, obtains witness statements, and documents investigations and agency follow-up requirements.

Cost Unit

The **Cost Unit** is responsible for collecting, analyzing, and reporting all costs related to an incident **(Table 7-5)**. The Cost Unit provides cost-analysis data for the incident in several ways. First, the Cost Unit ensures that equipment and personnel for which payment is required are properly identified and obtained. Second, the Cost Unit maintains records for all incident-incurred expenses and evaluates this cost data to prepare estimates for the Incident Commander and associated agencies. The Cost Unit also provides input on cost estimates for resource use to the Planning Section. The Cost Unit must maintain accurate information on the actual cost of all assigned resources.

> **Tip**
>
> Predetermined lines of financial authority and communication between Section Unit Leaders and supporting agencies and vendors allows for efficient and timely incident management and resource procurement. Preplanning also should include the creation of lists of vendor telephone numbers, contact telephone numbers, and addresses of key persons after normal business hours or on weekends, and identification of other communication methods in case telephones or wireless communications are out of service due to the incident or for other reasons.

Table 7-4 Responsibilities of the Compensation/Claims Unit
Review and understand the common NIMS and Unit Leader responsibilities.
Establish contact with the incident Safety Officer (SO) and the Medical Unit.
Determine the need for injury claims specialists.
Coordinate procedures for handling claims.
Ensure that all claim forms are complete, timely, accurate, and in compliance with required policies and procedures.
Brief the Finance/Administration Section Chief on Compensation/Claims Unit activities.
Maintain ICS activity logs.

Table 7-5 Responsibilities of the Cost Unit
Review and understand the common NIMS and Unit Leader responsibilities.
Coordinate with the IC regarding cost-reporting procedures.
Collect and record all cost data.
Develop incident-cost summaries.
Prepare resource-use cost estimates for the Planning Section.
Ensure that all cost-accounting documents are prepared.
Maintain a cumulative incident-cost report.
Brief the Finance/Administration Section Chief on the activities of the Cost Unit.
Maintain ICS activity logs.

The Finance/Administration Section provides an important NIMS function. One of the most important responsibilities of the Finance/Administration Section is management of the procurement process during an incident and the documentation of expenses for reimbursements. Preexisting procurement processes and resource agreements for equipment, rentals, supplies, and materials offer a systematic approach to obtaining such items during an incident. The Finance/Administration Section Chief operates closely with the Planning Section Chief and Logistics Section Chief on obtaining appropriate and accurate records and documents to monitor financial and cost data for available reimbursements.

Rural Case Study *Answers*

1. The Procurement Unit will be tasked with the purchase of shelter, food, and medical supplies.
2. The Finance/Administration Section may also handle civil tort claims involving property associated with or involved in the incident.

Urban Case Study *Answers*

1. The Finance/Administration Section will track and document personnel costs; the procurement and costs of materials, contracts, supplies, rental equipment, and food; and private-sector and nongovernmental costs associated with the incident.
2. The Finance/Administration Section has the responsibility to track, document, and brief the IC regarding personnel time, equipment usage time, commissary activities, procurement activities, injury compensation claims (as well as other claims not related to personnel), and cost accounting for the incident.

Wrap-Up

Summary

- The Finance/Administration Section is established when agencies involved in incident management activities require financial and administrative support services.
- Not all incidents will require a Finance/Administration Section. Do not assume that one must be established for every incident.
- The Finance/Administration Section may create units to support compensation and claims, cost management and analysis, procurement operations, and personnel time recording.
- The Finance/Administration Section should have preestablished agreements, contracts, and procedural processes with local vendors, suppliers, and contractors on equipment and/or supplies that may be required during a disaster.

Glossary

Compensation/Claims Unit: A functional unit within the Finance/Administration Section that oversees and handles injury compensation and claims. This unit coordinates activities with the Medical Unit for on-scene care.

Cost Unit: A functional unit within the Finance/Administration Section that is responsible for collecting, analyzing, and reporting all costs related to the management of an incident.

Finance/Administration Section: The functional section of the ICS responsible for financial reimbursement and administrative services to support incident management.

Finance/Administration Section Chief: A member of the General Staff who provides cost estimates and ensures that the Incident Action Plan (IAP) is within the financial limits established by the Incident Commander.

Procurement Unit: A functional unit within the Finance/Administration Section that is responsible for the purchase of goods or services.

Time Unit: A functional unit within the Finance/Administration Section that is responsible for ensuring the proper daily recording of personnel time. This unit also may track equipment usage time.

Wrap-Up Case Study

Your city has just experienced a small-magnitude earthquake. The damage is moderate and centered mainly in the downtown area. Emergency management has determined that 11 apartment buildings are in danger of structural collapse and orders their evacuation. The Finance/Administration Section Chief assigns you to be the Procurement Unit Leader. You begin to work with the Planning and Logistics Units, which are arranging and providing shelter for the evacuated residents. You are tasked with obtaining materials for these displaced citizens in the shelters.

1. Which of the following is *not* a unit of the Finance/Administration Section?
    A. Compensation/Claims Unit
    B. Ground Support Unit
    C. Cost Unit
    D. Procurement Unit

2. The Procurement Unit coordinates with local jurisdictions to:
    A. identify sources of equipment.
    B. prepare and sign equipment rental agreements.
    C. process all administrative requirements associated with equipment rental and supply contracts.
    D. all of the above.

3. As the Procurement Unit Leader, which of the following is *not* one of your responsibilities?
    A. Draft memoranda of understanding (MOU) as needed.
    B. Ensure proper accounting for all new property and assets.
    C. Maintain a cumulative incident-cost report.
    D. Maintain ICS activity logs.

CHAPTER 8

Intelligence/Investigations

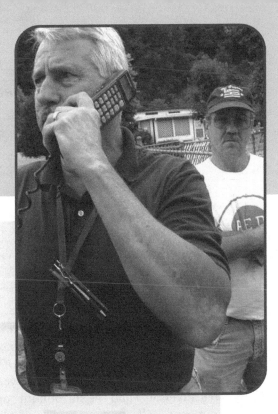

Rural Case Study

As teams and agencies begin the response process following the Stadtown F4 tornado incident, an Intelligence/Investigations Function is developed. Group members begin to collect and develop reports for the Incident Commander. One of the priorities for the Intelligence/Investigations Function is to work with the National Weather Service to determine if there is a continued threat of severe weather at the incident site. The Intelligence/Investigations Function is able to ascertain that continued storms will threaten the area over the next 24 hours.

The Intelligence/Investigations Function also begins working with various town and county agencies to determine the damage to critical infrastructure, such as the water supply, communications, and power and gas lines. The Intelligence/Investigations Function is informed that Stadtown's water supply is contaminated and that the water treatment plant has sustained damage, placing it out of service. They report this information to the Incident Commander to assist in the development of the Incident Action Plan (IAP).

1. List at least three other types of information and intelligence that may be gathered during this incident.
2. How should the Intelligence/Investigations Function be organized within the Incident Command System (ICS) for the Stadtown incident?

Urban Case Study

One of the first priorities for the responders at the Pleasantville incident is to determine the types, nature, and amount of chemicals that are or have the potential to be involved in the spill and fire. This information is essential in determining not only how to fight the fire, but also what type of protective measures need to be implemented at the scene and in the surrounding community. The initial responding units take this immediate responsibility; however, as the incident escalates and more resources become available, a hazardous materials specialist takes over the task.

Because of the highly toxic nature of this incident and the increasing hazard to individuals in the downwind areas, hazardous materials specialists and planners will need to supply a great deal of information to the Incident Commander. Weather data, plume modeling and geospatial information, toxic contaminate levels, and personnel medical surveillance are just a few examples of types of information that will be collected, analyzed, and reported to the Incident Commander and the Planning Section.

The incident quickly becomes more complicated with the report of possible terrorist involvement. The fact that it may be a terrorist incident means that specialized law enforcement officers from local, state,

(Continues)

and federal agencies will be activated and become engaged at numerous levels of this response. The need to manage the incident is complicated by concerns of secondary devices, the need to preserve critical evidence, and the management of intelligence data concerning terrorist activity. Law enforcement officers from several agencies will together collect sensitive intelligence and try to determine who committed this act of terrorism and what, if any, other threats may exist.

1. What is the most appropriate way to organize the law enforcement intelligence function for this incident?
2. Who determines the distribution of information and intelligence at the incident site?

Introduction

The **Intelligence/Investigations Function** strives to accomplish the critical objective of providing Incident Command/Unified Command (IC/UC) with accurate and timely knowledge about an adversary (or potential adversary) and the surrounding operational environment. The primary goal of the Intelligence/Investigations Function is to support decision making by reducing uncertainty about a hostile environment or situation to an acceptable level.

The analysis and distribution of information and intelligence are important elements of the ICS. Although this fundamental concept is not new for organizations that have previously accepted and implemented incident management systems, the type and amount of information and intelligence, as well as the process for handling and distributing it, may be somewhat new.

It is important that emergency response and emergency management organizations embrace the new concept that intelligence is not limited to just high-level national intelligence agency security data and other classified materials, nor is intelligence solely a law enforcement function. Rather, information and intelligence also includes incident operational information. Examples of incident-related information and intelligence include the following:

- Risk assessments
- Medical intelligence (i.e., surveillance)
- Weather information
- Geospatial data
- Preincident response plan data (e.g., structural designs, utilities and public works data)
- Agency response plans
- Special-event plans and details
- Toxic contaminant levels
- Personnel rosters and associated staffing data
- Incident after-action reports

This is just a fundamental sampling of the sensitive data that today's emergency response and emergency management organizations handle on a daily basis. The critical infrastructure and response data that many emergency personnel can be of great value to those who wish to do harm to a target community.

Tip

Because of the different types of information and intelligence that may be required for an incident, specialists from many different disciplines are required. It is essential that these different individuals work together and communicate using common terminology as reports are prepared for planners and Incident Commanders. These elements should be incorporated into drills and exercises and practiced as a team.

Implementation of the Intelligence/Investigations Function

Historically, the Intelligence/Investigations Function has been assigned to the Planning Section within the ICS. Nevertheless, in extraordinary situations, such as high impact/high yield disasters or terrorist attacks, the Incident Commander may delegate the Intelligence/Investigations Function to other components of the ICS. In the National Incident Management System (NIMS) ICS, a potential sixth functional area to cover Intelligence/Investigations can be established for gathering and sharing incident-related information and intelligence based upon unique incident characteristics and response requirements.

Whatever the case may be, the Intelligence/Investigations Function must appropriately analyze and distribute information in a timely manner to those who need it to sustain and advance the incident operation. Distribution of information and intelligence will occur only at the direction of the IC/UC to designated personnel who have the proper clearance (appropriate for the level of information to be disseminated) and an operational need to know in order to ensure that they can effectively support decision making and manage their resources and the incident.

Tip

Some incidents involve a great deal of sensitive information that does not need to be known by all responders on the scene. The release of this information over nonsecure communications networks may compromise operations and place personnel at risk. It is very important for the IC/UC to ensure that these communications are relayed and maintained via secure channels and networks.

The Intelligence/Investigations Function can be deployed in several different ways within the NIMS. Because ICS and NIMS call for flexible command systems and functions, a check-box mentality should be avoided. Flexibility is critical for incident management efficacy and for the efficient utilization of staff to achieve desired functional goals. Therefore, the

Intelligence/Investigations Function can be organized in several different ways, depending on the incident being addressed and the operational scope (Figure 8-1).

- *Within the Command Staff:* This configuration is appropriate for incidents with little need for tactical or classified intelligence. Incidents where event intelligence is provided by supporting Liaison Officers (LNOs) through real-time reach-back capabilities onsite or in an Incident Command Post (ICP) will employ this model.
- *Unit within the Planning Section:* This configuration is appropriate for incidents where the need for tactical intelligence exists to support operations and when the UC does not include a law enforcement entity.
- *Branch within the Operations Section:* This configuration is appropriate for incidents with a significant demand for tactical (predominantly classified) intelligence and when a law enforcement entity is a member of the UC. It also is appropriate when significant amounts of data from a criminal investigation are being analyzed.
- *Separate General Staff Section:* This configuration is appropriate for incidents that are heavily influenced by intelligence factors or

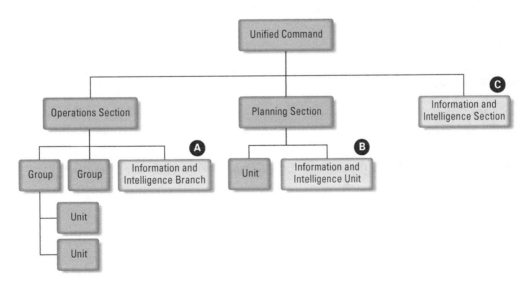

Figure 8-1 During an incident where there is a need for tactical or classified intelligence, the information and intelligence function can be organized as follows:

A. Branch within the Operations Section
B. Unit within the Planning Section
C. Separate General Staff Section

The type of organization used depends on the nature of the incident and the operational scope.

when there is a need to administer or analyze a large volume of classified or highly sensitive intelligence or information. This alternative is particularly appropriate in a terrorism incident for which sensitive intelligence plays a central role throughout the incident life cycle.

Irrespective of how this role is assigned and organized, the Intelligence/Investigations Function is responsible for developing, processing, and managing information related to security plans and operations as directed by the IC/UC. This responsibility might include information security (INFOSEC) functions and participating in operational security (OPSEC) activities. It could also include the complicated undertaking of guaranteeing that all sensitive information or data requiring protection (i.e., sensitive public safety or law enforcement information; classified information; personnel information; or preincident response plan data, such as structural designs and utilities and public works data) is managed in a manner that not only safeguards the information, but also establishes and sustains a means of distribution that delivers the product to those who need it in order to safely and effectively conduct their tasks.

The Intelligence/Investigations Function is also responsible for coordinating information and operational security matters with the Public Information Officer (PIO), who is responsible for the public awareness that can affect the security of sensitive information or the operational activities.

Rural Case Study *Answers*

1. Other types of information and intelligence that may be gathered during this incident include the following:
   - Risk assessments
   - Medical intelligence
   - Geospatial data
   - Preincident response plan data
   - Toxic contaminate levels
   - Personnel and associated staffing data
2. In this case, the Intelligence/Investigations Function should operate from within the Command Staff because there is little need for tactical or classified intelligence.

Urban Case Study *Answers*

1. In this case, the Intelligence/Investigations Function should be separate from the General Staff. This incident will generate a large volume of information and intelligence, some of which will be considered very sensitive or classified. Intelligence will play a large role throughout the entire incident life cycle.
2. The IC or UC determines the distribution of information and intelligence at the incident site.

Wrap-Up

Summary

- The analysis and distribution of information and intelligence are important elements of ICS and NIMS.
- The Intelligence/Investigations Function strives to accomplish the critical objective of providing the IC/UC with accurate and timely knowledge about an adversary and/or the surrounding operational environment.
- The primary goal of the Intelligence/ Investigations Function is to support decision making by reducing uncertainty about a hostile environment or situation to an acceptable level.

- The Intelligence/Investigations Function is typically assigned to the Planning Section. This may be modified based on the unique nature of the incident or the sensitivity of the intelligence.

Glossary

Intelligence/Investigations Function: The component of NIMS that strives to provide the IC/UC with accurate and timely knowledge about a potential adversary and the surrounding operational environment.

For several months, small brush fires have plagued a rural county. The fires have been contained and extinguished without any major difficulties. The Department of Forestry and the County Fire Marshall have determined that in every case, the fires have been set intentionally. A group of youths was seen leaving the area of the last fire, but witnesses were not able to provide conclusive information.

Two days ago another fire started; however, due to a very dry season and poor forest conditions, the fire rapidly spread into a second county and is now threatening two towns along its path. The same youths were seen in the area of the source of the fire, and a physical description of the car was provided along with a partial license plate number. A major incident response is underway to fight the fire, involving local, state, and US Forest Service personnel.

1. In which section of ICS is the Intelligence/Investigations Function usually placed?
    A. Operations
    B. Planning
    C. Logistics
    D. General Staff

2. For the smaller brush fires that occurred in the preceding months, who was responsible for the distribution of information?
    A. The County Fire Marshall
    B. The Planning Section Chief
    C. The Incident Commander
    D. Local law enforcement

3. How should the Intelligence/Investigations Function be organized for a larger incident, such as this one, that has a significant demand for tactical intelligence and where law enforcement is a member of the UC?
    A. As a unit within the Planning Section
    B. Within the Incident Command Staff
    C. As a separate General Staff position
    D. As a branch within the Operations Section

CHAPTER 9

Multiagency Coordination Systems

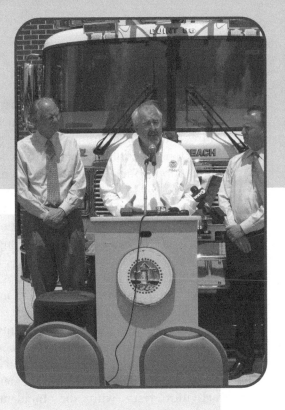

Rural Case Study

The tornado strike in Smith County has created a multi-incident disaster. Clearly, coordination among multiple response agencies over the large rural area is required immediately. The Smith County Emergency Operations Center (EOC) is activated because the operational and logistical demands of this incident require multiagency coordination. The small EOC facility is augmented by an adjoining boardroom and several small offices.

The EOC Logistics, Planning, and Finance/Administration Sections are integrated to form a Multiagency Coordination System (MACS). However, those sections are only partially staffed. By midnight, personnel from the State Emergency Management Office and the American Red Cross arrive to augment the MACS staffing. The MACS operations are severely hampered by inadequate communications. When additional Command personnel arrive, an Area Command is formed and located in the EOC.

1. Why was the MACS located in the EOC?
2. What model is used to organize the MACS?
3. Discuss the justification for establishing an Area Command.

Urban Case Study

The county EOC activation near Pleasantville is organized using the Incident Command System (ICS) template. The unified Operations Section has representatives from law enforcement, fire/rescue, and emergency medical services (EMS). The Operations Section serves as an operations liaison between the command post and the City of Metro.

Due to rapidly increasing incident demands, Logistics and Planning Sections are activated and staffed. Fiscal concerns are assigned to the Finance/Administration Section. The County Finance Director (Finance/Administration Section) is prepared to initiate prenegotiated contract agreements for equipment and supply resources. These three EOC sections become a MACS.

The EOC Planning Section is also responsible for maintaining a common operational picture (COP). The Planning Section displays scene information from the Incident Commander, as well as communications center information from response agencies in Pleasantville and Metro. The Director of Emergency Management (the EOC Commander) forms an Intelligence/Investigations Section that is directed by a Captain from the Metro Police Department who has a federal security clearance.

1. Discuss the rationale for activating the EOC.
2. What are the functions of the MACS in the EOC?
3. Why was an Intelligence/Investigations Section established?

Introduction

A **Multiagency Coordination System (MACS)** is a system of facilities, equipment, personnel, procedures, and communications integrated into a common system that is responsible for coordinating and supporting domestic incident management activities. A MACS is not simply a facility or physical location; the primary ICS functions of Logistics, Planning, and Finance/Administration are the foundation of the MACS. A MACS supports incident management policies and priorities, facilitates logistics support and resource tracking, facilitates resource allocation decisions using incident management priorities, coordinates incident-related information, and coordinates interagency and intergovernmental issues regarding incident management policies, priorities, and strategies. Direct tactical and operational responsibility for conducting incident management activities rests with the Incident Commander. Multiagency coordination systems contain multiagency coordinating entities and are usually located in an EOC.

A fully implemented MACS is critical for seamless multiagency coordination activities and is essential to the success and safety of the response whenever more than one jurisdictional agency responds. Moreover, the use of MACS is one of the fundamental components of Command and Management within the National Incident Management System (NIMS), because it promotes the scalability and flexibility necessary for a coordinated response.

Multiagency Coordination Entities

The primary function of MACS is to coordinate activities above the field level and to prioritize the incident demands for critical or competing resources, thereby assisting the coordination of operations in the field.

When incidents cross disciplinary or jurisdictional boundaries or involve complex incident management scenarios, a multiagency coordination entity, such as an emergency management agency, may be used to facilitate incident management and policy coordination (**Figure 9-1**). For example, an incident may occur at a city–county boundary and require coordination among city and county response agencies. A complex management scenario is illustrated by a major natural disaster or attack in which police, fire, EMS, and public works agencies must

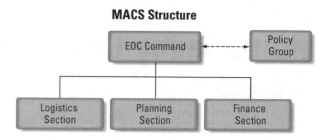

MACS Structure

Figure 9-1 MACS structure

coordinate their response activities. The situation, the ICS template, and the needs of the jurisdictions involved dictate the MACS structure and how these multiagency coordination entities conduct their business.

> **Tip**
>
> A MACS is a combination of the ICS Logistics, Planning, and Finance/Administration Functions and is usually located in an EOC.

Multiagency coordination entities typically consist of principals (or their designees) from organizations and agencies with direct incident management responsibility or with significant incident management support or resource responsibilities. These entities are sometimes referred to as crisis action teams, policy committees, incident management groups, executive teams, or other similar terms.

In most instances, an EOC becomes the multiagency coordination entity in major incidents. In other cases, the preparedness organizations discussed in Chapter 11 may fulfill this role. Regardless of the term or organizational structure used, these entities typically provide strategic coordination during domestic incidents. If constituted separately, multiagency coordination entities, preparedness organizations, and EOCs must coordinate and communicate with one another to provide uniform and consistent guidance to incident management personnel.

The principle functions and responsibilities of multiagency coordination entities typically include the following:

- Ensuring that each agency involved in incident management activities is providing appropriate situational awareness and resource status information (Resources Unit)

- Establishing priorities among incident and/or Area commands in concert with the Incident Command/Unified Command (IC/UC) involved (Command Staff)
- Acquiring and allocating resources required by incident management personnel in concert with the priorities established by the IC/UC (Logistics Section)
- Anticipating and identifying future resource requirements (Logistics and Planning Sections)
- Coordinating and resolving policy issues arising from the incident(s) (Policy Group)
- Providing strategic coordination as required (Command Staff)

Following incidents, multiagency coordination entities also are typically responsible for ensuring that improvements in plans, procedures, communications, staffing, and other capabilities necessary for improved incident management are acted upon. For example, a multiagency coordination entity analyzes after-action reports and lessons learned from a major incident and recommends additional communications networks and a new procedure for requesting mutual-aid units. These improvements are coordinated with appropriate preparedness organizations (see Chapter 11).

Figure 9-2 illustrates an overview of MACS as it transitions over the course of an incident. This figure shows how an incident begins with the on-scene single command. As it grows in size and complexity,

potentially developing into a UC, the incident may require off-scene coordination and support.

System Elements

A MACS includes a combination of facilities, equipment, personnel, and procedures integrated into a common system with responsibility for coordination of resources and support to emergency operations. These elements are defined as follows:

- *Facilities:* The need for location(s)—such as a communications/dispatch center, EOC, city hall, or virtual location—to house system activities will depend on the anticipated functions of the system.
- *Equipment:* Equipment (such as computers and phones) must be identified and procured to accomplish system activities.
- *Personnel:* Agency administrators/executives or their appointed representatives are needed. They must be authorized to commit agency resources and funds in a coordinated response effort. Personnel can also include authorized representatives from supporting agencies, nongovernmental organizations (NGOs), and the private sector, who assist in coordinating activities above the field level.
- *Procedures:* Processes, protocols, agreements, and business practices are needed that prescribe the activities, relationships, and functionality of the MACS.

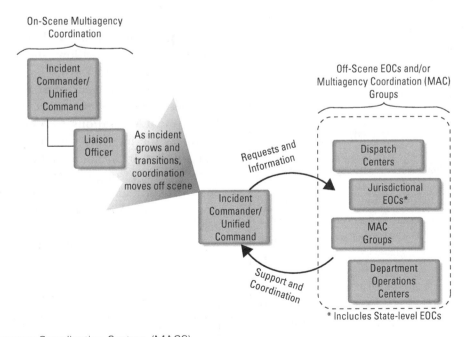

Figure 9-2 Multiagency Coordination System (MACS).

Emergency Operations Center

The two most commonly used elements of MACS are **Emergency Operations Centers (EOCs)** and MAC Groups (discussed in the next section). An EOC is a facility designed to serve as a local or regional incident support center **(Table 9-1)**. EOCs represent the physical location at which the coordination of information and resources to support incident management activities normally takes place. The Incident Command Post (ICP) located at or in the immediate vicinity of an incident site, although primarily focused on the tactical on-scene response, may perform an EOC-like function in smaller-scale incidents or during the initial phase of the response to larger, more complex events. Standing EOCs, or those activated to support larger, more complex events, are typically established in a more central or permanently established facility at a higher level of organization within a jurisdiction.

Table 9-1 Emergency Operations Center (EOC)
An EOC is activated
■ to support the on-scene response during an escalating incident by relieving the burden of external coordination and securing additional resources.
An EOC is
■ a physical location;
■ staffed with personnel trained and authorized to represent their agency/discipline;
■ equipped with mechanisms for communicating with the incident site and obtaining resources and potential resources;
■ managed through protocols;
■ applicable at different levels of government.
An EOC consists of
■ personnel and equipment appropriate to the level of incident.
An EOC is used
■ in varying ways within all levels of government and the private sector;
■ to provide coordination, direction, and support during emergencies.
An EOC may
■ facilitate MACS functions and may be needed to support Area Command, IC, or UC when resource needs exceed local capabilities.
An EOC does not
■ command the on-scene level of the incident.

EOCs may be organized by the following methods:

- Major discipline (e.g., fire, law enforcement, or EMS)
- Emergency support function (e.g., transportation, communications, public works and engineering, or resource support)
- Jurisdiction (e.g., city, county, or region)
- Some combination of these methods (which is most common)

ICPs need good communication links to EOCs to ensure effective and efficient incident management. For complex incidents, EOCs are staffed by personnel representing multiple jurisdictions and functional disciplines and a wide variety of resources. For example, a local EOC established in response to a bioterrorism incident should include a mix of law enforcement, emergency management, public health, and medical personnel (representatives of healthcare facilities, prehospital EMS, patient transportation systems, pharmaceutical repositories, laboratories, etc.).

EOCs may be permanent organizations and facilities, or they may be established to meet temporary, short-term needs. The physical size, staffing, and equipping of an EOC will depend on the size of the jurisdiction, the resources available, and the anticipated incident management workload. EOCs are organized and staffed as required. In smaller EOCs, individuals may be responsible for two or more ICS assignments because of staffing limitations. Regardless of the specific organizational structure used, EOCs should include the following support functions: coordination; communications; resource dispatch and tracking; and information collection, analysis, and dissemination. EOCs may also support multiagency coordination and joint information activities (see Chapter 10).

Governmental agencies or private organizations may also have operations centers referred to as **Department Operations Centers (DOCs)**. A DOC serves as the interface between the ongoing operations of that organization and the emergency operations it is supporting. The DOC may directly support the incident and receive information relative to its operations. In most cases, DOCs are physically represented in a combined agency EOC by authorized agent(s) for the department or agency.

Tip
Communications and information flow within the EOC is based on the ICS model.

On activation of a local EOC, communications and coordination must be established between the IC/UC and the EOC when they are not collocated. ICS field organizations must also establish communications with the activated local EOC, either directly or through their parent organizations. Additionally, EOCs at all levels of government and across functional agencies must be capable of communicating appropriately with other EOCs during incidents, including those maintained by private organizations.

Communications among EOCs must be reliable and contain built-in redundancies. Backup communications systems, such as satellite telephones or the use of ham radio operators, are effective when traditional systems fail.

The efficient functioning of EOCs most frequently depends on the existence of mutual-aid agreements and joint communications protocols among participating agencies. These issues must be continually addressed by the planning efforts of preparedness organizations.

EOC Implementation

Most counties and urban cities in the United States have an EOC. Each state has an EOC that serves as a state operations/coordination center and as a liaison with county and federal EOCs. An EOC must be designed to support a full staff and be organized using the NIMS ICS template. The key functions in the EOC are Finance/Administration, Planning, and Logistics, with a Command Staff. Operations functions are usually assigned to the appropriate command post; however, in many EOC structures, liaison personnel for different operations agencies are placed in a quasi-operations section. For example, in a hurricane, a public works supervisor is assigned to the EOC Operations Section to coordinate with fire, EMS, and police representatives. The primary operations agencies are fire/rescue, law enforcement, EMS, public works, public health, and public transportation. Their primary function is to coordinate operations between the DOCs and the EOC.

> **Tip**
>
> An EOC structure is based on the ICS functions of Command, Finance/Administration, Logistics, Planning, and Operations.

An EOC is often advised by a **Policy Group** that supports the EOC Command. The EOC usually is commanded at local or state levels by a **Director of Emergency Management**. The Policy Staff consists of chief executives and elected officials (e.g., county/city managers, mayors, commissioners, and council members).

A Legal Advisor is recommended for the Policy Group. The Legal Advisor provides guidance relating to interpretation of state statutes, curfew laws, and legal requirements for emergency legislation. It is important that formal legislative procedures be adopted to specify the responsibility and limitations of the Policy Group. In some cases, elected officials in the Policy Group may have to convene in an emergency session to formally declare an emergency or pass emergency legislation.

Policy Groups usually convene in boardrooms. The Policy Group should be restricted from making operational decisions or interfacing with ICS-level staffers. Policy Group members have little operational experience or training and hinder operations personnel if they attempt to micromanage operations decisions.

The major limitation of most EOCs is space. The structure must be large enough for seating five groups (i.e., the five ICS functions). Additional space is required for the Joint Information Center (JIC) and multiagency coordination entities. Additionally, meeting rooms and a communications center are required, along with a kitchen, a break room, and restrooms with showers. The Federal Emergency Management Agency (FEMA) has developed extensive standards and specifications for EOCs. Auditoriums with theater-like seating are not suitable EOC arrangements.

Most EOC facilities have multiple functions. During nondisaster operations (which is 99 percent of the time), the EOC is available for exercises, meetings, or classes. Avoid using the EOC for storage. Removing stored materials during short-notice activations is time consuming and ties up essential personnel.

Most communities cannot afford separate facilities for Area Commands, MACS, or JICs. Due to necessity, these functions are almost always located in a local EOC. Fortunately, many EOCs are in a government complex. Offices, boardrooms, and courtrooms provide temporary space for disaster operations.

> **Tip**
>
> EOCs require adequate space for multiple ICS functional groups and support organizations.

Table 9-2 Effective Message Tracking Methods
Use copied message forms (ICS form 213).
Prioritize all messages.
Distribute messages accordingly.
Establish a feedback loop to ensure reception of messages by the proper personnel.
Track message status (completed, in progress, and unable to complete).
Create a message archive system for postincident analysis.

EOC Functions

The primary functions of the EOC are resource support for various incident sites and the management of information and data. Most of the information that flows through an EOC deals with resource requests, resource tracking, resource allocation, and demobilization. There is also heavy message traffic relating to situation status, weather, damage assessment, and public information (see Chapter 10). Effective message procedures are critical in EOC operations **(Table 9-2)**. It is vital that message tracking procedures be implemented (see Appendix D for relevant ICS forms).

ICS is a good template for channeling and tracking information flow. The nature of the message determines the ICS function that receives it. For example, resource requests are directed to the MACS Logistics Section and coordinated with operational commands. Public information-related traffic is directed to the JIC, and policy issues are directed to the Policy Group. Use the ICS model; it is a guide for effective internal EOC communications and messages.

The EOC is an effective location for the **common operational picture (COP)**, such as information display, situation status, and resource status. The COP is a broad-based view of critical information from multiple sources. It gives an overview of an incident, including resource status and situation status. This is a function of the ICS Planning Section. In sophisticated and well-financed EOCs, information is displayed on large, wall-mounted computer screens. Most EOCs utilize wall charts or dry-erase boards. The displayed information should be visible from every point in the room. When the computers fail or wall charts are filled, a low-tech solution is to use poster boards or white paper taped to the walls.

The following information should be displayed at the EOC:

- Shelter status
- Damage assessments
- Incidents in progress
- Agencies present
- Safety and weather information
- Communications systems information
- Equipment status
- Hospital bed availability
- Security information
- Road and transportation status
- Mutual-aid resources
- EOC staffing charts

The EOC has multiple uses during nonemergency operations. An EOC is effective for supporting major planned events, such as festivals, sports events, religious ceremonies, and conventions. In any major preplanned event where resource support, coordination, and public information is required, consider activating the EOC.

Interoperability in the EOC

Interoperability is the ability of diverse organizations to work together effectively. This is a new word in the public safety arena. Interoperability is a difficult challenge for agencies at all levels. Agencies that are thrown together at a major incident are not proficient at interagency coordination. The equipment, people, language, and culture often are incompatible. The EOC is a focal point to ensure interoperability of support and command functions (via the ICS model).

The EOC is often the only location that maintains a COP. A COP is a broad-based view of an incident or group of incidents. In daily operations, agencies are focused on their own operations. It is not unusual for a county to have 10 or more police, fire, and EMS departments with separate, and sometimes incompatible, dispatch centers. For example, in the Washington, DC area, there are more than 25 separate police departments. The EOC is often the only area where information from diverse sources is collected, processed, and displayed as a COP.

Tip
A major function of NIMS is the development of an interoperability standard. This standard, released on March 10, 2004, from the US Department of Homeland Security (DHS), is called the Statement of Requirements for Public Safety Wireless Communications and Interoperability.

Multiagency Committees (MAC Groups)

A multiagency committee, or **Multiagency Coordination (MAC) Group** (also known as emergency management committees), is typically formed by agency administrators/executives or their designees who are authorized to represent or commit agency resources and funds. Personnel assigned to the EOC who meet the criteria for participation in a MAC Group may be asked to fulfill that role.

A MAC Group does not have any direct incident involvement and will often be located some distance from the incident site(s). In many cases, a MAC Group can function virtually to accomplish its assigned tasks.

A MAC Group may require a support organization for its own logistics and documentation needs; to manage incident-related decision support information, such as tracking critical resources, situation status, and intelligence or investigative information; and to provide public information to the news media and public. The number and skills of its personnel will vary by incident complexity, activity levels, the needs of the MAC Group, and other factors identified through agreements or by preparedness organizations. A MAC Group may be established at any level (e.g., national, state, or local) or within any discipline (e.g., emergency management, public health, critical infrastructure, or private sector).

Primary Functions of the Multiagency Coordination System (MACS)

MACS should be both flexible and scalable to be efficient and effective. MACS will generally perform common functions during an incident; however, not all of the system's functions will be performed during every incident, and functions may not occur in any particular order.

Situation Assessment

This assessment includes the collection, processing, and display of all needed information. This may take the form of consolidating situation reports, obtaining supplemental information, and preparing maps and status boards.

Incident Priority Determination

Establishing the priorities among ongoing incidents within the defined area of responsibility is another component of MACS. Typically, a process or procedure is established to coordinate with Area or Incident Commands to prioritize the incident demands for critical resources. Additional considerations for determining priorities include the following:

- Life-threatening situations
- Threat to property
- High damage potential
- Incident complexity
- Environmental impact
- Economic impact
- Other criteria established by the MACS

Critical Resource Acquisition and Allocation

Designated critical resources will be acquired, if possible, from the involved agencies or jurisdictions. These agencies or jurisdictions may shift resources internally to match the incident needs as a result of incident priority decisions. Resources available from incidents in the process of demobilization may be shifted (e.g., to higher-priority incidents). Resources may also be acquired from outside the affected area. Procedures for acquiring outside resources will vary, depending on such things as the agencies involved and written agreements.

Support for Relevant Incident Management Policies and Interagency Activities

A primary function of MACS is to coordinate, support, and assist with policy-level decisions and interagency activities relevant to incident management activities, policies, priorities, and strategies.

Coordination with Other MACS Elements

A critical part of MACS is outlining how each system element will communicate and coordinate with other system elements at the same level, the next higher level, and the next lower level. Those involved in multiagency coordination functions following an incident may be responsible for incorporating lessons learned into their procedures, protocols, business practices, and communications strategies. These improvements may need to be coordinated with other appropriate preparedness organizations.

Coordination with Elected and Appointed Officials

Another primary function outlined in MACS is a process or procedure to keep elected and appointed officials at all levels of government informed. Maintaining the awareness and support of these officials, particularly those from jurisdictions within the affected area, is extremely important because scarce resources may need to move to an agency or jurisdiction with higher priorities.

Coordination of Summary Information

By virtue of the situation assessment function, personnel implementing the multiagency coordination procedures may provide summary information on incidents within their area of responsibility.

DHS Office for Interoperability and Compatibility

The DHS has established the Office for Interoperability and Compatibility (OIC). The goals of the OIC are as follows:

- To strengthen research and development, testing and evaluation, standards, technical assistance, training, and grant funding related to interoperability
- To become an information resource on interoperability issues
- To reduce duplication in public safety programs
- To identify and promote interoperability best practices

The OIC will enhance the ability of critical response systems or products to work with other systems or products without special demands on the user. The initial priorities of the OIC are communications, equipment, and training.

ICS Forms in the EOC

A by-product of the original wildland-fire ICS is the official ICS forms. These forms have been adopted by the NIMS. ICS forms are an effective organizational and interoperability tool for EOC functions, as well as command post functions. There is a simple rule: each agency uses official ICS forms.

Critical ICS forms include the following:

- ICS 202: Incident Objectives
- ICS 203: Organization Assignment List
- ICS 204: Assignment List
- ICS 205: Incident Radio Communications Plan
- ICS 206: Medical Plan
- ICS 207: Organizational Chart
- ICS 209: Incident Status Summary
- ICS 211: Check-in List
- ICS 213: General Message
- ICS 220: Air Operations Summary
- ICS 221: Demobilization Check-out and Instructions

Copies of ICS forms are provided in Appendix D.

Tip

Use official ICS forms during EOC and incident operations.

EOC Security and Force Protection

An EOC is a critical infrastructure. It is vulnerable in natural disasters and is a target for terrorist attacks. The EOC has to be housed in a robust building. In some instances, EOCs have not fared well in real-world incidents.

The EOC must be heavily secured. Access to it must be controlled. In terrorism scenarios, force protection must be strictly enforced. This includes buffer zones for protection against vehicle bombs. During an attack alert (red threat level), heavily armed tactical teams must be deployed to protect the EOC.

Communications and information flowing through the EOC must be secured, especially during terrorism incidents. Most civilian agencies do not have the capability to secure communications and information to military standards. Encrypted communications are a new public safety venture. The National Integration Center is in the process of developing national encryption and data protection standards. New hardware, software, and training are required. This hardware, software, and training can be costly for local and state agencies that frequently experience budget shortages.

Hurricane Opal

In October 1995, Hurricane Opal formed near the Yucatan Peninsula. The storm was on a northern track and was projected to make landfall along the Mississippi–Alabama gulf coast. During the night, the storm increased in intensity and forward speed and shifted its track toward Destin, Florida.

The Okaloosa County EOC went from partial activation to full activation at 3:30 A.M. and was structured using ICS procedures. At dawn, citizens who failed to heed the previous night's evacuation orders flooded the roadways. Damage reports began flowing into the EOC at about 11:00 A.M. At one point, there were reports of 35 tornado touchdowns.

Emergency responses for accidents, medical emergencies, and downed wires escalated to record levels. At 1:00 P.M., all responses ceased due to high winds. As expected, the community lost power, and telecommunications ceased.

The following morning, initial assessments revealed horrendous coastal damage due to a 14-foot storm surge. The EOC became the focal point for interoperability and the COP. EOC functions included the following:

- A Policy Group was formed and supported by the county manager, and it was directed by the chairman of the Board of County Commissioners.
- A Command Staff was created under the director of Emergency Services.
- An Area Command was established in the Operations Section. The Operations Section acted as a liaison with DOCs located in adjacent courtrooms.
- The Logistics Section supported shelter operations and resource requests.
- A liaison from the Florida Division of Emergency Management provided coordination between the local and the state EOC.
- Message tracking and status displays were maintained by the Planning Section.
- The American Red Cross and the Salvation Army were assigned to the Logistics Section, as were coordinators for volunteers and donations.
- The JIC played a major role in the dissemination of evacuation orders and reentry procedures, as well as the issuing of advisories.

ICS forms were used to organize, chart, and maintain all EOC functions.

Area Command

An Area Command is established when the complexity of the incident and the incident management span-of-control considerations so dictate. Generally, the administrator(s) of the agency who has jurisdictional responsibility for the incident makes the decision to establish an Area Command.

The purpose of an Area Command is to oversee the management of multiple incidents managed by a separate ICS organization or to manage a very large or complex incident with multiple incident management teams. This type of command is generally used when there are several incidents in the same area and of the same type, such as two or more HazMat spills or fires. In this sense, acts of biological, chemical, radiological, and/or nuclear terrorism represent particular challenges for the traditional ICS structure and require extraordinary coordination. These are usually the kinds of incidents that may compete for the same resources.

When incidents are of different types and/or do not have similar resource demands, they are usually handled as separate incidents or are coordinated through an EOC. If the incidents under the authority of the Area Command span multiple jurisdictions, a **Unified Area Command** should be established. This allows each jurisdiction involved to have appropriate representation in the Area Command.

An Area Command integrates with the functions performed by an EOC. An Area Command oversees management of the incident(s) in the Operations Section. The MACS supports the Area Command. MAC Groups are often confused with Area Command; **Table 9-3** highlights some of the primary differences.

Area Commands are particularly relevant to public health emergencies that are not site specific, that are not immediately identifiable, and that are geographically dispersed. Oftentimes such incidents

Table 9-3 Differences Between a MAC Group and Area Command

MAC Group	Area Command
The group is an off-scene coordination and support organization with no direct incident authority or responsibility.	The group assumes the management function of ICS with oversight responsibility and authority of Incident Management Teams (IMTs) assigned at multiple incidents. Area Command may be established as Unified Area Command.
Members are agency administrators/executives or designees from the agencies involved or heavily committed to the incident.	Members are the most highly skilled incident management personnel.
The organization generally consists of multiagency coordination personnel (including agency administrators/executives), the MAC Group coordinator, and an intelligence and information support staff.	The organization generally consists of an Area Commander, Assistant Area Commander (Planning), and Assistant Area Commander (Logistics).
Members are agency administrators/executives or designees.	Authority for a specific incident(s) is delegated from the agency administrator/executive.
The group allocates and reallocates critical resources through the communications/dispatch system by setting incident priorities.	The command assigns and reassigns critical resources allocated to it by MACS or the normal communications/dispatch system organization.
The group makes coordinated decisions at the agency administrator/executive level on issues that affect multiple agencies.	The command ensures that incident objectives and strategies are complementary among IMTs.

evolve over days or weeks. Such emergencies, as well as acts of biological, chemical, radiological, and nuclear terrorism, require a coordinated intergovernmental, private-sector, and NGO response, with large-scale coordination typically conducted at a higher jurisdictional level.

Area Command Responsibilities

The Area Command does not have direct operational responsibilities. For the incidents under its authority, the Area Command does the following:

- Sets overall incident-related priorities at the agency level
- Allocates critical resources according to the established priorities
- Ensures that incidents are properly managed
- Ensures effective communications
- Ensures that incident management objectives are met and do not conflict with one another or with agency policies
- Identifies critical resource needs and reports them to the interagency coordination system (generally EOCs)
- Ensures that short-term emergency recovery is coordinated to assist in the transition to full recovery operations
- Provides for personnel accountability and a safe operating environment

The Area Command and the Planning Section develop an action plan detailing incident management priorities, needs, and objectives. This plan should clearly state policies, objectives, and priorities; provide a structural organization with clear lines of authority and communications; and identify incident management functions performed by the Area Command.

Area Command Organization

The Area Command organization operates under the same basic principles as ICS. The key positions in an Area Command are as follows:

- Area Commander
- Area Command Logistics Chief
- Area Command Planning Chief
- Area Command support positions

Area Commander

The **Area Commander** (also Unified Area Command) is responsible for the overall direction of the incident management teams assigned to the same incident or to incidents in close proximity. This responsibility includes ensuring that conflicts are resolved, that incident objectives are established, and that strategies are selected for the use of critical resources. The Area Commander also is responsible for coordinating with federal, state, local, tribal, and participating private organizations.

Area Command Logistics Chief

The **Area Command Logistics Chief** provides facilities, services, and materials at the Area Command level and ensures the effective allocation of resources and supplies among the incident management teams.

Area Command Planning Chief

The **Area Command Planning Chief** collects information from various incident management teams to assess and evaluate potential conflicts in establishing incident objectives, strategies, and priorities for allocating critical resources.

Area Command Support Positions

The following Area Command support positions are activated as necessary:

- The Resources Unit Leader tracks and maintains the status and availability of resources assigned to each incident under the Area Command.
- The **Situation Unit Leader** monitors the status of objectives for each incident or IMT assigned to the Area Command.
- The Public Information Officer (PIO) provides public information coordination among incident locations and serves as the point of contact for media requests to the Area Command.
- The Liaison Officer (LNO) helps maintain off-incident interagency contacts and coordination.
- An **Aviation Coordinator** is assigned when aviation resources are competing for common airspace and critical resources. The Aviation Coordinator also works in coordination with incident aviation organizations to evaluate potential conflicts, develop common airspace management procedures, and prioritize resources **(Figure 9-3)**.

> **Tip**
>
> The previously discussed Area Command support sections and units are present in a fully staffed EOC. There is no need to create additional positions for the Area Command; use the EOC team.

Location of the Area Command

The following guidelines should be followed when locating an Area Command: To the extent possible, the Area Command should be established in close proximity to the incidents under its authority. This makes it easier for the Area Commander and the Incident Commanders to meet and otherwise interact. It is, however, best not to collocate an Area Command with any individual ICP. Doing so might cause confusion with the command and management activities associated with that particular incident.

Area Commands must establish effective, efficient communications and coordination processes and protocols with subordinate ICPs, as well as with other incident management organizations involved in incident operations. The facility used to house the organization should be large enough to accommodate a full Area Command staff. It should also be able to accommodate meetings among the Area Command Staff, the Incident Commanders, and agency executive(s), as well as news media representatives. Area Commands are most often located at an EOC or, less frequently, at a DOC.

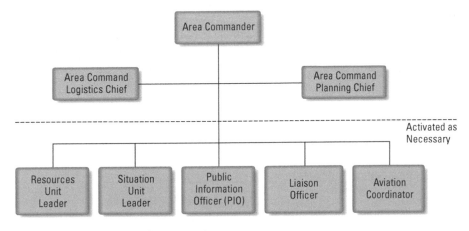

Figure 9-3 Chain of command for the area of command.

Reporting Relationships

When an Area Command is involved in coordinating multiple incident management activities, the following reporting relationships will apply:

- The Incident Commanders for the incidents under the Area Command's authority report to the Area Commander.
- The Area Commander is accountable to the agency(ies) or to the jurisdictional executive(s) or administrator(s).

- If one or more incidents within the Area Command are multijurisdictional, a unified Area Command should be established. In this instance, Incident Commanders report to the Unified Area Commander for their jurisdiction.

Rural Case Study *Answers*

1. The Smith County EOC has the space (although limited) and communications capabilities that are essential for an effective MACS. The EOC also provides a means for communications with the state EOC and the county's public safety dispatch center.

2. The MACS is organized using the ICS template. Logistics and Planning Sections are required to establish communications and to order, allocate, and track resources. The Finance/Administration Section contracts for and purchases resources.

3. The natural disaster in Smith County is a series of incidents, each having an ICP and an ICS structure. An Area Command is a tool for prioritizing resources and coordinating the various Incident Command Posts. The Area Command becomes unified with the additions of the Sheriff and the Director of Emergency Management, and it is located in the EOC.

Urban Case Study *Answers*

1. The incident has escalated beyond the ICP level. The large-scale evacuations, along with a terrorist attack threat, present interoperability problems and COP requirements that are addressed by a fully activated EOC.

2. This incident requires complex coordination between multiple police, fire, and EMS agencies. State assistance and federal law enforcement support must be interoperable with the local effort. In this incident, the primary functions of the MACS are as follows:

- Logistics support and resource tracking
- Coordination of information and interagency issues
- Implementation of preparedness plans

3. The initial explosion and the threat of another attack classify this as a national security incident. Intelligence information must be protected and effectively utilized for strategic planning. This is accomplished by elevating the Intelligence/Investigations Function to the Section level in the EOC.

Wrap-Up

Summary

- A MACS supports incident management activities.
- MACS provides Logistics, Planning, and Finance/Administration functions (ICS template).
- MACS is usually located in the EOC during major incidents. It facilitates logistics support and resource tracking.
- The EOC coordinates operations among ICPs and DOCs and is organized around the ICS structure.
- The EOC should maintain a COP of an incident and facilitate interoperability among agencies.
- An Area Command with multiple ICPs is utilized for large-scale incidents, such as biological, chemical, or radiological attacks.

Glossary

Area Command Logistics Chief: Provides logistics support to the Area Commander and the related Incident Commander.

Area Command Planning Chief: Provides planning support for the Area Commander and the related Incident Commanders.

Area Commander: Responsible for the direction of incident management teams in a given area.

Aviation Coordinator: Coordinates aviation activities, including airspace management and resource prioritization, with the Area Commander.

Common operational picture (COP): A broad-based view of critical information from multiple sources that is processed by the Planning Section. It gives an overview of an incident, including resource status and situation status.

Department Operations Center (DOC): An agency-specific center that coordinates with the EOC Operations Section.

Director of Emergency Management: The senior manager of a local, county, or state emergency management agency.

Emergency Operations Center (EOC): A facility that serves as an incident support center. It displays a common operational picture of an incident or event.

Interoperability: The ability of diverse organizations to effectively coordinate and integrate command and support functions during routine incidents, events, or disasters.

Multiagency Coordination (MAC) Group: Committee that manages incident-related decision support information, such as tracking critical resources, situation status, and intelligence or investigative information. Also provides public information to the news media and public.

Multiagency Coordination System (MACS): A combination of facilities, equipment, personnel, procedures, and communications integrated into a common system for incident coordination and support. Usually located at an EOC and structured via the ICS template.

Policy Group: Elected officials and senior executives who give policy advice to the EOC Command.

Situation Unit Leader: Monitors the status of objectives for each incident.

Unified Area Command: An Area Command that spans multiple jurisdictions and gives each jurisdiction appropriate representation.

Wrap-Up Case Study

Wilson County has a population of 85,000 and is 60 miles from Metro City. A large Woodstock-style open-air rock concert with 150,000 fans is in progress. The concert location is protected by a volunteer fire department, a private EMS agency, and the Wilson County Sheriff's Department. Off-duty police officers from Metro City have been contracted by the concert promoters to provide on-site security.

A decision was made to utilize the Wilson County EOC to support the logistics and operational demands of the concert. The EOC remains partially activated for a period of 3 days. The preplanned organization includes the core functions of the ICS. A MACS and a JIC are established within the EOC.

1. Why is the EOC being used for a nonemergency event?
   A. EOCs are for emergencies only and should not be used for planned events.
   B. The EOC is a good facility for storing concert equipment.
   C. The EOC can be used as a makeshift casualty collection center.
   D. The EOC is effective for coordinating logistics, communications, and support functions for a multi-agency event that could easily evolve into an emergency situation for law enforcement and EMS.

2. What multiagency coordination functions are most likely required?
   A. Interoperability and maintenance of a COP
   B. Coordination of preevent plans with operations agencies
   C. Logistics support and resource tracking
   D. All of the above

3. What ICS core functions should be staffed in the EOC?
   A. Command, Operations, Planning, Logistics, and Finance/Administration
   B. Intelligence/Investigations
   C. Tactical networks, hospital operations, and Task Forces
   D. Directors, Section Chiefs, Supervisors, and Unit Leaders

The Message

The three basic categories of public information are narrative information, advisories and warnings, and action messages.

Narrative Information

Narrative information provides general information or an overview of an event or incident. The following are examples of narrative information:

- "The flood now extends to three states."
- "The terrorists are from . . ."
- "The mayor has announced an investigation into . . ."

Narratives usually are audio sound bites, video clips, or newspaper articles. This information is important because it keeps the public informed and paints a general picture of the magnitude and progress of an unfolding scenario. Accuracy and timeliness are important but not critical. In essence, inaccurate information is embarrassing, but it does not hurt anyone or affect the outcome of the response effort.

Advisories and Warnings

Advisories and warnings inform the public of a concern or hazard and provide instructions relating to specific procedures that should be followed. The following are examples of advisory and warning messages:

- "Avoid the Bayshore Road area."
- "Boil all water before drinking."
- "Do not fuel generators while they are running."

Advisory and warning messages are time sensitive. Accuracy is important. Warnings often contain technical information that must be written using common language that is free of acronyms. The JIC must have access to official publications or electronic data and have established coordination with technical experts to ensure accuracy. Multiple warnings cannot conflict.

Action Messages

Action messages prompt the public to take immediate action. Timeliness and accuracy can literally mean life and death. Action messages require a media blitz that uses radio, television, and public warning systems, as well as nonmedia systems, such as reverse 911. Reverse 911 systems can call citizens in a designated area with an automated action message. It is an information blitz from a 911 center to the public. The following are examples of action messages:

- "Residents in Hanover should take cover immediately."
- "An evacuation has been ordered for all areas south of Highway 98."

Joint Information Procedures

The JIS requires clear, concise, written procedures to ensure that the right message goes to the right audience at the right time. Messages may originate from many sources, including JICs; PIOs; EOCs; agency offices (local, state, and federal); NGOs, such as the Salvation Army and the American Red Cross; and private-sector agencies. **Table 10-2** lists key NIMS joint information procedures.

Table 10-2 Key NIMS Joint Information Procedures

Public information must be formally approved by the Incident Commander and the JIS manager.

A system for prioritizing public information is essential. Action messages have the highest priority.

A system must be in place for coordination with elected officials and private organizations.

Distribution procedures and media contacts must be identified.

The JIS must identify and have access to technical experts and reference sources.

Specific media procedures must be established for media briefings, identification and clearances, escorted media tours, and pool reporting.

Local, state, and federal information protocols must be formalized.

Elected officials and their staffs (Policy Group) must be integrated into the JIS.

NIMS specifies that NGOs and corporate entities are important components in the JIS.

Postincident evaluation and corrections are valuable tools for information operations.

Elected officials can project leadership and calmness, as Governor Frank Keating did during the Oklahoma City bombing. On the negative side, officials running for office can complicate a disaster incident. After Hurricane Andrew, presidential candidates were leapfrogging in helicopters from one site to another. This delayed cleanup efforts because resources were diverted to securing and assisting the presidential candidates.

Nonofficial Information Sources

During a disaster, not all information filters into the JIC through formal means. Often the public calls the EOC with information. This information often includes rumors that must be investigated and clarified. Newspaper offices, television stations, radio news stations, and hospitals are flooded with calls. This information often gets relayed to the EOC. The JIC will get frequent calls from reporters following up on information they received from the public. In essence, public information goes from the media back to the JIC as well as the traditional model of public messages going out from the JIC.

It is not unusual for ICS staffers to get incident information from CNN before it comes in by official channels. EOCs, Area Commands, and state/federal command centers should monitor the national television media. Consider the national media to be good overview sources that are sometimes inaccurate.

National Media Support

When a local incident escalates to national media coverage, the JIS must respond to a new set of demands. National-level news reporters expect time, access, and celebrity treatment. Media news trucks place high demands on local communications systems. Cellular telephone systems are quickly overloaded (referred to as *hot cell sites*). Computer bandwidth becomes overloaded. Satellite trucks require space, facilities, food, and water. JIS procedures should incorporate plans for logistics support for national and regional news crews, including additional PIOs, facilities, and communications.

Tip
National coverage places high demands on the JIS.

Operational Security and Force Protection

Operational security (OPSEC) encompasses procedures that prevent sensitive information from being released (intentionally or unintentionally) that may compromise tactical operations. OPSEC is critical in criminal or terrorism-related incidents. Discussions about strategy/tactics or video of weapons, protective equipment, or tactical deployments must not be broadcast. The enemy is most likely watching television along with the public.

Information relating to a victim's medical status or condition also must be secured and not released. The Health Insurance Portability and Accountability Act of 1996 (HIPAA) addresses the security and privacy of health data. National security information, official-use-only information, and law enforcement information in the EOC also must be properly secured and archived or disposed of.

Force protection is the protection of key personnel and facilities to prevent losses in the event of an attack. The JIC, especially if it is located in the EOC, must be protected. Force-protection procedures are scalable based on the national alert level and the type of incident. Law enforcement agencies should have force-protection procedures that can be implemented immediately.

Key Points in Implementing a JIS

The following points, as provided by NIMS, should be kept in mind when developing a JIS:

- JIC facilities should have adequate space, communications capabilities, and auxiliary power.
- Assign a PIO to each command center.
- Develop formal JIS procedures.
- Develop technical reach-back capabilities.
- Prioritize messages.
- Implement interagency coordination.
- Coordinate with NGOs and private-sector agencies.
- Maintain a media contacts database.
- Plan for national media support.
- Develop an OPSEC plan.
- Implement a force-protection protocol based on the threat level.
- Protect medical and national security information.

Rural Case Study *Answers*

1. Smith County officials did not anticipate a disaster and did not plan accordingly. Officials were aware of NIMS but did not implement a JIS. Namely, they lacked information procedures and trained personnel.
2. The message priorities are advisories and action messages. The advisory messages include information about safety procedures, such as those for downed power lines. The action messages are instructions for taking immediate shelter and emergency flood information.
3. Smith County's inadequate planning results in an inability to support national media crews. Demands for logistics support, communications, and press briefings will have to be met by state officials after they arrive.

Urban Case Study *Answers*

1. The JIC requires communications equipment, supplies, food, and water from the Logistics Section. The Planning Section supplies the COP, the situation status, and technical information. All public messages are coordinated with the EOC Commander (Command Staff).
2. The JIC provides for the following:
   - Interagency coordination
   - A coordinated message system
   - Crisis communications
   - National media support
3. A liaison from each federal agency must be assigned to the JIC. Federal agencies can still maintain autonomy. However, messages and public instructions are coordinated jointly with local agencies, ensuring continuity and clarity of information.

Wrap-Up

Summary

- A PIO is a key member of the ICS Command Staff.
- A PIO coordinates information from the incident site with the JIS.
- Public information functions must be coordinated across jurisdictions and with private-sector agencies and NGOs.
- The JIC provides a location for joint coordination of public information.
- Public messages may be narratives, advisories and warnings, or action messages.
- Information coordination with elected officials and corporations presents challenges.
- A JIS must process information from unofficial sources and respond to rumors.
- National media coverage results in additional support requirements from the JIC and ICS.

Glossary

Action messages: Information that prompts the public to take immediate action.

Advisories and warnings: Information that informs the public and provides specific instructions.

Force protection: Protection of key personnel and facilities to prevent losses in the event of an attack.

Joint Information System (JIS): An integrated and coordinated mechanism to ensure the delivery of timely and accurate information.

Narrative information: General information that informs the public about the nature and progress of an incident or event.

Operational security (OPSEC): The protection of information that would compromise security or tactical operations.

In Okaloosa County, Florida (the Fort Walton Beach/Destin area), a single case of bacterial meningitis has resulted in the death of a child. Within a week, the outbreak escalates to several additional cases. Public concern rises to almost panic levels, and parents keep their children out of school and consider sending children to relatives outside the area.

Misinformation and rumors escalate. Physicians' offices, hospitals, and 911 centers are flooded with calls. The public perceives the disease to be like Ebola or smallpox. In reality, meningitis transmission requires constant contact (8 hours or more per day) for several weeks. This misconception has to be corrected.

The key strategy, drafted by the Public Health Department, emergency medical services (EMS), and the Emergency Management Office, is to establish an inoculation program and a public information plan. The EOC is activated and establishes 20 additional telephone lines. Physicians draft an accurate and carefully worded information packet using layman's language. Call center personnel are given a crash course on facts about meningitis and basic preventive measures.

The EOC becomes a JIC. Other agencies, such as media offices and hospitals, forward calls to the JIC. At the height of the event, the JIC receives more than 200 calls per hour.

The JIC also conducts press conferences and media briefings on a scheduled basis (two per day). The incident receives national media coverage as well. The informed public is calmed by the information it receives, participates in the inoculation program, and follows prevention procedures as instructed. The successful outcome of this incident is mainly due to an effective JIS.

1. How were inaccurate rumors corrected?
    A. It is not an ICS or a NIMS function to correct rumors.
    B. Questions were answered by the JIC call center, and information was broadcast in layman's language.
    C. Correcting rumors and information is synonymous in the JIS.
    D. None of the above.
2. What ICS functions were utilized in this case?
    A. The Command Staff PIO function was utilized.
    B. Because response agencies were not utilized, no ICS functions were utilized.
    C. EMS was the only function utilized due to the medical nature of the event.
    D. A Planning Section and a Logistics Section supported the Command Staff and the JIC.
3. Why was the JIC located in the EOC?
    A. Both NIMS and ICS require that all information be disseminated from the EOC.
    B. The EOC has communications equipment (telephone and radio), a system for information display, the common operational picture (COP), and a facility with available space.
    C. The JIC should have been located at the County Commissioner's Office because elected officials should approve all messages.
    D. The national media usually prefers to get information from an EOC.

CHAPTER 11

Preparedness

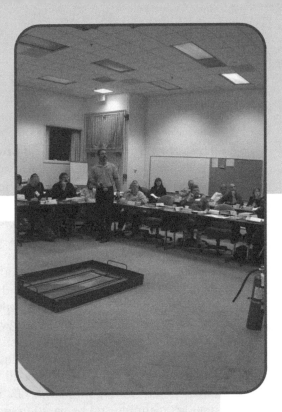

Rural Case Study

Since the mid-1960s, several major storms that have spawned tornadoes have passed through Smith County. Many people in the region have taken measures to prepare for such events, and so have the local public safety agencies. When the National Weather Service notifies the Smith County Emergency Operations Center (EOC) of the approaching storm, a Tornado Watch is issued for the area. Upon confirmation of a funnel cloud on the ground by local law enforcement, the EOC activates the tornado alert sirens, notifying citizens to seek emergency shelter.

Following the storm, the Smith County EOC is activated. It notifies the state EOC regarding its status. Reports come in from all over the county reporting major damage at multiple sites. The Smith County agencies have conducted emergency planning over the years, but they have never taken into account the possibility of a catastrophic series of storms striking at once. The Smith County Emergency Operations Plan (EOP) is put into action as units begin to deploy into the area.

1. List five elements of preparedness planning for the Smith County incident.
2. Describe the role of the National Incident Management System (NIMS) in preparedness planning.

Urban Case Study

As the incident in Pleasantville begins to evolve, local resources and response capabilities are greatly reduced. Fortunately, the city has a standing mutual-aid agreement with the surrounding jurisdictions. The Incident Commander requests additional resources from the dispatch center to augment and backfill the Pleasantville area. The Pleasantville dispatch center requests units through the mutual-aid procedures.

As the incident escalates to include the terrorist activity and threat to the surrounding downwind community, all regional resources are called into service. The EOCs are activated and the state terrorism warning point is notified. The state activates its EOC, and local EOPs are utilized to mobilize all community and regional resources to begin the evacuation effort. Recently, a regional field operations guide (FOG) was created; however, training and implementation were not completed. The Unified Command (UC) center, in conjunction with the regional and state EOCs, begins a massive effort to carry out the response plans.

1. List four types of preparedness plans that may be called into service for this incident.
2. What types of mitigation activities would be beneficial in this incident?

Introduction

Major or complex incidents are not uncommon to emergency responders; in fact, they occur on a daily basis. However, high-impact catastrophic incidents are very unusual. Because of the lower probability of a catastrophic incident, there is a tendency toward complacency or underestimation of their effects. Unfortunately, there is evidence that the numbers and costs of these incidents may be increasing.

When catastrophic incidents occur, citizens expect public safety agencies and other members of the response community to act and assist immediately. The preservation of life and reduction of injury are without a doubt important; however, these cannot be accomplished without the assistance of many additional well-trained and coordinated resources. For this reason, it is critical that all resources function together during all phases of an incident. This requires planning and preparation by all members of the response community for all types of hazards and events.

The emergency management of large-scale or technically complicated incidents presents tremendous hazards to responders and represents the single greatest challenge facing the emergency response community. Recurring scene factors and difficulties are frequently encountered during these incidents. These are lessons learned, and they contribute to developing solutions before the next incident. In this chapter, we will explore and describe specific actions that jurisdictions and agencies can develop and incorporate into a systems approach to enhance their preparedness for incident management of all hazards.

Essential Principles and Concepts of Preparedness

Various methods have been described and developed over the years to assist planners in major incident responses. In some cases, the effects of major or catastrophic incidents can be reduced before the actual event. Most incidents are broken into four phases: mitigation, planning, response, and recovery. Preparedness affects each of these phases and has deep roots in the first two: mitigation and planning.

Oftentimes preparedness planning focuses on a singular event or does not include all of the response community partners. When developing, refining, and expanding preparedness programs and activities within a jurisdiction or agency, incident manage-

ment officials and planners must seek out and incorporate the entire response community into existing preparedness efforts and partnerships. The operational preparedness of our nation's incident management capabilities is distinct from the preparedness of individual citizens and private industry. Public preparedness (citizen training and community resilience) for domestic incidents is beyond the scope of the NIMS but is an important element of homeland security.

Within the NIMS, preparedness is based on the following core concepts and principles:

- Levels of capability
- Unified approach
- NIMS publications
- Mitigation

Levels of Capability

Preparedness involves actions to establish and sustain determined levels of response necessary to execute a full range of incident management operations. Preparedness is implemented through a continuous and systematic process of planning, training, equipping, exercising, evaluating, and taking action to correct and mitigate. Paper planning is an excellent component of preparedness; however, without deliberate practice and feedback with error correction and remediation, preparedness activities will not be as efficient or effective as they could be.

Tip
Effective incident responses by teams within the NIMS do not just happen. Furthermore, teamwork does not necessarily occur simply because of team formation or planning. Effective team structure is defined by team size, membership, leadership, formation, roles, and communication. Teamwork is the result of deliberate planning and practice; assemble response community partners and prepare them for an effective response. Deliberate practice is a critical step in developing a highly effective response community.

Unified Approach

Preparedness requires a unified approach. A major objective of preparedness efforts is to ensure mission integration and interoperability in response to emergent crises across functional (specific disciplines) and jurisdictional (geographic) lines, as well as between public and private organizations and the citizens for whom the response system works.

NIMS Publications

The NIMS provides or establishes processes for providing guidelines; protocols; standards for planning, training, qualifications, and certification; and publication management. National-level preparedness standards related to the NIMS are maintained and managed through the National Integration Center (discussed in Chapter 2) using a collaborative process.

Mitigation

Mitigation refers to activities, planning, or developing codes that lessen the severity of an incident. These actions may occur before or during an incident and may be the result of lessons learned from previous or similar events. Mitigation activities are an important element of preparedness. Mitigation activities provide a critical foundation across the incident management spectrum, from prevention through response and recovery.

Examples of key mitigation activities include the following:

- Ongoing public education and outreach activities designed to reduce loss of life and destruction of property
- Structural retrofitting to deter or lessen the effects of incidents and reduce loss of life, destruction of property, and effects on the environment

- Code enforcement through such activities as zoning regulation, land management, and building codes
- Flood insurance and the buyout of properties subject to frequent flooding
- Evacuation drills and predesignated emergency shelters for known natural and potential man-made disasters

Achieving Preparedness

Federal, state, and local jurisdictions are responsible for implementing the preparedness cycle in advance of an incident and appropriately including private-sector and nongovernmental organizations (NGOs). The preparedness cycle can easily be remembered with the acronym POTEE **(Figure 11-1)**:

- Plan
- Organize
- Train
- Exercise
- Evaluate

In the sections that follow, we will review and discuss the tools that the NIMS provides to ensure and enhance preparedness. These tools include preparedness organizations and programs that provide or establish processes for planning, training, and exercises; personnel qualification and certification;

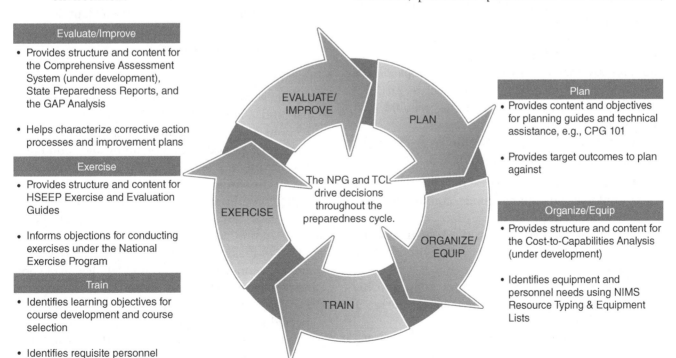

Evaluate/Improve
- Provides structure and content for the Comprehensive Assessment System (under development), State Preparedness Reports, and the GAP Analysis
- Helps characterize corrective action processes and improvement plans

Exercise
- Provides structure and content for HSEEP Exercise and Evaluation Guides
- Informs objections for conducting exercises under the National Exercise Program

Train
- Identifies learning objectives for course development and course selection
- Identifies requisite personnel competencies

The NPG and TCL drive decisions throughout the preparedness cycle.

Plan
- Provides content and objectives for planning guides and technical assistance, e.g., CPG 101
- Provides target outcomes to plan against

Organize/Equip
- Provides structure and content for the Cost-to-Capabilities Analysis (under development)
- Identifies equipment and personnel needs using NIMS Resource Typing & Equipment Lists

Figure 11-1 Preparedness cycle.

equipment certification; mutual aid; and publication management.

The role of engaging the entire community in the overarching preparedness effort cannot be understated. For a community to respond to and recover from a large-scale incident, they must have developed a clear planning process informed by the role of the emergency management community and based on the capability and capacity of the community-wide response organizations.

Preparedness Organizations

Preparedness is the responsibility of all members of the response community as well as its citizens. This responsibility includes coordinating preparedness activities among all agencies within a jurisdiction, across jurisdictions, and with private organizations. This coordination is affected by entities ranging from individuals, to small committees, to large organizations. For the purposes of the NIMS, these entities are called preparedness organizations. These groups are ongoing forums for coordinating preparedness activities in advance of an incident.

Preparedness organizations represent a wide variety of committees, planning groups, and other organizations that meet regularly and coordinate to ensure an appropriate focus on planning, training, equipping, and other preparedness requirements within a jurisdiction and/or across jurisdictions. The needs of the jurisdictions involved dictate how frequently such organizations must conduct their business and how they are structured. When preparedness activities are routinely accomplished across jurisdictions, preparedness organizations should be multijurisdictional.

The essential roles of preparedness organizations at all jurisdictional levels are as follows:

- Establish and coordinate emergency plans and protocols, including public communications and awareness.
- Integrate and coordinate the activities of the jurisdictions and functions within their purview.
- Establish standards, guidelines, and protocols to promote interoperability among member jurisdictions and agencies.
- Adopt standards, guidelines, and protocols for providing resources to requesting organizations, including protocols for incident support organizations.

- Set priorities for resources and other requirements.
- Ensure the establishment and maintenance of multiagency coordination mechanisms, including EOCs, mutual-aid agreements, incident information systems, NGO and private-sector outreach, public awareness and information systems, and mechanisms to deal with information and operations security.

Preparedness Programs

Individual jurisdictions establish programs that address the requirements for each step of the preparedness cycle (planning, training, equipping, exercising, evaluating, and taking action to correct and mitigate). These programs should adopt relevant NIMS standards, guidelines, processes, and protocols.

Planning and Problem Solving

Planning and problem solving are shared responsibilities throughout the NIMS. Teams feed valuable information to key leadership positions for decision making. Teams also play a valuable role in monitoring plans and decisions to detect potential errors in the execution of Incident Action Plans (IAPs). Remember, everyone in the response community has a responsibility to provide critical incident decision-making information that informs the public and ensures responder safety.

Planning

For the NIMS teams to function effectively, they must understand the IAP. This includes essential directions and the goals and objectives for the team during work periods. Team planning and action plan coordination are key elements in teamwork and reduce errors in execution and improve safety.

Planning during an incident response takes one of two basic forms: long term or situational. Long-term planning addresses complex issues requiring analysis of incident data and conditions to develop a course of action. This involves a high degree of coordination among all levels of the NIMS. Long-term planning typically focuses on the common or expected issues during incident phases.

Situational planning is used to adapt to an unexpected or emergency situation requiring immediate action. This type of planning adapts the long-term plan to these unique, event-specific problems.

Situational plans require immediate communication with the team and leadership.

Problem Solving

Problem solving is accomplished by a variety of methods. At incidents, individuals frequently want to get to work immediately. It can be difficult to convince them to discuss, plan, and reach consensus. The response community can undertake several steps to enhance its ability to solve problems.

Critical Steps to Problem Solving

The critical steps to problem solving are as follows:

1. *Define the incident issues.* The first step in the problem-solving process is to define the issues. Collect all available information regarding the incident threats, challenges, and potential opportunities. This process helps to identify the response community partners needed for incident management.

2. *Develop the IAP.* The second problem-solving step is to develop an IAP. An IAP is simply a list of proposed outcomes. It is critical for informing and reminding all of the response community partners about the goals and recommended actions. Action plans are organized as topics, dates, priorities, geographic areas, or responsibilities. Each step within the plan clearly defines what, who, when, and how. Part of this process includes setting priorities for each of the goals. Do not implement the plan unless you are ready to act and know the issues, goals, and alternatives and have the needed resources and personnel for the mission.

3. *Communicate the plan to the response community.* Ensure that each Incident Command System (ICS) subgroup is briefed and understands its role. Remember that communications flow in both directions. When a team is deployed for a specific task, it communicates its status and leadership changes so that necessary adjustments can be made.

Consensus Building

Consensus building is a decision-making process that is vital to any multiagency planning effort. Consensus building allows all participants to raise issues, understand one another's views, and cooperatively develop courses of action. This is an essential process to building a strong response community within the NIMS. Consensus building is part of the NIMS preparedness planning process and plays a part in large-scale responses involving multiple agencies or jurisdictions.

Tip

Consensus means a generally agreed-upon plan. Consensus does not represent a unanimous opinion of response community partners. It is a majority judgment.

Preparedness Planning

Plans describe how personnel, equipment, and other governmental and nongovernmental resources support incident management requirements. Plans represent the operational core of preparedness and provide mechanisms for setting priorities, integrating multiple entities and functions, establishing collaborative relationships, and ensuring that communications and other systems effectively support the complete spectrum of incident management activities. An unfortunate belief is that response and management is accomplished simply because of a written plan. This phenomenon is well researched and documented and is called the *paper plan syndrome*. Although written plans are an essential element for incident preparedness, successful plans must relate to the spectrum of preparedness activities.

Preparedness plans include the following:

- The National Response Framework (NRF)
- EOPs
- Standard operating procedures (SOPs)
- Preparedness plans
- Corrective action and mitigation plans
- Recovery plans

Relation of NIMS to the NRF

In complex incidents, the NIMS serves to establish structure, concepts, principles, processes, and language for the efficient and effective utilization of all capabilities. The NRF was designed to build on the NIMS process and elucidates the specific roles and structures that the federal government will employ during a large or complex incident.

This framework, which has replaced the National Response Plan, ensures an overall doctrinal process by which the federal government will engage with local, state, and tribal jurisdictions to ensure that a cohesive, coordinated, and seamless national response occurs. NIMS and the NRF are based upon the guiding principle that all disasters are best managed at the local level. NIMS creates the capability for local and state emergency management officials to engage federal resources as required without giving up the inherent responsibility of the local and state jurisdictions to retain command, control, and authority of the overall response. Chapter 15 provides further details on this subject.

Relationship of the NIMS to National Preparedness

Integral to the NIMS is the national preparedness process that, under Homeland Security Presidential Directive/HSPD-8, establishes a comprehensive approach to planning. In this strategy, target capabilities are identified based on the needs of a large-scale response to the National Planning Scenarios. Each community can integrate these target capabilities into their unique planning process to develop a cohesive all-hazards response plan to all of the scenarios that they may face within their respective communities. NIMS provides an operational construct to escalate and deescalate these plans as needed.

Emergency Operations Plan

Each agency or jurisdiction develops an **Emergency Operations Plan (EOP)** that defines the scope of preparedness and incident management activities necessary for that organization. The EOP also describes organizational structures, roles and responsibilities, policies, and protocols for providing emergency support. The EOP facilitates response and short-term recovery activities (which set the stage for successful long-term recovery). It drives decisions on long-term prevention and mitigation efforts or risk-based preparedness measures directed at specific hazards.

An EOP should be flexible for use in all emergencies. It should also contain Federal Emergency Management Agency (FEMA) emergency support functional annexes, hazard-specific appendices, and a glossary. EOPs should assign jurisdictional and/or functional area representatives to the Incident Commander or UC to facilitate responsive and collaborative incident management. Although the preparedness of the public is generally beyond the scope of the NIMS, EOPs should also include preincident and postincident public awareness, education, and communications plans and protocols.

Key components of an EOP include the following:

- Description of the purpose of the plan
- Situation and assumptions
- Concept of operations

- Organization and assignment of responsibilities
- Administration and logistics
- Plan development and maintenance
- Authorities
- References

Standard Operating Procedures

Each organization in the EOP should develop **standard operating procedures (SOPs)** that describe the EOP organizational tasks and specify action-oriented checklists for incident management. They include predesignated procedures for how organizations accomplish assigned tasks.

Examples of SOPs and resource materials include the following:

- Procedural checklists and documents
- Mechanisms for notifying staff
- Processes for obtaining and using equipment, supplies, and vehicles
- Methods of obtaining mutual aid
- Mechanisms for reporting information to organizational work centers and EOCs
- Communications operating instructions, including connectivity with private-sector organizations and NGOs
- Resource listings
- Maps
- Charts and other pertinent data

The development of SOPs is required in accordance with the law for certain risk-based, hazard-specific programs. There are four standard levels of procedural documents:

- *Overview.* A brief concept summary of an incident-related function, team, or capability
- *SOP or operations manual.* A complete reference document that details the procedures for performing a single function or a number of interdependent functions
- *FOG or handbook.* A durable pocket or desk guide that contains essential information required to perform specific assignments or functions
- *Job aid.* A checklist or other aid that is useful in performing or training for a job

Ideally, these documents should be distributed to all responders of that agency or jurisdiction.

Preparedness Plans

Preparedness plans describe the process and schedule for identifying and meeting training needs. These plans are linked to the expectations outlined in the EOP. Preparedness plans should include the following components:

1. The process and schedule for developing, conducting, and evaluating exercises and correcting identified deficiencies
2. Arrangements for procuring or obtaining required incident management resources through mutual-aid mechanisms
3. Plans for facilities and equipment that withstand the effects that threaten a jurisdiction

Corrective Action Plans and Mitigation Plans

Corrective action plans are designed to implement procedures that are based on lessons learned from incidents or from training and exercises. **Mitigation plans** describe activities taken before, during, or after an incident to reduce or eliminate risks to persons or property or to lessen the actual or potential effects or consequences of an incident. One of the most important features of corrective-action planning is continuous feedback. A strong feedback system enhances error correction and increases safety.

Tip

A noted shortcoming in major incident preparedness is a lack of accurate information concerning actual disasters and major incidents. Use the following areas as a guide to communicate your lessons learned from training exercises and incidents:

- *Documentation.* Provide enough information regarding the drill or incident to allow others to sense and understand the scope of the problem. Avoid merely describing the EOP or the incident attributes. Analyze the effectiveness of the plan against the response and report what did happen rather than what should have happened.
- *Objectivity.* Avoid a singular perspective. Use and report on the findings from all members of the response community. Describe impartial evaluations of the actions taken instead of justifications or defenses. Avoid biases held by your community or agency. Report the analysis beyond the benefit of your in-house system. Remember, this is designed to assist other responders.
- *Perspective.* The more individuals involved in the documentation of the incident, the greater the view of the overall event. Be sure to include the interrelations among the various response disciplines.

Recovery Plans

Recovery plans describe actions beyond rapid damage assessment and life support for victims. Long-term recovery planning involves identifying strategic priorities for restoration, improvement, and growth. For example, say your community incurred flooding during a large storm. In the recovery planning phase, you should incorporate the assets of public works, private construction companies, and public health and administration into the operation.

Training and Exercises

Incident management organizations at all levels of government must be trained to improve all-hazards incident management capabilities nationwide. This comprehensive response community must participate in realistic training exercises. These events include multidisciplinary and multijurisdictional incidents that interface with and incorporate private-sector organizations and NGOs. The ultimate goal of these activities is to improve integration and interoperability.

Tip

All exercises and training should engage the full spectrum of resources within a community that affect children, and they should integrate the issues of children across the operational spectrum to ensure preparedness.

Training activities vary from small focused courses to large-scale regional drills incorporating thousands of responders and participants. Training involving standard courses on incident command and management, incident management structure, and operational coordination processes and systems—together with courses focused on discipline- and agency-specific subject-matter expertise—ensure that personnel at all jurisdictional levels and across disciplines function effectively during an incident.

The Role of the National Integration Center in Training Exercises

The National Integration Center is a focal point for the development, assessment, and evaluation of training exercises across all disciplines, government agencies, and private-sector organizations throughout the United States. The National Integration Center has developed the following goals:

- Facilitate the development and dissemination of national standards, guidelines, and protocols for incident management training and exercises, including consideration of existing exercises and training programs at all jurisdictional levels.
- Facilitate the use of modeling and simulation capabilities for training and exercise programs.
- Facilitate the definition of general training requirements and approved training courses for all NIMS users. These requirements are based on mission-to-task analysis. They address critical elements of an effective national training system, including field-based training, specification of mission-essential tasks, and requirements for specialized instruction. They also cover fundamental administrative matters, such as instructor qualifications and course completion documentation.
- Review and approve discipline-specific requirements and training courses, with the assistance of national professional organizations and with input from federal, state, local, tribal, private-sector, and nongovernmental entities.

The training that was developed for the ICS is a model for course curricula and materials applicable to other components of the NIMS. ICS training is organized around four course levels: ICS-100, Introduction to ICS; ICS-200, Basic ICS; ICS-300, Intermediate ICS; and ICS-400, Advanced ICS. Course materials are developed nationally and are shared by a number of federal, state, local, tribal, and other specialized training providers. This allows the use of a broad set of training providers and ensures that programs relate to federal, state, and local agencies and public-sector organizations.

Personnel Qualification and Certification

Under the NIMS, preparedness is based on national standards for the qualification and certification of the entire response community. Standards will help to ensure that field personnel in participating agencies and organizations possess the minimum knowledge, skills, and experience necessary to execute incident management and emergency response activities safely and effectively. Standards typically include

training, experience, credentialing, currency, and physical and mental fitness.

Personnel who are certified for employment in support of an incident that transcends interstate jurisdictions through the Emergency Management Assistance Compact (EMAC) system are required to meet national qualification and certification standards. Federal, state, local, and tribal certifying agencies; professional organizations; and private organizations should credential their personnel for their respective jurisdictions.

The role of the National Integration Center in personnel qualification and certification is as follows:

- Facilitate the development and/or dissemination of national standards, guidelines, and protocols for qualification and certification.
- Review and approve (with national professional organizations and with input from federal, state, local, private-sector, and nongovernmental entities) the discipline-specific requirements submitted by incident management organizations and associations.
- Facilitate the establishment of a data maintenance system to provide incident managers with the detailed qualification, experience, and training information needed to credential personnel for prescribed incident management positions.

Elected and Appointed Officials

Every official who is elected or appointed to a leadership position at the local, state, tribal, or federal level must be familiar with the NIMS and be capable of utilizing it to provide policy guidance during times of a large-scale incident. These officials are frequently to whom that the public looks for answers when there has been a disaster. For officials to serve their constituents well during a disaster, they should do the following:

- Understand, commit to, and receive training on NIMS and participate in exercises.
- Maintain an understanding of basic emergency management, continuity of operations, continuity of government plans, jurisdictional response capabilities, and initiation of disaster declarations.
- Lead and encourage preparedness efforts within the community, agencies of the jurisdiction, NGOs, and the private sector, as appropriate.

- Help to establish relationships with other jurisdictions and, as appropriate, NGOs and the private sector.
- Support and encourage participation in mitigation efforts within the jurisdiction and, as appropriate, with NGOs and the private sector.
- Provide guidance to their jurisdictions, departments, and/or agencies, with clearly stated policies for NIMS implementation.
- Understand laws and regulations in their jurisdictions that pertain to emergency management and incident response.
- Maintain awareness of critical infrastructure and key resources (CIKR) within their jurisdictions, potential incident impacts, and restoration priorities.

Equipment Certification

Incident management and emergency responder organizations at all levels rely on equipment to perform mission-essential tasks. A critical component of operational preparedness is the acquisition of equipment that will perform to certain standards, including the capability to be interoperable with equipment used by other jurisdictions.

The role of the National Integration Center in equipment certification is to set standards to facilitate the development and/or publication of national standards, guidelines, and protocols for equipment certification. This effort includes the incorporation of standards and certification programs already in use by incident management and emergency response organizations nationwide. Additionally, the National Integration Center must review and approve (with the assistance of national professional organizations and with input from federal, state, local, private-sector, and nongovernmental entities) lists of emergency responder equipment that meets national certification requirements.

Mutual-Aid Agreements

Mutual-aid agreements are the means for one jurisdiction to provide resources, facilities, services, and other required support to another jurisdiction during an incident. Each jurisdiction should be party to mutual-aid agreements (such as the EMAC) with jurisdictions they expect to coordinate with. This normally includes all neighboring or nearby jurisdictions and relevant private-sector organizations and NGOs. States should participate in interstate compacts and establish intrastate agreements that encompass all local jurisdictions. Mutual-aid agreements also are needed with private organizations, such as the American Red Cross, to facilitate the timely delivery of private assistance at the appropriate jurisdictional level during incidents. Mutual-aid agreements may also be developed with private industry. These agreements facilitate immediate movement of resources and assets during an incident and reduce contract difficulties and time delays. Authorized officials from each of the participating jurisdictions will collectively approve all mutual-aid agreements.

The essential elements of mutual-aid agreements include:

- Definitions of key terms used in the agreement
- Roles and responsibilities of individual parties
- Procedures for requesting and providing assistance
- Procedures, authorities, and rules for payment, reimbursement, and allocation of costs
- Notification procedures
- Protocols for interoperable communications
- Relationships with other agreements among jurisdictions
- Workers' compensation
- Treatment of liability and immunity
- Recognition of qualifications and certifications
- Sharing agreements, as required

Publication Management

The NIMS focuses on five areas regarding publication management:

1. Development of naming and numbering conventions
2. Review and certification of publications
3. Methods for publications control
4. Identification of sources and suppliers for publications and related services
5. Management of publication distribution

The NIMS produces the following types of products:

- Qualifications information
- Training course and exercise information
- Task books
- ICS training and forms
- Job aids
- Guides
- Computer programs

- Audio and video resources
- Templates
- Best practices

The role of the National Integration Center in publication management is to facilitate the development, publication, and dissemination of national standards, guidelines, and protocols for a NIMS publication management system and to facilitate the development and issuance of general publications for all NIMS users via the NIMS publication management system. Additionally, the National Integration Center will review and approve (with the assistance of appropriate national professional standards-making, certifying, and accrediting organizations, and with input from federal, state, local, private-sector, and nongovernmental organizations) the discipline-specific publication management requirements and training courses submitted by professional organizations and associations.

Procedures and Protocols

Many have argued that prevention is the simplest, most cost-effective way to manage a problem.

Unfortunately, we know that it is not possible to prevent disasters and emergencies. Therefore, it is essential to create preparedness plans that address these potential problems. The NIMS outlines and provides structure for these activities.

Preparedness plans transcend traditional paper plans. Preparedness planning includes the development of guidelines, exercises and training, personnel qualifications, equipment certifications, and standardized publication management.

Preparedness is a continuous process, not a singular event. Your response community should develop a systematic method for planning, training, equipping, evaluating, and improving the plan to ensure a unified, coordinated, and professional response (Table 11-1).

Tip
Remember, planning is a continuous process, not a singular act!

Table 11-1 Preparedness Planning

Plan
- Determine the types of major, complicated, or catastrophic incidents that can occur in your agency, jurisdiction, and surrounding area. In this assessment, remember that natural disasters involve all of the response community partners.
- Assemble and review all current plans. Ask the following questions:
  - Do the plans focus on size-specific events?
  - Do they focus on likely events?
  - Can the response plans be expanded in stages?
  - Do the plans include provisions for cost sharing?
  - Do the plans indicate resources and incorporate all response partners?
  - Do the plans incorporate training exercises, feedback, and error correction?

Train
- Review current training within your response community.
- Develop a training matrix utilizing appropriate courses (a training-course matrix is available from the US Department of Homeland Security Office for Domestic Preparedness).
- Implement training within your response community and ensure that all agencies, partners, and professionals are included.
- Ensure opportunities for ongoing training.

Equipment
- Provide the equipment appropriate to the level of training or operational mission requirements.
- Ensure the proper and continued working order of all equipment.
- Ensure that all partners of the response community have access to the necessary tools, technologies, and supplies required to respond.
- Ensure equipment interoperability across disciplines and agencies.

(Continues)

Table 11-1 Preparedness Planning *(Continued)*

Exercise

- Plan, develop, and execute annual training exercises in your region that involve the entire response community.
- Conduct mission-, agency-, or profession-specific exercises focusing on specialized tasks (e.g., trench rescue, bomb disposal, flood management, etc.).

Evaluate

- Obtain information concerning the evaluation of other events (after-action reports) that provide insight and lessons learned to assist in refining and critiquing your plans, training, and exercises.
- Develop exercise-assessment tools and train the evaluators in their correct use.
- Involve all response community partners in the evaluation of drills and exercises. This avoids a single perspective and gives a clearer picture of the event.
- Provide a feedback mechanism for operational personnel concerning the plans, exercises, training, and equipment.

Improve

- Use the feedback mechanisms, lessons learned, and evaluations to refine all aspects of your response community's preparedness.
- Ensure appropriate notification of changes in the response community.

Rural Case Study *Answers*

1. The following elements should be involved in preparedness planning:
   - Development of planning guidelines, protocols, and standards
   - Exercise development and training
   - Personnel qualification and certification
   - Equipment certification
   - Publication management
2. The NIMS provides a framework for a systematic approach to preparedness activities. It ensures levels of capability, a unified approach, and overall guidance for achieving preparedness.

Urban Case Study *Answers*

1. Any four of the following preparedness plans may be called into service for this incident:
   - The National Response Plan
   - EOPs
   - SOPs
   - Preparedness plans
   - Corrective action and mitigation plans
   - Recovery plans
2. The following mitigation activities may be beneficial:
   - Evacuation plans and drills
   - Predesignated emergency sheltering
   - Public education and outreach activities
   - Code enforcement activities

Wrap-Up

Summary

- Preparedness activities occur during all phases (mitigation, planning, response, and recovery) of a major incident.
- Preparedness activities are a continuous quality management process.
- The essential elements of NIMS preparedness are the following:
  - Development of guidelines, protocols, and standards
  - Exercise development and training
  - Personnel qualification and certification
  - Equipment certification
  - Publication management
  - Engagement of elected and appointed officials
- The preparedness cycle can easily be remembered with the acronym POTEE (plan, organize, train, exercise, evaluate).
- The National Response Framework, which has replaced the National Response Plan, ensures an overall doctrinal process by which the federal government will engage with local, state, and tribal jurisdictions.
- Preparedness activities require the involvement of the entire response community, including NGOs, to ensure a unified approach.
- Training and exercises are an essential element of planning for a major incident.
- Preparedness activities facilitate the development of mutual-aid agreements and cooperation of the response community.

Glossary

Corrective action plans: Implemented solutions that result in the reduction or elimination of an identified problem.

Emergency Operations Plan (EOP): A systematic process to initiate, manage, and recover from any emergency in a similar manner to improve preparation and response.

Mitigation: Reduction of harshness or hostility.

Mitigation plans: Proposals to reduce or alleviate potentially harmful impacts. Any sustained action taken to reduce or eliminate the long-term risk to human life and property from hazards.

Mutual-aid agreements: Intergovernmental or interagency agreements that provide shared and common assistance when requested by member agencies. The equipment and personnel provided by a mutual-aid request may be predetermined for a particular type of incident or it may be determined at the time of the request in consideration of available resources.

Recovery plans: Guides for the activities to be undertaken by federal, state, or private entities to direct recovery efforts in areas affected by disasters.

Standard operating procedures (SOPs): Detailed written procedures for the uniform performance of a function.

Wrap-Up Case Study

Thomas County is a coastal community comprising five islands that are connected to the mainland by the north island and six major bridges. In late October, a severe storm strikes Thomas County, causing loss of power throughout the county and structural damage and destruction of two of the main bridges, isolating the lower islands. Many citizens are stranded, and transportation among the islands has been halted. County officials request resources from surrounding counties to assist in the recovery of critical infrastructure and evacuation of stranded citizens. This is the second time in the past 20 years a severe storm has struck the area.

Following the first major destructive storm, the Thomas County EOP was revised to address several deficiencies that were noted in the after-action report. Plans were developed to provide alternative methods to evacuate citizens and improve communications prior to and following a storm. Additional equipment was purchased, and training was completed in the response community. Thomas County also implemented several agreements with ferry services to provide emergency transportation of its citizens.

1. A document that allows for one jurisdiction to provide Thomas County resources, facilities, services, or other support is called a(n):
   A. corrective action plan.
   B. mutual-aid agreement.
   C. SOP.
   D. emergency recovery plan.

2. Public education activities, such as those that would inform the citizens of Thomas County how to behave during and after a major storm, that are designed to reduce loss of life and destruction of property is an example of what type of activity?
   A. Recovery
   B. Corrective action
   C. Mitigation
   D. Mutual aid

3. Which of the following would include a specific, action-oriented, predesignated procedure checklist to be used during incident management operations in Thomas County?
   A. Concept of operations
   B. Corrective action plan
   C. Mitigation plan
   D. SOPs

CHAPTER 12

Communications and Information Management

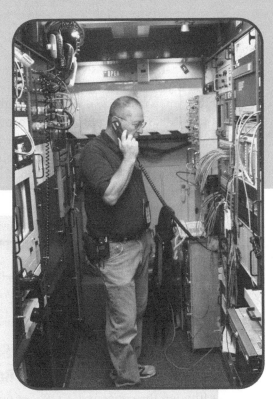

Rural Case Study

The communications infrastructure in Stadtown has been severely damaged by the tornado. Telephone, radio, cable TV, and cellular systems are all offline and will not be available for weeks. The Emergency Operations Center (EOC) does not have any good reference materials or plans for this eventuality.

1. Who can be called for assistance regarding communications options?
2. What local volunteer organizations might be helpful in dealing with this problem?
3. What other options, besides traditional communications tools, exist to share information?

Urban Case Study

The Metro Mobile Communications Unit has responded and is on the scene of the HazMat incident. Additional resources from the state and federal government are en route, as are representatives of the railroad.

1. What interoperable voice communications issues exist at this incident? How can they be addressed?
2. To establish a common operational picture (COP) between the scene and the EOC, what technologies should be deployed by the Communications Unit?

> **Tip**
>
> Communications and Information Management within the National Incident Management System (NIMS) is extremely dependent on computer systems. Information technology personnel should be involved in incident management activities, including reporting to the incident scene and to your jurisdiction's operations and communications centers.

Introduction

Communications and Information Management continues to be one of the most rapidly evolving areas of the NIMS and of domestic incident management in general. Substantial resources at all levels of gov-

ernment and private industry are addressing the issues outlined within this section of the NIMS.

Concepts and Principles

> **Tip**
>
> Communications interoperability is the ability to get the right information to the right people in the right time frame.

Common Operational Picture

Common operational picture (COP) is a formal term describing the more familiar concept of **situational awareness**. In the past, emergency response organizations discussed and taught situational awareness with an emphasis on specific tactical aspects of emergency response operations. In the framework of the NIMS, COP is a broader concept. The concept is simple, even though it appears to be complicated. Incident management personnel should see, hear, and read the same information whether at the Incident Command Post (ICP), a local EOC, or a state or federal command facility.

More formally, COP is defined by the NIMS as an overview of an incident created by collating and gathering information—such as traffic, weather, actual damage, and resource availability—of any type (voice, data, etc.) from agencies/organizations in order to support decision making.

Interoperability, Reliability, Scalability, Portability, Resiliency, and Redundancy

Although the concept of COP is simple, the supporting technology enabling it is not **(Figure 12-1)**. The development of a successful COP requires interoperable, redundant communications systems. Such systems allow communications across dissimilar radio, data collection, and transmission systems and operate using common standards across different computing platforms (e.g., Windows, Mac, Linux). These systems must be able to collect and transmit high-quality multimedia information, such as pictures, video, audio, and graphics, and maintain all of these capabilities even when the traditional community infrastructure (i.e., power, telephone, fiber optic networks, cellular systems, public safety radio, and data systems) has been disrupted. These systems

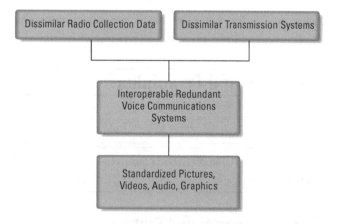

Figure 12-1 Technological components of a COP. Interoperable, redundant communications systems enable all incident management personnel to see, hear, and read the same information.

should be designed for quick deployment and for operations in hostile environments. In addition, they should be able to be used by personnel in personal protective equipment (PPE). The systems should require minimal training to eliminate dependence on highly-skilled technical personnel.

Currently, few public safety organizations maintain COP capabilities on a routine basis; they usually depend on mutual-aid assistance from state or federal organizations to bring this type of capability to incident locations. Although COP capabilities do not currently exist in many locations, it is easy to understand why COP is a priority. The ability to share real-time information and reference materials among the scene, operations centers, and other incident management facilities or control centers creates possibilities that substantially improve local, state, and federal prevention, preparedness, and response capabilities. It also gives responding mutual-aid organizations situational awareness.

Operationally, this means being able to electronically send the incident site map, with accurate locations of apparatus and Incident Command System (ICS) facilities, to incoming command personnel from Urban Search and Rescue Teams (USAR) along with still and video images of the areas that are a high priority during initial search operations. Plume models developed at the scene by the HazMat science officer can be immediately sent to the EOC and media organizations to allow for the initiation of an evacuation. Additionally, the same map may automatically activate an Emergency Notification System (ENS), which calls each residence and business in the impacted area and advises them of the evacuation and shelter locations.

More routinely, the Incident Commander from a local fire department makes real-time notations on his or her electronic map indicating the progression of the fires they are battling. This same map may also be displayed at the EOC and the local communications center, allowing incoming resources to be routed around changing road closures for quick access to the incident staging area. The state Fire Coordination Center can watch the fire in real time through video and electronic mapping as well as the current electronic Incident Action Plan (IAP). This information is also shared with federal officials who can anticipate the needs of this evolving incident and balance them against other incidents nationwide.

These capabilities and many more currently exist as components of the COP concept. A COP (and the technology to support it successfully) ensures consistency at all levels of incident management across jurisdictions and among various governmental agencies, the private sector, and nongovernmental entities that are responders or are potentially impacted by the events.

Management Characteristics

As organizations nationwide have attempted to integrate advanced, interoperable communications technologies into their organizations and communities, many have learned a critical lesson. The most important component within the realm of interoperable communications is the operator of the device.

Standardized Communications Types

Successful communications and information management require that emergency management/ response personnel and their affiliated organizations use standardized communications types. The determination of the individual or agency/organization responsible for these communications is discussed in the Command and Management component of the NIMS and in Appendix E. The following is a list of standardized communication types:

- *Strategic communications.* High-level directions, including resource priority decisions, roles and responsibilities determinations, and overall incident response courses of action
- *Tactical communications.* Communications among command and support elements and, as appropriate, cooperating agencies and organizations
- *Support communications.* Coordination in support of strategic and tactical communications (for example, communications among hospitals concerning resource ordering, dispatching, and tracking from logistics centers; and traffic and public works communications)
- *Public address communications.* Emergency alerts and warnings, press conferences, etc.

Policy and Planning

Progressing further, the NIMS specifically defines the objectives and key measures associated with the need to undertake a detailed, comprehensive planning process regarding interoperable communications by specifically addressing *how* (which technologies), *who* (which personnel in which situations), *what*

(type of information), and *when* (temporal requirements and guidelines). For many organizations, this will be the most difficult aspect of developing a true interoperable capability because it is a cultural change within each organization and requires dedicated and committed leadership to achieve.

The final outcome—the interoperable communications policies and procedures—should incorporate the following:

- Information needs as defined by the jurisdiction/organization; these needs are often met at the federal, state, tribal, and local levels in concert with nongovernmental organizations (NGOs) and the private sector, primarily through preparedness organizations
- Guidance, standards, and tools to enable the integration of information needs into a COP when needed
- Procedures and protocols for the release of warnings, incident notifications, public communications, and other critical information disseminated through a defined combination of networks used by EOCs; notifications are made to the appropriate jurisdictional levels and to NGOs and the private sector through defined mechanisms specified in Emergency Operations Plans (EOPs) and IAPs
- Effective and efficient use of information management technologies (e.g., computers, networks, and information-sharing mechanisms) to integrate all command, coordination, and support functions involved in incident management and to enable the sharing of critical information and the cataloging of required corrective actions
- Agreements to ensure that the elements within plans and procedures will be in effect at the time of an incident; agreements should specify all of the communications systems and platforms through which the parties agree to use or share information

It is also critical that organizations review and adopt equipment standards and develop appropriate training to support these technologies within the constellation of organizations that will be using the systems. The specific limitations and applications of each technology need to be fully understood by those who are responsible for using them. Integrating the realistic, consistent use of the various technologies into drills, exercises, and daily routine operations also assures that personnel are well prepared to operate during periods of high stress. Organizations such as the DHS SAFECOM Program and the Organization for the Advancement of Structured Information Standards (OASIS) oversee all initiatives and projects pertaining to public safety communications and interoperability and continuously develop and publish interoperability standards. The focus of the SAFECOM Program is wireless communications interoperability, while OASIS promotes the development and adoption of e-business and web service standards.

Organization and Operations

Incident Information

During the course of an incident, information is vital to assist the Incident Command (IC), Unified Command (UC), and supporting agencies and organizations in making decisions. Much of the information is used for diverse functions within the Incident Command System. For example, the same piece of information may accomplish the following:

- Aid in the planning process to develop an IAP.
- Be a key point in the release of public information.
- Assist the Finance/Administration Section in determining the incident cost.
- Determine the need for additional involvement of NGOs or private-sector resources.
- Identify a safety issue.
- Follow-up on an information request.

The following sections outline examples of information generated by an incident that can be used for decision-making purposes.

Incident Notification, Situation, and Status Reports

Incident reporting and documentation procedures should be standardized to ensure that situational awareness is maintained and that emergency management/response personnel have easy access to critical information. This standardization is one of the most powerful aspects of incorporating the use of defined, exercised Incident Management Teams (IMTs) into organizations' major incident response plans. Situation reports (known within ICS as SitStat) offer a snapshot of the past operational period and contain confirmed or verified information regarding the explicit details (who, what, when, where, and how) relating to the incident. Status reports, which

may be contained in situation reports, relay information specifically related to the status of resources (e.g., availability or assignment of resources).

The information contained in incident notification, situation, and status reports must be standardized to facilitate processing; however, the standardization must not prevent the collection or dissemination of information that is unique to a reporting organization. Transmission of data in a common format enables the passing of pertinent information to appropriate jurisdictions and organizations and to a national system that can handle data queries and information/intelligence assessments and analysis.

Analytical Data

Data such as information on public health and environmental monitoring should be collected in a manner that observes standard data collection techniques and definitions. The data should then be transmitted using standardized analysis processes and data surety procedures. During incidents that require public health and environmental sampling, multiple organizations at different levels of government often collect data, so standardization of data collection and analysis is critical. Additionally, standardization of sampling and data collection enables more reliable analysis and improves the quality of assessments provided to decision makers.

Geospatial Information

Geospatial information is defined as information pertaining to the geographic location and characteristics of natural or constructed features and boundaries. It is often used to integrate assessments, situation reports, and incident notification into a COP and as a data fusion and analysis tool to synthesize many kinds and sources of data and imagery. The use of geospatial data (and the recognition of its intelligence capabilities) is increasingly important during incidents. Geospatial information capabilities (such as nationally consistent grid systems or global positioning systems based on lines of longitude and latitude) should be managed through preparedness efforts and integrated within the command, coordination, and support elements of an incident, including resource management and public information. This also has key implications in terms of making sure that field response personnel have sufficient, accurate global positioning system (GPS) devices to allow for the most effective use of this data in developing a COP.

The use of geospatial data should be tied to consistent standards because it has the potential to be misinterpreted, transposed incorrectly, or otherwise misapplied, causing inconspicuous yet serious errors. Standards covering geospatial information should also enable systems to be used in remote field locations or devastated areas where telecommunications may not be capable of handling large images or may be limited in terms of computing hardware.

Communications Standards and Formats

Communications and data standards, related testing, and associated compliance mechanisms are necessary to enable diverse organizations to work together effectively. These include a standard set of organizational elements and functions, common typing of resources to reflect specific capabilities, and common identifiers for facilities and operational locations to support incident operations.

Common terminology, standards, and procedures should be established and detailed in plans and agreements, where possible. Jurisdictions may be required to comply with national interoperable communications standards. Standards appropriate for NIMS users will be designated by the National Integration Center (NIC) in partnership with recognized standards development organizations.

Radio Usage Procedures

Procedures and protocols for incident-specific communications and other critical incident information should be set forth in agreements or plans prior to an incident, where possible (Figure 12-2). These procedures and protocols form the foundation for the development of the communications plan during an incident. The receiving center should be required to acknowledge receipt of the emergency information. Additionally, each agency/organization should be responsible for disseminating this information to its respective personnel. All emergency management/response personnel participating in emergency management and incident response activities should follow recognized procedures and protocols for establishing interoperability, coordination, and command and control.

| INCIDENT RADIO COMMUNICATIONS PLAN | | | 1. Incident Name

Stadtown Flood | 2. Date/Time Prepared

9-15-2009/1630 | 3. Operational Period Date/Time

9-15-2009/1630–2230 |
|---|---|---|---|---|---|
| 4. Basic Radio Channel Utilization | | | | | |
| System/Cache | Channel | Function | Frequency/Tone | Assignment | Remarks |
| VHF | 4 | City Wide, Ops | 155.750 | Ops | |
| VHF | 6 | North Div-Rescue | 155.950 | Rescue | |
| | | | | | |
| | | | | | |
| | | | | | |
| | | | | | |
| | | | | | |
| | | | | | |
| 5. Prepared by (Communications Unit)

Planning Section | | | | | |

Figure 12-2 ICS form 205: sample incident communications plan.

Common Terminology

The ability of emergency management/response personnel from different disciplines, jurisdictions, organizations, and agencies to work together depends greatly on their ability to communicate with each other. Common terminology enables emergency management/response personnel to communicate clearly with one another and effectively coordinate activities, no matter the size, scope, location, or complexity of the incident.

The use of plain language (clear text) in emergency management and incident response is a matter of public safety, especially the safety of emergency management/response personnel and those affected by the incident. It is critical that all those involved with an incident know and use commonly established operational structures, terminology, policies, and procedures. This will facilitate interoperability across agencies/organizations, jurisdictions, and disciplines.

All communications among organizational elements during an incident, whether oral or written, should be in plain language; this ensures that information dissemination is timely, clear, acknowledged, and understood by all intended recipients. Codes should not be used, and all communications should be confined to essential messages. The use of acronyms should be avoided during incidents that require the participation of multiple agencies or organizations. Policies and procedures that foster compatibility should be defined to allow information sharing to the greatest extent possible among all emergency management/response personnel and their affiliated organizations.

Encryption or Tactical Language

When necessary, emergency management/response personnel and their affiliated organizations need to have a methodology and the systems in place to encrypt information so that security can be maintained. Although plain language may be appropriate during response to most incidents, tactical language is occasionally warranted due to the nature of the incident (e.g., during an ongoing terrorist event). The use of specialized encryption and tactical language should be incorporated into any comprehensive IAP or incident management communications plan. The use of encryption is not seamless, however, and organizations should completely and thoroughly test the configuration and programming of encrypted communications prior to deployment during any incident. Organizations should also incorporate a fail-safe process into operations involving encrypted communications to ensure the personnel do not become isolated if their encryption system or key fails during a mission.

Joint Information System and Joint Information Center

The Joint Information System (JIS) and the Joint Information Center (JIC) are designed to foster the use of common information formats. The JIS integrates incident information and public affairs into a cohesive organization designed to provide consistent, coordinated, accurate, accessible, and timely information during crisis or incident operations.

The JIC provides a structure for developing and delivering incident-related coordinated messages. It develops, recommends, and executes public information plans and strategies; advises the IC, UC, and supporting agencies or organizations concerning public affairs issues that could affect a response effort; and controls rumors and inaccurate information that could undermine public confidence in the emergency response effort. It is the central point of contact for all news media at the scene of an incident. Public information officials from all participating agencies/organizations should collocate at the JIC. This should include key private-sector partners (e.g., utilities, hospitals, major employers/facility owners).

Internet/Web Procedures

The Internet and other Web-based tools can be used, as appropriate, during incidents to help with situational awareness and crisis information management. These tools can be resources for emergency management/response personnel and their affiliated organizations. For example, they can be used prior to and during incidents as a mechanism to offer situational awareness to organizations/agencies involved in the incident or to the public, when appropriate.

New and evolving technologies (such as Twitter) have proven useful during recent incidents and allow for transmission of limited amounts of data with very low bandwidths. Organizations will need to be acutely aware of the most current trends in communications or social networking and leverage these technologies to allow for rapid communication of key data.

Procedures for use of these tools during an incident should be established to leverage them as valuable communications system resources. Information posted or shared during an incident through these applications should follow planned and standardized methods and generally conform to the overall standards, procedures, and protocols.

Information Security

Procedures and protocols must be established to ensure information security. Inadequate information security can result in the untimely, inappropriate, and piecemeal release of information, which increases the likelihood of misunderstanding and can compound already complicated public safety issues. The release of inappropriate classified or sensitive public health or law enforcement information can jeopardize national security, ongoing investigations, or public health. Misinformation can place persons in danger, cause public panic, and disrupt the critical flow of proper information. Correcting misinformation wastes the valuable time and effort of incident response personnel.

Individuals and organizations that have access to incident information and, in particular, contribute information to the system (e.g., situation reports) must be properly authenticated and certified for security purposes. This requires a national authentication and security certification standard that is flexible and robust enough to ensure that information can be properly authenticated and protected. Although the NIC is responsible for facilitating the development of these standards, all levels of government, NGOs, and the private sector should collaborate on the authentication process.

As information technology professionals become more involved in supporting advanced incident management technologies, they need to become more familiar with the language of domestic incident management and the ICS. In turn, successful incident management personnel will learn the language of information technology as well.

Table 12-1 identifies communication and information systems. This information is technical and specifically intended to lay the groundwork for technology personnel within organizations so that they understand the requirements of compliance.

Table 12-1 Communications and Information Systems
NIMS communications and information systems enable the essential functions needed to provide a COP and interoperability for incident management at all levels in two ways: incident management communications and information management.
Incident Management Communications
Preparedness organizations must ensure that effective communications processes and systems support a complete spectrum of incident management activities. The following principles apply:
■ *Individual jurisdictions.* They are required to comply with national interoperable communications standards, when such standards are developed. Standards appropriate for NIMS users are designated by the NIC in partnership with recognized standards development organizations (SDOs).
■ *Incident communications.* They are required to follow ICS standards. The ICS manages communications at an incident using a common communications plan and an incident-based communications center established solely for use by the command, tactical, and support resources assigned to the incident. All entities involved in managing the incident will utilize common terminology, prescribed by the NIMS, for communications.
Information Management
The NIC facilitates the definition and maintenance of the information framework required to guide the development of NIMS-related information systems. This framework consists of documented policies and interoperability standards:
■ *Policies.* The documented policies are as follows:
• *Preincident information.* Preincident information needs are met at the federal, state, local, and tribal levels in concert with private-sector organizations and NGOs, primarily through the preparedness organizations described in Section III.B.1.
• *Information management.* The information management system provides guidance, standards, and tools to enable federal, state, local, tribal, and private-sector and nongovernmental entities to integrate their information needs into a COP.

(Continues)

Table 12-1 Communications and Information Systems *(Continued)*

- *Networks.* Indications and warnings, incident notifications and public communications, and the critical information that constitute a COP are disseminated through a combination of networks used by EOCs. Notifications are made to the appropriate jurisdictional levels, private-sector organizations, and NGOs through the mechanisms defined in EOPs and IAPs at all levels of government.
- *Technology use.* Agencies must plan for the effective and efficient use of information management technologies (e.g., computers and networks) to link all command, tactical, and support units involved in incident management and enable these entities to share information critical to mission execution and the cataloging of required corrective actions.

■ *Interoperability standards.* Facilitating the development of data standards for the following functions, including secure communications when required, is the responsibility of the NIC described in Chapter VII. Standards will be developed in accordance with the following design goals:

- *Incident notification and situation report.* Incident notification takes place at all levels. Although notification and situation report data must be standardized, it must not prevent information unique to a reporting organization from being collected or disseminated. Standardized transmission of data in a common format enables the passing of appropriate notification information to a national system that processes data queries, information and intelligence assessments, and analysis.
- *Status reporting.* All levels of government initiate status reports (e.g., Situation Reports [SITREPS] and Pollution Reports [POLREPS]) and disseminate them to other jurisdictions. A standard set of data elements is defined to facilitate this process.
- *Analytical data.* Analytical data, such as information on public health and environmental monitoring, is collected in the field in a manner that observes standard data definitions. It is then transmitted to laboratories using standardized analysis processes. During incidents that require public health and environmental sampling, multiple organizations at different levels of government often respond and collect data. Standardization of sampling and data collection enables more reliable laboratory analysis and improves the quality of assessments provided to decision makers.
- *Geospatial information.* Geospatial information is used to integrate assessments, situation reports, and incident notification into a coherent COP. Correct utilization of geospatial data is increasingly important to decision makers. The use of geospatial data must be tied to consistent standards because of the potential for coordinates to be transformed incorrectly or otherwise misapplied, causing inconspicuous, yet serious, errors. Geospatial information standards should be robust and enable systems utilization in remote locations. Telecommunications systems may not have sufficient bandwidth to process large images and may have limited computer hardware.
- *Wireless communications.* To ensure that incident management organizations can communicate and share information with one another through wireless systems, the NIMS includes standards to ensure that wireless communications and computing are interoperable between federal, state, local, tribal, public safety, and nongovernmental organizations.
- *Identification and authentication.* Individuals and organizations that access the NIMS Communication and Information Management system and those that contribute information to the system (e.g., situation reports) must be properly authenticated and certified for security purposes. Although the National Integration Center is responsible for facilitating the development of these standards, different levels of government and private organizations must collaborate to administer the authentication process.
- *National database of incident reports.* Through the National Integration Center, federal, state, local, and tribal organizations responsible for receiving initial incident reports are developing a national database of incident reports that support incident management efforts.

Rural Case Study *Answers*

1. In these situations, it is easy to forget the layers of response within our country. The next options available to a local government are either a regional organization or the state.

2. Most local communities have active amateur radio users. These individuals, even if they have not been previously organized, can be mobilized to provide both voice and data links between incident locations and key facilities. Even if your jurisdiction has not actively worked with these communications experts, they need to be a key resource in your communications plan.

3. In addition to considering amateur radio operators, don't forget the simplest method of sharing information: runners. Though they are not timely or efficient, they provide an alternative when the communications infrastructure has been damaged.

Urban Case Study *Answers*

1. The response of state, federal, and private resources creates substantial challenges due to different technology standards used by each. Radio-system-patching units (known as black boxes) can sometimes be used to interconnect systems. Alternatively, the ICS Communications Unit (within the Logistics Section) can assign personnel to monitor and transmit information between systems. Many organizations are developing field dispatch teams that consist of communications professionals who are deployed to large incidents to assist with on-scene communications.

2. In addition to voice communications, many communications vehicles have the capability to deploy a wide area computer network with associated computers to enable the collection and recording of incident information. These units also routinely have high-quality video cameras. This information is combined at the scene to ensure that IC personnel have a COP. Additionally, with data transmission capabilities, information can be shared with other incident management facilities, such as Department Operations Centers (DOCs) and EOCs.

Wrap-Up

Summary

- The two primary goals of the Communications and Information Management section of the NIMS are as follows:
  - Develop technologies that support organizations at the local, state, and federal level to operate with a COP.
  - Develop common standards for communications and data to support incident management technologies.
- COP is defined by the NIMS as an overview of an incident created by collating and gathering information. The development of a successful COP requires interoperable, redundant communications systems.
- Standardized communication types are divided into strategic, tactical, support, and public address communications.

- Information is vital to assist the Incident Command (IC), Unified Command (UC), and supporting agencies and organizations in making decisions, including incident notification, situation, and status reports; analytical data; and geospatial information.
- During incident response activities, radio traffic should be restricted to those messages necessary for the effective execution of emergency management/response personnel tasks.

Glossary

Situational awareness: The ability to access all required information for effectively managing an incident. It is similar to the common operational picture (COP).

The Chief Technology Officer (CTO) of your city has been tasked by the City Manager to develop a new voice and data communications system for the city. The system will serve the public safety and public works organizations and other city offices and operations. The CTO was recently hired from a local computer manufacturer and is known for his efficiency.

The project has been placed on the fast track, and the CTO has assembled a team to develop the system. Your role on the team is to represent the public safety organizations. The team also includes several members from the local technology community who bring a private-sector perspective to the development effort.

1. During the initial development of ideas related to capabilities and system design, you are asked what components public safety needs. Based on your desire to achieve compliance with the NIMS, which of the following would you include?

   A. A wireless data network that supports real-time video transmission

   B. A dedicated satellite transmission system among all public safety facilities

   C. A single radio system for all response agencies that simultaneously supports multiple tactical channels and incidents

   D. Both A and C

2. To ensure interoperable communications, who should you collect radio and data system information from prior to designing your system?

   A. The state government

   B. Regional governments and response organizations

   C. The federal government

   D. All of the above

3. After the initial design has been completed, the CTO confronts you during a meeting and states, "There is no federal requirement for interoperability. This is an expensive folly." What federal organization can assist and support you?

   A. The Federal Communications Commission (FCC)

   B. The US Department of Homeland Security (DHS) Office for Interoperability and Compatibility (OIC)

   C. The DHS NIC

   D. Both B and C

CHAPTER 13

Resource Management

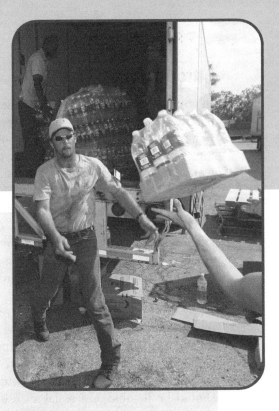

Rural Case Study

In the initial hours following the tornado, departments and responders from several counties are activated and dispatched to assist in the rescue and recovery process. The Incident Commander has developed a General Staff, and the Logistics and Planning Sections have established staging areas and have deployed personnel and equipment into several incident areas.

As the incident progresses, more responders and equipment are requested by the Incident Commander through the Emergency Operations Center (EOC) as they begin to realize the magnitude of the disaster throughout the county. The Planning Section establishes a Resources Unit and assigns a Resources Unit Leader. The Resources Unit Leader is briefed by the Logistics and Planning Section Chiefs as to the current deployment status and available resources at their disposal.

The Resources Unit develops a status board that identifies all known resources at the incident site as well as those that have been requested and are responding to the staging area. An accountability system is established, and a report is completed and sent to the Planning Section Chief to update the Planning Section on the current status of incident resources.

1. What types of incident resources should the Resources Unit track?
2. How should incident resources be categorized?

Urban Case Study

The incident in Pleasantville requires a complicated response involving many resources and highly specialized responders. It is unlikely that the average department will have all of the required specialists and equipment. In this incident, resources are requested from neighboring cities and counties by activating mutual-aid agreements. The Incident Commander requests these resources through the county EOC. As these responders and equipment deploy to the incident area, they are directed to report to the staging area.

The requests received by the EOC from the Pleasantville Incident Commander are processed by the Multiagency Coordinating System (MACS) that has been activated. This facilitates appropriate direction of limited resources to both the Pleasantville incident and to the Metro areas that are now being evacuated.

Because this incident has been declared a potential terrorism event, the State Warning Point has been notified. This notification activates additional state and federal resources that will begin to deploy to the incident area. This incident shows the many different agencies, disciplines, resources, and levels of government that must work together in an organized fashion to meet operational objectives.

1. What principles of resource management will benefit this incident?
2. What are the primary tasks for the Resources Unit and the Resources Unit Leader?

Introduction

In any incident, regardless of its size, scope, or complexity, effective **resource management** is critical. Emergency management and incident response activities require an array of resources (e.g., personnel, teams, facilities, equipment, and supplies) to meet incident needs. Resources consist of all of the actual and potential personnel and equipment that are activated, in service, out of service, or available for assignment. The ability to select the most appropriate resource for a particular mission or task is essential for the operation to proceed in a safe, efficient manner.

Utilization of the standardized resource management concepts, such as typing, inventorying, organizing, and tracking, will facilitate the dispatch, deployment, and recovery of resources before, during, and after an incident. Resource management should be flexible and scalable in order to support any incident and be adaptable to changes. Efficient and effective deployment of resources requires that resource management concepts and principles be used in all phases of emergency management and incident response.

Resource management involves coordination, oversight, and procedures that provide timely and appropriate resources during any incident, from local, contained events to large-scale incidents that require a coordinated federal response. Resources may support incident response through the Incident Command Post (ICP) or as a function within the MACS serving at an EOC.

Maintenance of the status of these resources is a difficult task and requires a great deal of attention, especially when the incident size is large, covers multiple jurisdictions, or is occurring at multiple sites within a region. As incident priorities are established, needs are identified, and resources are ordered, resource management systems are used to process the requests. Typically during the initial response to an incident, the majority of resources are requested and managed locally or through mutual-aid agreements. As an incident grows in size or complexity, or in cases of large-scale incidents, resource needs may need to be met by state, tribal, federal, or private sources. Further, in large-scale incidents, there may be competition for critical resources. In this case, MACS can be used to prioritize and coordinate resource allocation and distribution based on need, availability, and incident considerations.

Resources are managed by the Resources Unit, under the direction of a Unit Leader, within the Planning Section of the General Staff. This chapter provides an in-depth look at the function and role of incident resource management.

The Resources Unit

The **Resources Unit** is a component of the Planning Section in the Incident Command System (ICS) structure. This unit includes the primary managers of all assigned personnel or other resources that have checked in at an incident site. The unit is responsible for keeping track of the location and status of all assigned, available, or out-of-service resources.

Basic concepts and principles guide the resource management process used in the National Incident Management System (NIMS). By standardizing the procedures, methodologies, and functions involved in these processes, the NIMS ensures that resources move quickly and efficiently to support incident managers and emergency responders. Resource management within the NIMS should provide a uniform method of identifying, acquiring, allocating, and tracking resources. Resource management must incorporate effective mutual-aid and donor assistance, including resources contributed by private-sector and nongovernmental organizations (NGOs).

This assistance is further enabled by the standardized classification of kinds and types of resources, across all agencies and disciplines, required to support the incident management organization. Resource management uses a credentialing system tied to uniform training and certification standards to ensure that requested personnel resources are successfully integrated into ongoing incident operations. The coordination of resources is the responsibility of EOCs or MACS as well as the Resources Unit of the Planning Section.

The **Resources Unit Leader** is responsible for maintaining the status of all resources at an incident. The most basic method of accomplishing this task is simply by checking in and checking out all resources at an incident (like a librarian). A more efficient system is for the Resources Unit to maintain a master list of all resources that indicates each resource's current location and status (i.e., in use, available, at staging, or out of service). At small-scale incidents, this task may be accomplished by a single person; at larger incidents, an entire team may be required.

Table 13-1	Essential Resource Management Concepts	
Consistency	Provision of a standard method for identifying, acquiring, allocating, and tracking resources
Standardization	Resource classification to improve the effectiveness of mutual-aid agreements or assistance agreements
Coordination	Facilitation and integration of resources for optimal benefit
Use	Incorporating available resources from all levels of government, NGOs, and the private sector, where appropriate, in a jurisdiction's resource management planning efforts
Information management	Provisions for the thorough integration of communications and information management elements into resource management organizations, processes, technologies, and decision support
Credentialing	Use of criteria that ensure consistent training, licensure, and certification standards

Resource Management Concepts

Resource management centers around six essential concepts (Table 13-1). The first is for planners and resource managers to apply *consistency* by providing a standardized method for identifying, acquiring, allocating, and tracking resources. These systems should also be interoperable among other responder groups and agencies when possible. Second, a *standardized* approach to resource classification must be employed to improve the effectiveness of mutual-aid and assistance agreements. Third, *coordination* should be assured for all resources at an incident to facilitate the integration and optimal benefit. Fourth, resource *use* ensures incorporation and common planning efforts of all available resources from all levels of government, NGOs, and the private sector. Fifth, provisions must be made for the thorough integration of communications and *information management* elements into overall resource management processes, technologies, and decision support. And finally, a *credentialing* system must be used to ensure consistent training, licensure, and certification standards for resources that may be used during incident response. Some of these concepts and activities occur prior to an incident taking place; others occur at the time of or immediately following an incident. In

either case, these concepts and their application to resource management is a primary responsibility of the Planning Section.

Resource Management Principles

Resource management within the NIMS is founded and based on these five principles: planning, use of agreements, categorizing resources, resource identification, and effective management of resources. The following sections review each of these in the context of incident resource management.

Planning

Coordinated planning, training to common standards, and inclusive exercises provide a foundation for the interoperability and compatibility of resources throughout an incident. Jurisdictions should work together in advance of an incident to develop plans for identifying, ordering, managing, and employing resources. The planning process should include identifying resource needs based on the threats to and vulnerabilities of the jurisdiction and developing alternative strategies to obtain the needed resources.

Planning may include the creation of new policies or procedures to encourage positioning of resources near the expected incident site in response to anticipated resource needs. Plans should anticipate conditions or circumstances that may trigger a specific reaction based on prior information and modeling when possible, such as the restocking of supplies when inventories reach a predetermined minimum. Organizations and jurisdictions should continually assess the status of their resources to have an accurate list of resources available at any given time. Additionally, emergency management/response personnel (and all organizations and individuals who assume an emergency management role) should be familiar with the National Response Framework (NRF) and should be prepared to integrate and coordinate with federal resources.

Use of Agreements

Agreements between and among parties providing or requesting resources are necessary to enable effective and efficient resource management during incident operations. Standing mutual-aid agreements between departments, agencies, and jurisdictions are a common practice in public safety. A mutual-aid agreement is simply an arrangement made between two or more entities to assist each other and enhance response capabilities. Mutual-aid agreements and Emergency Management Assistance Compacts (EMACs) are frequently established among agencies to ensure the employment of standardized, interoperable equipment and other incident resources during incident operations. These agreements also enable effective and efficient resource management during incident operations.

It is unrealistic for each agency, department, or jurisdiction to have one of every type of resource that may be required to manage an incident. Neighboring or regional areas must develop agreements to share and efficiently use these valued resources. The goal of these agreements is to facilitate a turnkey mechanism to request resources at the moment of need without having to negotiate the terms of use during incident response, and they should routinely be evaluated during planning periods.

Categorizing Resources

To optimize the use and management of resources during incident response, resources are categorized by size, capacity, capability, skill, and other characteristics. These criteria are used to describe a vast array of resources, from personnel and teams to hand tools and heavy equipment. This process of resource categorization facilitates the requisition process and ensures that the person making the request and the person delivering the resource are speaking about the same type of resource. Large incidents frequently require resources from within jurisdictions, across jurisdictions, and between governmental and nongovernmental entities. Resource-typing definitions provide emergency managers with the tools they need to request and receive the resources they need during an emergency or disaster. This common language for describing resources makes the resource-ordering and dispatch process within and across jurisdictions—and among all levels of governments, NGOs, and the private sector—more efficient and ensures that needed resources are received.

Resource Identification and Ordering

Resource managers and Resources Unit Leaders use a standardized process to order, identify, mobilize, dispatch, and track the resources required to support incident management activities. Resource managers perform these tasks either at an Incident Commander's request or in accordance with planning requirements.

The NIMS encourages the development of systems that will inventory preidentified, credentialed, categorized, and capability-typed resources. Such a system will greatly improve the efficiency of a response group in getting the right resource for a particular incident objective. Preidentified resource listings also save a great deal of time in locating specialized or uncommon resources. The NIMS provides a *National Mutual Aid Glossary of Terms and Definitions* that provides a basic understanding of the resources that are employed in incident management. This guide provides definitions regarding the capabilities of federal, state, and local entities.

> **Tip**
>
> The NIMS *National Mutual Aid Glossary of Terms and Definitions* is a valuable resource guide that provides definitions regarding the capabilities of federal, state, and local entities. It is designed to provide a basic understanding of the resources that are employed in incident management.

In some cases, the identification and ordering process is compressed, where an Incident Command (IC) has determined the resources necessary for the task and specifies a resource order directly. However, in larger, more complex incidents, the IC may not be fully aware of resources available. At this point, the IC may identify needs based on incident objectives and use the resource management process to fill these needs.

Effective Management of Resources

Resource management involves acquisition procedures; management information; and redundant systems and protocols for ordering, mobilizing, dispatching, and demobilizing resources. The NIMS provides guidance for the individuals involved in the management of resources. Resource managers and Unit Leaders are encouraged to use these validated practices in the performance of tasks. Examples include systematic and efficient approaches to acquisition procedures, management information systems, redundant information systems, and ordering, mobilization, dispatching, and demobilization protocols. Each of these will be discussed in the following paragraphs.

Acquisition Procedures

Acquisition procedures are used to obtain resources to support operational requirements. Preparedness organizations should develop these tools and related standardized processes to support acquisition activities during their community planning process. Examples include mission tasking, contracting, drawing from existing stocks, and making small purchases.

A key aspect of the inventory process is determining whether an organization needs to warehouse specific items prior to an incident. Some types of commonly needed resources may be acquired well in advance of an incident and stored (stockpiled) for times of need. Other types of resources cannot be stockpiled and must be obtained on demand (just in time), usually through prearranged contracts and agreements. Individuals in charge of resource management responsibilities must determine which resources fall into these categories of supply. This decision must take into account the urgency of the need, speed of procurement, and sufficient quantities to meet the typical demand.

Another important consideration in the process of stockpiling and managing resource inventories is the resource-specific shelf life and special maintenance considerations. Strict reliance on stockpiling raises issues concerning shelf life and durability; however, strict reliance on just-in-time resources raises its own concerns related to timely delivery. Just-in-time assets need to be accurately accounted for to ensure that multiple jurisdictions or private-sector organizations are not relying solely on the same response asset, which can lead to shortages during a response. Those with resource management responsibilities should build sufficient funding into their budgets for periodic replenishments, preventive maintenance, and capital improvements.

An integral part of acquisition procedures is developing methods and protocols for the handling and distribution of donated resources.

Management Information Systems

Management information systems are used to collect, update, and process data; track resources; and display their readiness status. These tools range from simplistic status boards to highly sophisticated computer network systems capable of real-time resource status data transfer across wide areas. All of these tools enhance information flow, provide data among incident managers, and are especially useful when different jurisdictions and functional agencies are managing various aspects of the incident in a coordinated effort. Examples of such systems include geographical information systems (GIS), resource tracking systems, transportation tracking systems, inventory management systems, and reporting and display terminal systems. The selection and use of systems for resource management should be based on the identification of the information needs within a jurisdiction.

Redundant Information Systems

Resource managers should be able to identify and activate backup systems to manage resources in the event that the primary resource management information system is disrupted or unavailable. Management information systems should also have sufficiently redundant and diverse power supplies and communication capabilities. If possible, the backup storage should not be collocated, and the information should be backed up at least every 24 hours during the incident to avoid catastrophic data loss.

Ordering, Mobilization, Dispatching, and Demobilization Protocols

Ordering, mobilization, dispatching, and demobilization protocols are used to request resources, prioritize requests, activate and dispatch resources to incidents, and return resources to normal status and their donor organizations. Many preparedness organizations have developed standard protocols within their jurisdictions. Expansion of current protocols may be necessary as communities expand and enhance their response capabilities. All of these protocols must work within the guidelines of NIMS to ensure an efficient, effective process. Examples include tracking systems that identify the location and status of mobilized or dispatched resources and procedures to demobilize resources and return them to their original locations and status.

Managing Resources

To implement the concepts and principles of resource management, NIMS includes standardized procedures, methodologies, and functions in its seven-step resource management process. The seven steps are as follows:

1. Identifying resource requirements
2. Ordering and acquiring resources
3. Mobilizing resources
4. Tracking and reporting resources
5. Recovering and demobilizing resources
6. Reimbursing resources
7. Inventorying resources

This process reflects functional considerations, geographic factors, and validated practices within and across disciplines. It is important for responders to keep in mind that these processes will likely be adjusted as new lessons are learned.

Maintenance of resources is important during all aspects of resource management. Maintenance prior to resource deployment ensures availability and capability. Maintenance during the deployment phase ensures continued capabilities, such as adequate fuel supplies during use. Postoperational inspection and maintenance ensures future availability.

The foundation for resource management provided in this component will be expanded and refined over time in a collaborative cross-jurisdictional, cross-disciplinary effort led by the National Integration Center (NIC).

The resource management process can be separated into two parts: resource management as an element of preparedness and resource management during an incident. The preparedness activities (i.e., resource typing, credentialing, and inventorying) are conducted on a continual basis to help ensure that resources are ready to be mobilized when they are called to an incident. Resource management during an incident is a defined process with a distinct begin-

ning and ending specific to the needs of the particular incident **(Figure 13-1)**.

Identifying Resource Requirements

Responders and planners at an incident site are constantly evaluating and determining which resources are required during the incident life cycle. This process involves accurately identifying (1) what and how much of a particular resource is needed to accomplish the objectives of the incident, (2) where and when these resources are needed, and (3) who will be receiving or using the resource(s). Identified resources may include supplies, equipment, facilities, and incident management personnel or emergency response teams. If a requestor is unable to describe an item by resource type or classification system, the resource manager should provide technical advice to define and develop a specification for the given resource. Because resource availability and requirements will constantly change as the incident evolves, all entities participating in an operation must coordinate closely in this process. Specific resources for critical infrastructure and key resources may need to be identified and coordinated through mutual-aid agreements or assistance agreements

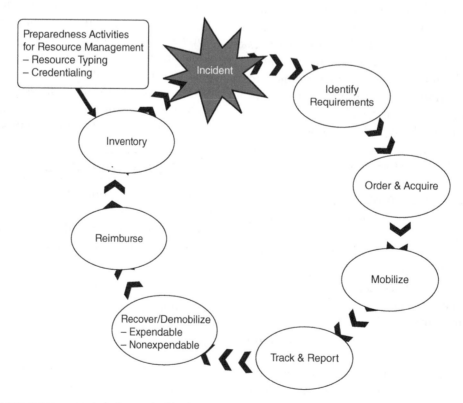

Figure 13-1 Resource management during an incident

unique to those sectors and should be accessible through preparedness organizations or MACS.

Resource availability and requirements will constantly change as the incident evolves. Consequently, all emergency management/response personnel and their affiliated organizations involved in an operation should coordinate closely throughout this process. Coordination should begin as early as possible, preferably prior to the need for incident response activities.

In situations when an incident is projected to have catastrophic implications (e.g., a major hurricane or flooding), states and/or the federal government may position resources in the anticipated incident area. In cases where there is time to assess the requirements and plan for a catastrophic incident, the federal response will be coordinated with state, tribal, and local jurisdictions, and the positioning of federal resources will be tailored to address the specific situation. The flow of requests and assistance is shown in **Figure 13-2.**

Ordering and Acquiring Resources

Requests for items that cannot be obtained locally are submitted through the local EOC or MACS using established ordering procedures. If the servicing EOC is unable to fill the order locally, the order is forwarded to the next level—generally an adjacent local, state, or regional EOC or multiagency coordination entity. A series of standardized ICS forms are used to accomplish this process.

The decision cycles for placing and filling resource orders are different for incident (field) personnel with resource management responsibilities and resource coordination processes such as MACS. Generally the IC will develop resource requests based on priorities that consider current and successive operational periods. Decisions regarding resource allocation are based primarily on organizational or agency protocol and possible resource demands of other incidents. Requested resources will be mobilized only with the consent of the jurisdiction that is

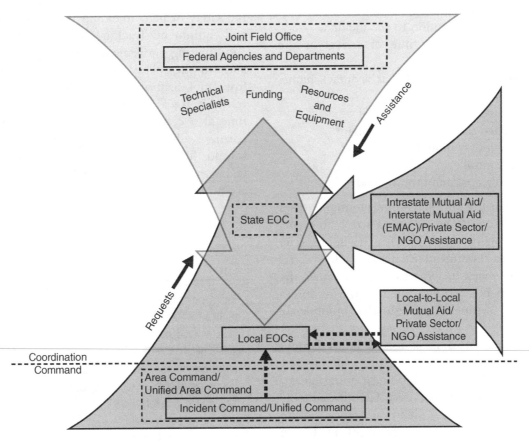

Figure 13-2 Flow of requests and assistance during large-scale incidents.

being asked to provide the resources. Discrepancies between requested resources and those available for delivery must be communicated to the requestor.

Personnel involved in the management of resources should be cautious of the practice of requesting resources by circumventing the official resource coordination process, a method sometimes referred to as *bypass requisitioning*. This method creates substantial limitations to the overall resource management operation and multiagency coordination system supporting the incident. These requests do not proceed within the context of orderly resource management and typically result in inefficient resource use or lack of accountability for overall incident resources.

Mobilizing Resources

Emergency management, response personnel, and incident personnel begin mobilizing when notified through established channels. I condensed these two sentences into one to avoid excessive repetition. A standardized process is established in the ICS for mobilizing resources. At the time of notification, personnel should be notified of the following:

- Date, time, and place of departure
- Mode of transportation to the incident
- Estimated date and time of arrival at the incident
- Reporting location (address, contact name, and phone number)
- Anticipated incident assignment
- Anticipated duration of deployment
- Resource order number
- Incident number
- Applicable cost and funding codes

The resource tracking and mobilization processes are directly linked. When resources arrive on scene, they must formally check in with the appropriate section of the command structure. This starts the on-scene check-in process and validates the order requirements. Notification that the resources have arrived is made through the appropriate channels.

The mobilization process also includes deployment planning based on existing interagency mobilization guidelines; equipping; training; designating assembly points that have facilities suitable for logistical support; and obtaining transportation to deliver resources to the incident most quickly, in line with priorities and budgets. Mobilization plans should also recognize that some resources are fixed facilities, such as laboratories, hospitals, EOCs, shelters, and waste management systems. These facilities assist operations without moving into the incident area in the way that other resources are mobilized. Plans and systems to monitor resource mobilization status should be flexible enough to adapt to both types of mobilization.

Managers should plan and prepare for the demobilization process well in advance, often at the same time they begin the resource mobilization process. Early planning for demobilization facilitates accountability and makes transportation of resources efficient, cost-effective, and timely.

Tracking and Reporting Resources

Resource tracking is a standardized, integrated process conducted prior to, during, and after an incident by all emergency management/response personnel and their affiliated organizations, as appropriate. Resource tracking provides incident managers with a clear picture of where resources are located and their current status (available, in service, out of service, etc.). Tracking and reporting also helps incident staff prepare to receive resources and protect the safety of personnel and the security of supplies and equipment. Tracking is an essential process for coordinating movement of personnel, equipment, and supplies. This process should be continuous, from mobilization through demobilization. Ideally, resource tracking information is displayed in real time at a centralized point accessible to all NIMS partners, allowing total visibility of assets. Managers should follow all procedures for acquiring and managing resources, including reconciliation, accounting, auditing, and inventorying.

Tip
Radio and cellular communications provide an excellent method for tracking and reporting resources, but historical disaster incident reviews have identified that failures of such communication devices have caused major incident management problems. Make sure your NIMS plan has alternative backup systems that can track and report resources in a timely manner. In many major disasters, radio and cellular communication systems fail due to damage to towers and land-based electrical systems.

Recovering and Demobilizing Resources

Resource recovery takes place during and following an incident. During an incident, resources are frequently recovered and prepared for another use. Ultimately, each resource that is activated and deployed to an incident site must be recovered, restored, and returned to the donor agency. During this process, resources are rehabilitated, replenished, disposed of (when appropriate), and retrograded. This process is closely tied to resource inventory maintenance. Accurate inventorying will result in a final list of resources requiring restocking, cleaning, or preventive maintenance.

Demobilization is the orderly, safe, and efficient return of an incident resource to its original location and status. It can begin at any point of an incident, but it should begin as soon as possible to facilitate accountability. For large-scale incidents, the demobilization process should coordinate between the incident(s) and MACS to reassign resources, if necessary, and to prioritize critical resource needs during demobilization.

The Demobilization Unit in the Planning Section develops an Incident Demobilization Plan, containing specific demobilization instructions, as part of the Incident Action Plan (IAP). Demobilization planning and processes should include provisions addressing the safe return of resources to their original location and status and notification of return. Demobilization should also include processes for tracking resources and for addressing applicable reimbursement. Furthermore, documentation regarding the transportation of resources should be collected and maintained for reimbursement, if applicable. Demobilization provisions may need to meet specific organizational requirements.

There are two major categories of resources that must be accounted for in the recovery and demobilization process: nonexpendable and expendable. **Nonexpendable resources** are those resources that are not normally used up or consumed in service or those that are generally easy to recover and make ready for continued service. In these cases, the resource is serviced fully to normal functioning condition and returned to storage for the next mobilization. Broken and/or lost items should be replaced through the Supply Unit by the organization with invoicing responsibility for the incident or as defined in preincident agreements. Examples of nonexpendable resources include firearms, firefighting equipment, water supply lines, and patient monitoring equipment. In the case of human resources, adequate rest and recuperation time and facilities should be provided according to established guidelines. Important occupational health and mental health issues also must be addressed, including monitoring how events affect emergency responders over time.

Expendable resources are those resources that are normally used up or consumed in service or those that are more easily replaced than rescued, salvaged, or protected. Examples of expendable resources include medical gloves, water filters, and bandages. Disposal of certain types of expendable resources that require special handling and disposition (e.g., biological waste and contaminated supplies, debris, and equipment) should be dealt with according to established regulations and policies. Another important issue related to expendable resources is managing inventories that have a shelf life or special maintenance considerations (e.g., temperature storage requirements). Resource managers must build sufficient funding into their budgets for periodic replenishments, preventive maintenance, and special storage requirements.

Returned resources that are not in restorable condition, whether expendable or nonexpendable, must be declared as excess according to established regulations and policies of the controlling jurisdiction, agency, or organization. Waste management is of special note in the process of recovering resources because resources that require special handling and disposition (e.g., biological waste and contaminated supplies, debris, and equipment) are handled according to established regulatory guidelines and policies.

Reimbursing Resources

Reimbursement provides a mechanism to recover funds expended for incident-specific activities. Processes for reimbursement play an important role in establishing and maintaining the readiness of resources and should be in place to ensure that resource providers are reimbursed in a timely manner. They should include mechanisms for billing and accessing reimbursement programs, such as the Public Assistance Program and the Emergency Relief Program. Reimbursement mechanisms should be included in preparedness plans, mutual-aid agreements, and assistance agreements. It is important to remember, however, that some resources may not be reimbursable based on regulations or agreements established before the incident.

Inventorying Resources

The use of inventory systems is a key tool for resource managers in assessing the assets available or provided to an incident. These systems should include all resources deployed to the incident location regardless of their origin. During the planning and identification process, organizations should submit and enter all resources available for activation and deployment into resource tracking systems. Ideally, the systems should be maintained at local, regional, state, and national levels using common terminology, categorization, and typing. This data is made available to appropriate resource managers in times of need. Resources identified within an inventory system are not an indication of automatic availability. The jurisdiction and/or owner of the resources have the final determination on availability.

Inventory systems for resource management should be adaptable and scalable and should account for the potential of double counting of personnel or equipment. In particular, resource summaries should clearly reflect any overlap of personnel across different resource pools. Personnel inventories should reflect single resources with multiple skills, taking care not to overstate the total resources. For example, many fire fighters also have credentials as emergency medical technicians (EMTs). A resource summary, then, could count a fire fighter as a fire fighter or as an EMT, but not both. The total should reflect the number of available personnel, not simply the sum of the fire fighter and EMT counts.

Deployable resources have different inventory, ordering, and response profiles depending on their primary use during the response or recovery phases of an incident. Planning for resource use, inventory, and tracking should recognize the fundamental difference in resource deployment in the response and recovery phases. The response phase relies heavily on mutual-aid agreements and assistance agreements, and recovery resources are typically acquired through contracts with NGOs and the private sector.

As part of the inventory management process, several key concepts need to be considered: credentialing systems and identification and typing systems. These will facilitate the process of creating accurate inventories using a common language that, ideally, any resource manager requesting or disbursing resources will understand. This helps ensure that the resource requested matches the resource delivered.

Credentialing Personnel

The credentialing process includes the objective evaluation and documentation of an individual's current certification, license, degree, training, and experience. The process also considers the individual's competence or proficiency to meet nationally accepted standards, provide particular services and functions, or perform specific tasks under specific conditions during an incident. For the purpose of NIMS, credentialing is the administrative process for validating personnel qualifications, providing authorization to perform specific functions, and granting specific access to an incident involving mutual aid. **Figure 13-3** illustrates the following NIC-recommended process for credentialing under NIMS.

When a request for mutual aid or assistance is received, the supporting department or agency evaluates its capacity to accommodate the anticipated loss of the resources that would be deployed without compromising mission performance. For example, a fire department receives a request for personnel to assist in a large wildfire. The department must consider if it can allow 20 percent of its equipment and personnel to be deployed to another jurisdiction for 30 days and still meet its own community's needs.

If the supporting department or agency determines that it can accommodate the requested deployment of resources, it must next identify specific personnel who will be deployed. The department or agency then submits applications for each member selected for deployment to an authorized accrediting agency identified by the credentialing authority of the state to which the mutual aid will be provided.

The accrediting agency evaluates each application and determines whether the applicant meets the established criteria for the positions required by the mission. Applications that fail to meet established criteria are returned to the submitting department or agency, and they may be resubmitted with additional documentation or when the applicant's qualifications change. For applications that are approved by the authorized accrediting agency, the following steps are taken:

1. The applicant's department or agency is notified.
2. A record of the individual is created in the official credentialing database.
3. An identification card or other credential is issued to the individual. (The identification card or credential should include an expiration date and be reissued as appropriate.)
4. Information on the applicant is uploaded to the incident management infrastructure.

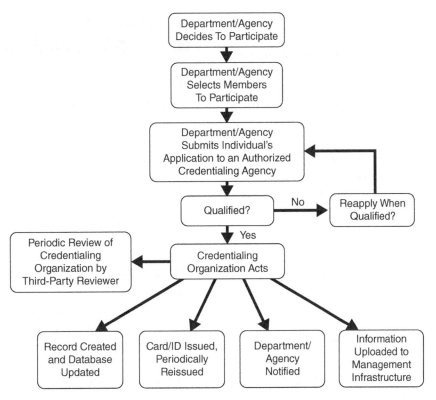

Figure 13-3 Recommended NIMS personnel credentialing process.

Although credentialing includes the issuing of identification cards or credentials, it is separate and distinct from the incident badging process. When access to a site is controlled through special badging, the badging process must be based on verification of identity, qualifications, and deployment authorization.

Organizations utilizing volunteers, especially spontaneous volunteers, are responsible for ensuring each volunteer's eligibility to participate in a response. These organizations—governmental agencies responsible for coordinating emergency responses; volunteer management agencies, such as the American Red Cross, Emergency System for Advance Registration of Volunteer Health Professionals, and Medical Reserve Corps; as well as hospitals, fire, and police departments—must develop protocols governing the activation and use of volunteers. Careful coordination is required to ensure the provision of services is not hindered by unaddressed safety and security considerations or legal or regulatory issues.

Remember, the goal of credentialing personnel is to ensure a standardized process whereby responders from a wide array of disciplines document and establish their professional abilities. This entails authoritatively attesting that an individual meets professional standards for training, experience, and performance that are required for key incident management functions or professional licensure and certification. This process helps to ensure that personnel representing various jurisdictional levels and functional disciplines possess a minimum common level of training, currency, experience, physical and mental fitness, and capability for the incident management or emergency responder position they are tasked to fill. Ideally, this information will be registered in a database that is accessible at the regional, state, and federal level to facilitate the identification and activation of personnel resources.

Identifying and Typing Resources

Resource typing is categorizing, by capability, the resources requested, deployed, and used in incidents. Measurable standards that identify resource capabilities and performance levels serve as the basis for typing categories. Resource users employ these standards to identify and inventory resources. Types of resources may be divided into subcategories to define more precisely the capabilities needed to meet specific requirements. Resource typing facilitates frequent use and accuracy in obtaining needed resources.

To allow resources to be deployed and used on a national basis, the NIC (with input from federal, state, tribal, local, private-sector, nongovernmental, and national professional organizations) is responsible for facilitating the development and issuance of national standards for resource typing and ensuring that these typed resources reflect operational capabilities. Proposals for additions to the NIMS Typed Resources Definitions may be submitted to the NIC's Incident Management Systems Integration Division for consideration if you discover you have specialized needs for resource typing that do not appear on the established definitions.

Resources are generally identified by four properties in the national resource-typing protocol: category, kind, type, and additional information.

Table 13-2 Sample Categories for National Resource Typing	
Transportation	Health and medical
Communications	Search and rescue
Public works and engineering	Hazardous materials response
Firefighting	Food and water
Information and planning	Energy
Law enforcement and security	Public information
Mass care	Animals and agricultural issues
Resource management	Volunteers and donations

Tip

By identifying and typing resources, resource managers can more effectively work with multiple agencies and jurisdictions. The system creates advantages in the following areas:

- *Planning.* Knowing the specific capabilities of the various kinds of resources helps planners decide the type and quantity of resource best suited to perform a specific mission function required by the incident.
- *Ordering.* Ordering resources by type saves time, minimizes errors, indicates exactly what is needed, and reduces unnecessary communications.
- *Monitoring use.* This allows managers to evaluate capabilities and make changes as needed. This may lead to enhanced efficiency and reduced cost of a resource and eliminate excessive and insufficient ordering.

Category

This is the function for which a resource would be most useful. **Table 13-2** outlines some examples of national resource-typing categories.

Kind

Kind refers to broad descriptors that characterize similar resources, such as teams, personnel, equipment, supplies, vehicles, etc. Remember, these are broad descriptions that describe a range of similar items, not a specific item or model. At times there is need to further define a kind of resource, in which case the resource is generally categorized by its components and measures.

Components

Components are the elements that make up a resource. For example, an engine company may have the following components: pump, water tank, ladder, hose 2.5 inch, hose 1.75 inch, master stream, hand tools, and personnel. Another example of this type of description is an Urban Search and Rescue Team (USAR), which consists of two 31-person teams, four canines, and a comprehensive specialized equipment cache.

Measures

Measures are standards that identify resource capability or capacity. The specific measures to define a kind of resource depend on the resource being typed and the expected operational conditions. Measures should be in terms that are useful in describing a resource's capability. For example, a measure for a disaster medical assistance team (DMAT) might be the number of ambulatory patients it can care for per day. Another example might be the gallons per minute a water pump can move.

Type

Type refers to the level of resource capability. Typing provides resource managers and planners with additional information that aids in selecting the most appropriate resource for a given operation. Types are described with a numeric value. For example, assigning a Type 1 label to a resource designates that it has a greater level of capability than Type 2 of the same resource. For example, the US Coast Guard has typed oil skimmers based on barrels per day. An oil skimmer might have the following types:

- Type 1: 9600 bbls/day
- Type 2: 2880 bbls/day

- Type 3: 480 bbls/day
- Type 4: Not applicable

Type values are assigned from 1 to 4, with 1 being the highest capability and 4 being the lowest capability. In some isolated cases, a resource may have fewer than or more than four types. In such cases, additional types are identified or described as *not applicable*.

Additional Information

The national resource-typing protocol will also provide the capability to use additional information that is pertinent to resource decision making. For example, if a particular set of resources can be released to support an incident only under particular authorities or laws, the protocol should alert responsible parties to such limitations.

Rural Case Study *Answers*

1. The Resources Unit should track all personnel and equipment that are activated, in service, out of service, or available for assignment.
2. Incident resources should be categorized based on developed national standards for the descriptions of resources and their capabilities. Resources are classified by category and kind, which refers to the resource's function. Further quantitative descriptions for each category provide information about the resource's level of capability, or type, which is a measure of minimum capabilities of a resource to perform a particular function.

Urban Case Study *Answers*

1. The following principles of resource management that will benefit this incident are the following:
   - Advanced planning
   - Resource identification and ordering
   - Categorization of resources
   - Use of agreements
   - Effective management of resources
2. The following are the primary tasks of the Resources Unit and the Resources Unit Leader:
   - Review and understand the common NIMS and Unit Leader responsibilities.
   - Establish a check-in and check-out system for incident resources.
   - Prepare and maintain a display system for incident resources.
   - Monitor and maintain the current status and location of incident resources.
   - Brief the Planning Section Chief on all resource management issues.
   - Maintain appropriate NIMS/ICS forms.

Wrap-Up

Summary

- The NIMS resource management process provides a uniform method of identifying, accruing, allocating, and training resources.
- Resource management within NIMS uses standardized classifications of types of resources to support the incident management organization.
- Resource management within NIMS uses a credentialing system involving uniform training and certification standards to ensure that personnel will integrate with ongoing incident operations.
- Resource management centers around six essential concepts: consistency, standardization, coordination, use, information management, and credentialing.
- Resource management is the responsibility of the Resources Unit of the Planning Section, the EOC, and MACS; it should encompass resources contributed by private-sector organizations and NGOs.
- The use of standardized NIMS forms is helpful in managing resources at an incident.
- Resource management involves coordinating and overseeing the application of tools, processes, and systems that provide incident managers with timely and appropriate resources during an incident.
- Resource management involves five principles: planning, use of agreements, categorizing resources, resource identification, and effective management of resources.
- The basic concepts and principles that guide the resource management processes used in NIMS allow these tasks to be conducted effectively.
- By standardizing the procedures, methodologies, and functions involved in these processes, NIMS ensures that resources move quickly and efficiently to support incident managers and emergency responders. ICS forms assist in the appropriate overseeing of resources used during an incident.

Glossary

Expendable resources: Equipment, supplies, or tools that are normally used up or consumed in service or those that are easier to replace than rescue, salvage, or protect.

Management information systems: Tools used to collect, update, and process data; track resources; and display readiness status.

Nonexpendable resources: Equipment that is not normally used up or consumed in service or that can be easily recovered and made ready for continued service.

Resource management: The coordination and oversight of assets that provide incident managers with timely and appropriate mechanisms to accomplish operational objectives during an incident.

Resources Unit: The component of the Planning Section (in the ICS structure) that serves as the primary manager of all assigned personnel or other resources that have checked in at an incident site.

Resources Unit Leader: The individual responsible for maintaining the status of all resources at an incident.

Wrap-Up Case Study

A Category 4 hurricane has struck the coast of the Carolinas, causing major damage to coastal communities and those up to 150 miles inland. The two states are declared a Federal Disaster Area, encompassing thousands of square miles. State and federal resources are moving into the area to assist in the recovery effort through the activation of mutual-aid agreements. A series of staging areas have been designated by each state's EOC, working with the multiagency coordinating systems. Incident Management Teams (IMTs) are being deployed to the command areas. In two coastal areas, access to the mainland has been cut off, stranding several communities.

1. Mutual-aid agreements and EMACs help to:
   A. spread the costs of emergency response around a region.
   B. facilitate the timely delivery of assistance during incidents.
   C. coordinate the full documentation of incidents.
   D. establish the command structure for incidents.

2. Resource typing involves categorizing resources based on which of the following?
   A. Availability
   B. Cost
   C. Manufacturer
   D. Kind

3. How does NIMS ensure that all personnel possess a minimum level of training, experience, fitness, capability, and currency?
   A. It maintains a database of personnel who have been trained for specific positions.
   B. It provides training to personnel who will be assigned to Command Staff positions.
   C. It oversees a national training and exercise program.
   D. It establishes certification and credentialing standards for key personnel.

4. Resource managers use established procedures to track resources continuously from _____ through demobilization.
   A. mobilization
   B. recovery
   C. typing
   D. purchase

CHAPTER 14

Supporting Technologies

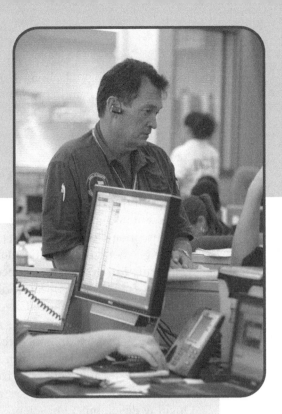

Rural Case Study

As Smith County begins to receive support from the regional and state resources in response to its Emergency Operations Center (EOC) requests, it is important that the requested resources are of the right type and are staged or positioned in needed areas. Smith County has not implemented computerized resource tracking software. The state EOC has software that tracks real-time requests, deployment status, and resource locations. Unfortunately, due to misguided priorities and internal squabbling, Smith County had not complied with the state's implementation schedule. Another major problem for Smith County is the loss of radio towers and interoperable communications throughout the region. Smith County will have to request mobile communication systems from the state EOC.

1. What technology systems should have been implemented before the incident?
2. List three benefits achieved by the standardization and typing of incident management technology.

Urban Case Study

The incident in Pleasantville has several issues that depend on supporting technologies. The HazMat teams will be using a great deal of equipment to monitor the incident, to protect responders, and to provide mission management. Because of the magnitude of the incident and the spread of contamination to the surrounding communities, it is critical that all responders work together and share this information.

Multiple EOCs need to communicate seamlessly to assist with establishing and sustaining an Area Command for this incident. Responders from different agencies (e.g., local, regional, and state) need to communicate on common channels. Responders from different agencies need to support one another with common equipment and materials to safely and effectively manage this complex incident. All of these tasks are accomplished by assuring the existence of a high degree of interoperability through supportive technologies.

1. List four types of response equipment that should share common characteristics across agencies and disciplines.
2. List three key National Incident Management System (NIMS) principles to improve response capabilities through supportive technologies.

Introduction

Previous chapters have illustrated the enormous amount of data and requisite information produced during an incident. Systems that review, catalog, analyze, communicate, and store incident information are highly effective and valued command assets. Small-scale incidents usually are managed with pen, paper, verbal communication, and scene indicators; however, in the case of complex or large-scale incidents, technology facilitates the actions of responders, planners, and commanders at the incident site and at local, state, and federal support agencies.

Supporting Technologies

Technology and technological systems provide capabilities essential to implementing and supporting NIMS. These include voice and data communications systems (e.g., mobile radios and mobile data terminals), information systems (e.g., recordkeeping and resource-tracking systems), and display systems. They also include specialized technologies that facilitate incident operations (e.g., monitoring and personal protective equipment technologies) and incident management activities in situations that call for unique technology-based capabilities (e.g., incident-modeling and tracking systems).

Ongoing development of science and technology is necessary for continual improvement and refinement of NIMS. Strategic research and development (R&D) ensures that this development takes place. NIMS also relies on scientifically based technical standards that support the nation's ability for preparation, prevention, response, and recovery from domestic incidents. Maintaining an appropriate focus on science and technology solutions relating to incident management involves a long-term collaborative effort among NIMS partners.

Concepts and Principles Related to Supporting Technologies

A major focus of NIMS is to improve scientific capabilities and lower costs. Five key principles are observed by NIMS to support the use of technology:

- Interoperability and compatibility
- Technology support
- Technology standards
- Broad-based requirements
- Strategic planning for research and development

Interoperability and Compatibility

For effective integration, systems must be compatible; they cannot interfere with one another across multiple jurisdictions, organizations, and NIMS functions. Interoperability and compatibility are achieved through the use of common communica-

tions, data standards, digital data formats, equipment standards, and design standards. These standards must be applied in both the public and private sectors to ensure the continuity of data transfer.

Tip
Common communications within NIMS goes beyond a common set of terminology at the incident scene. The digital information that passes from agency to agency must adhere to common rules and standards so that it is available to assisting agencies in the response community. It is critical to involve the entire local response community when implementing and transitioning to new data management systems.

Technology Support

Technology support permits NIMS organizations to enhance incident management and emergency response. Technology support facilitates incident operations and sustains the R&D programs that strengthen the long-term investment in the nation's future incident management capabilities.

Technology Standards

Supporting systems and technologies are based on requirements developed through preparedness organizations at various jurisdictional levels. National standards for key systems are required to facilitate the interoperability and compatibility of major systems across jurisdictional, geographic, and functional lines. For example, many respiratory protective devices use a similar technology to supply or filter air. Many of the filtering devices use a similar type of cartridge. The threads on the cartridge that connect into the breathing device use the same specifications, making the cartridges interchangeable between different products and response agencies.

Tip
It is not uncommon for new technologies to be developed by experts who are not the end users. It is critical for the interested community (e.g., fire, police, public health, dispatchers, etc.) to provide feedback to the developers and be involved in the testing of new technologies. This feedback is extremely valuable in accelerating the design, production, and field implementation of advancing technologies. A formalized system of product development testing and feedback ensures that new technologies are designed with the end user in mind.

Broad-Based Requirements

Needs for new technologies, procedures, protocols, and standards to facilitate incident management are identified at both the field and the national levels. Because these needs will most likely exceed available resources, NIMS provides a mechanism for combining and prioritizing them from the local to the national level. These needs will be met across the incident life cycle by coordinating basic, applied, developmental, and demonstration research, as well as testing and evaluation activities.

Strategic Planning for R&D

Strategic **research and development (R&D)** planning identifies future technologies that can improve preparedness, prevention, response, and recovery capabilities or lower the cost of existing capabilities. Again, responders need to become actively involved in providing feedback to ensure that their concerns and recommendations are considered during all phases of technology development.

To ensure effective R&D, the National Integration Center, in coordination with the US Department of Homeland Security (DHS) Undersecretary for Science and Technology, will integrate into the national R&D agenda the incident management science and technology needs of departments, government agencies, functional disciplines, private-sector entities, and nongovernmental organizations (NGOs) operating within NIMS. Additionally, these strategies are supported by end user responder group input via advisory bodies, such as the DHS Security Science and Technology Directorate First Responder Research, Development, Test and Evaluation Coordinating Working Group; the InterAgency Board (IAB); and research conducted by a variety of entities such as the national labs and academic institutions.

Supporting Incident Management with Science and Technology

Supporting technologies enhance incident management capabilities, facilitate responder capabilities and safety, and lower costs. This is accomplished through three principal activities: operational scientific support, technology standards support, and R&D support.

Operational Scientific Support

Operational scientific support identifies and, on request, mobilizes scientific and technical assets that can be used to support incident management activities. For example, DNA sampling and testing can be performed to positively identify victims of large-scale catastrophes. This type of activity is usually outside of local capabilities and relies on specialized scientific laboratories. Operational scientific support draws on the scientific and technological expertise of federal agencies and other public and private organizations.

Planning for this category of support is done at each level of government through the NIMS preparedness organizations. Operational scientific support is requisitioned and provided via NIMS through various programs coordinated by the DHS and other organizations and agencies.

Technical Standards Support

Technical standards support enables the development and coordination of technology standards for NIMS to ensure that personnel, organizations, communications and information systems, and other equipment perform consistently, effectively, and reliably together without disrupting one another. The National Integration Center coordinates the establishment of technical standards for NIMS users. Four principles are used in defining these technical support standards:

- Performance measurements as a basis for standards
- Consensus-based performance standards
- Testing and evaluation by objective experts
- Technical guidelines for training emergency responders on equipment use

Performance Measurements as a Basis for Standards

Performance measurement—collecting hard data on how things work in the real world—is the most reliable basis for standards that ensure the safety and mission effectiveness of emergency responders and incident managers. Within the technology-standards process, a performance measurement infrastructure develops guidelines, performance standards, testing protocols, personnel certification, reassessment tools, and training procedures to help incident management organizations use equipment systems effectively.

Tip

It is critical for users of supporting technologies to report their findings regarding the effectiveness and safety of the technologies used. This includes lessons learned from their use as well as tips and tricks for their enhanced use and implementation.

Consensus-Based Performance Standards

A consensus-based approach to technology performance builds on existing approaches to standards for interoperable equipment and systems and takes advantage of existing **standards development organizations (SDOs)** with long-standing interest and expertise. These SDOs include the following:

- National Institute of Justice (NIJ)
- National Institute of Standards and Technology (NIST)
- National Institute for Occupational Safety and Health (NIOSH)
- American National Standards Institute (ANSI)
- American Society for Testing and Materials (ASTM)
- National Fire Protection Association (NFPA)

NIMS, through the National Integration Center, establishes working relationships among these SDOs and incident management organizations at all levels to develop performance standards for incident management technology.

Testing and Evaluation by Objective Experts

NIMS technology criteria rely on private- and public-sector testing laboratories to evaluate equipment against NIMS technical standards. These organizations are selected in accordance with guidelines that ensure testing organizations are technically proficient and objective (free from conflicting interests) in their testing. The National Integration Center establishes appropriate guidelines as part of its standards-development and facilitation responsibilities.

Technical Guidelines for Training Emergency Responders on Equipment Use

Feedback and general guidance information from vulnerability analysts, equipment developers, users, and standards experts are employed to develop scientifically based technical guidelines for training emergency responders on proper equipment use. Based on incident management protocols, instruments, and instrument systems, these training guidelines take into account threat and vulnerability information, equipment and systems capabilities, and a range of expected operating conditions. In addition, performance measures and testing protocols developed from these training guidelines provide a reproducible method of measuring the effectiveness of equipment and systems.

R&D Support

R&D planning is based on the operational needs of the entire range of NIMS users. These needs represent key inputs as the nation formulates its R&D agenda for developing new and improved incident management capabilities. Because operational needs will usually exceed the resources available for research to address them, these needs must be validated, integrated, and prioritized. The preparedness organizations described in Chapter 11 perform these functions. The DHS is responsible for integrating user needs at all levels into the national R&D agenda.

US Department of Homeland Security

The DHS uses the best national scientific and technological resources to improve response capabilities to high-impact terrorist events and catastrophic natural disasters. Its primary focus is terrorism; however, DHS findings apply to any event that may result in large-scale human loss and economic impact. The main focus is centered on weapons of mass destruction, information and infrastructure, laboratories, and research facilities technologies.

The DHS Science and Technology Directorate established the Homeland Security Institute (HSI), a government think tank focused on related research and technology issues. The HSI employs an integrated systems approach to its mission through the following activities:

- *System evaluations* support homeland security program planning and execution. This includes systems analyses, risk analyses, vulnerability analyses, and the creation of strategic technology development plans to reduce vulnerabilities in the nation's critical infrastructure and key resources.
- *Operational assessments* are related to systems development, operational performance, and homeland security strategy. This includes the use of metrics to evaluate the effectiveness of programs and the design and support of exercises and simulations.
- *Technology assessments* provide scientific, technical, and analytical support for the identification, evaluation, and use of advanced technologies.
- *Resource and support analyses* are used to develop methods, techniques, and tools for

analyzing improved means for addressing resource issues. This includes economic policy analysis to assess the costs and benefits of alternative approaches to enhancing security.

- *Analysis supporting the SAFETY Act* provides analytical and technical evaluations used to support DHS determinations concerning new technologies.
- *Field operations analyses* provide personnel to field activities for operations analysis, systems evaluations, and other technical and analytical support.

Tip

The responsibilities of the HIS are as follows:
- System evaluation
- Operational assessments
- Technology assessments
- Resource and support analysis
- Analysis supporting the SAFETY Act
- Field operations analysis

Rural Case Study *Answers*

1. Smith County should have employed the following systems:
   - Logistical support-tracking software systems
   - Recordkeeping systems
   - Mobile radio stations and data terminals
   - Water purification systems
   - Damage assessment tools
   - Incident-tracking systems
2. The following are three benefits resulting from the standardization of incident management technology:
   - The equipment and technology used by all of the coordinating agencies are interoperable.
   - Cross-functionality is established across multiple disciplines or agencies.
   - Capabilities are improved, and new technology costs are reduced.

Urban Case Study *Answers*

1. The following are some examples of response equipment that should share common characteristics across agencies and disciplines:
   - Respiratory protective equipment
   - Communications equipment
   - Incident-monitoring equipment
   - Resource-tracking equipment
   - Public information technologies
   - Decontamination equipment
   - HazMat equipment

2. The key principles that NIMS provides to improve response capabilities through supportive technologies are as follows:
   - Interoperability and compatibility
   - Technology support
   - Technology standards
   - Broad-based requirements
   - Strategic planning for R&D

Wrap-Up

Summary

- Advanced technologies are absolutely necessary given the magnitude and complexity of responding to large-scale incidents.
- Large amounts of data are produced during an incident, requiring sophisticated systems to effectively manage the scene and ensure responder safety. Comprehensive, standardized systems to store, review, analyze, catalog, and communicate data are essential tools in NIMS.
- As threats against responders have become complicated by the possibility of weapons of mass destruction, tools and technologies must be developed and used to assist responders in reacting to such threats.
- The ongoing development of science and technology is necessary for improvement of NIMS.
- Technology systems must work together without interference.
- Technology support allows organizations to enhance incident management and emergency response.
- Technology standards are essential to ensure interoperability.
- New NIMS technologies should meet broad-based requirements to facilitate all levels of response.
- Performance measurements regarding the use of current and new technologies are essential.
- Research and development of new NIMS technologies will be based on the operational needs of all users.

Glossary

Research and development (R&D): The collection of information about a particular subject to create an action, process, tool, or result.

Standards development organizations (SDOs): Organizations with long-standing interest or expertise on existing approaches to establish standards for equipment and systems. Examples include the National Institute of Standards and Technology (NIST), the National Institute for Occupational Safety and Health (NIOSH), the American National Standards Institute (ANSI), and the National Fire Protection Association (NFPA).

Wrap-Up Case Study

The Black River runs through several states and many counties and is a major shipping thoroughfare. In the early spring, two container ships collide during the night, causing a large spill of petrochemicals and debris. Response agencies from seven counties and the state and federal government arrive to find a downstream spill area affecting almost 90 miles. The petrochemicals present an extreme health and safety hazard; citizens along the river are ordered to evacuate. Local HazMat teams are on site monitoring the incident, and private companies have been requested to begin the cleanup process.

1. How do the supporting technologies facilitated by NIMS provide a communications system for all of the responding agencies?
   A. By providing all of the responding agencies with portable radios
   B. By local response agencies giving private companies their radios
   C. By requiring interoperable and compatible communications equipment
   D. By mandating an emergency responder radio code system

2. Validation and establishment of technical guidelines for training emergency responders on equipment used at this incident will be coordinated by which of the following?
   A. The National Integration Center
   B. The NFPA
   C. The Standards Development Office
   D. Local and state training academies

3. NIOSH, ANSI, and the NFPA are examples of _____. These types of entities have long-standing expertise on existing standards for equipment and systems that may be used to respond to this incident.
   A. performance measures offices
   B. standards development organizations
   C. national science directorates
   D. technology development organizations

Utilizing the National Incident Management System

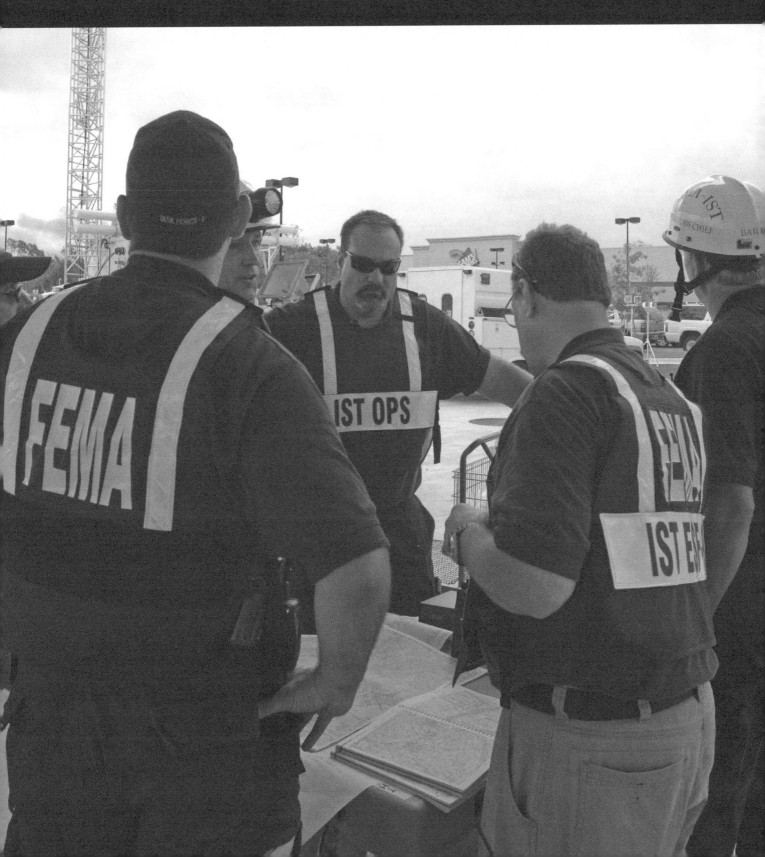

CHAPTER 15

National Response Framework

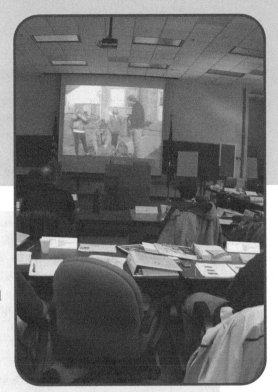

Rural Case Study

The Stadtown tornado incident is a classic example of a rural disaster that immediately overwhelmed local and regional resources. As a result, state and federal resources were deployed and integrated with local responders. A major component of the state and federal response was the establishment of a Multiagency Coordination System (MACS) that coordinated resource management at local, state, and federal levels.

1. Based on the rural case study information from previous chapters, describe the key National Response Framework (NRF) cycle that appears to be deficient in Smith County.
2. Define Emergency Support Functions (ESFs), and list five or more ESFs that may be activated for this disaster.

Urban Case Study

The response to the Pleasantville attack escalated from a local and regional response to a state and federal response. The NRF defined the local, state, and federal roles. In addition, the incident was a suspected terrorist attack. As a result, this incident became a crime with national and international implications. The terrorism implications also triggered immediate national media coverage. Because of these factors, the NRF complemented the National Incident Management System (NIMS) and served as a template for multiple levels of government.

1. How was the NRF triggered or initiated in this incident?
2. What NRF federal entities might be initiated for this incident?
3. What key goals in the national security strategy apply to this incident?

Introduction

The **National Response Framework (NRF)** is a coherent strategic framework (not a series of functional plans) for senior emergency response chiefs, emergency management practitioners, and senior executives in the private sector and nongovernmental organizations (NGOs). The NRF supersedes the National Response Plan (NRP).

The NRF is a complex document and operational concept. This chapter presents only a review of the key points and concepts in the framework, not a comprehensive or in-depth examination. Practitioners and other interested persons should continue to research and inspect the NRF, especially the varying roles agencies and personnel will be called upon to institute. The complete NRF and related annexes are available from the NRF Resource Center (www.fema.gov/NRF).

> **Tip**
>
> The NRF is a response template that replaces the NRP.

Key Characteristics of the NRF

The foundation of the NRF is its scalability, flexibility, and adaptable coordinating structures that align key roles and responsibilities for national emergency response and planning efforts. It articulates best practices and specific authorities for managing incidents ranging from locally controlled events to major disasters.

Scalability means that the framework is contracted or expanded according to the scope (or size) of the incident. For example, the NRF applies to incidents as small as a pipe bomb in a rural community or as large as anthrax attacks that concurrently impact several states, multiple jurisdictions (e.g., federal, state, county, and local), and numerous agencies are supported appropriately within the scalability context of the NRF.

The NRF **adaptability**, by design, establishes a responsive strategic framework to support response efforts for local responder requirements to any type of hazard or attack. This means that any response—especially those that present large and complex issues, such as a chemical leak, a terrorist attack, or a pandemic—are all adaptable within the NRF.

Adaptable coordinating structures in the NRF are incident management templates that provide a common language and organization for agencies and disciplines to integrate effectively. The integrated flexibility provides for the framework to align with all communities and disciplines. It is not a framework of rigid rules and structures. A small volunteer fire department, a suburban emergency medical services (EMS) agency, or an urban police department can apply the NRF to its mission.

Response is defined as immediate actions to save lives, protect property and the environment, and meet basic human needs. This definition is broadened in the NRF to include the execution of emergency plans and operations or actions that support short-term recovery. The emphasis of the NRF is multiagency engagement through a tiered response. This definition intentionally reflects the widely agreed upon belief that all disasters are local—that is, the response begins at the local emergency response level and then expands through regional, state, and federal governments. The overarching philosophy of the NRF is a *unified effort*, a *quick surge* capability, and a *readiness to act*.

A readiness to act posture reflects the intention of the NRF design to enable a rapid and timely response capacity to an attack or disaster. This readiness philosophy begins and progressively advances from the individual citizen, household, and community levels upward through county, state, tribal, and federal governments. This concept is described in the NRF as a forward-leaning posture because many incidents have the capability of rapidly expanding in size, severity, or complexity.

Relationship of the NRF and NIMS

When the response mode is initiated, all activities are governed by NIMS. The NIMS structure ensures Unified Command (UC) and a cohesive operational system to provide safety for all entities engaged in the incident. The NRF and NIMS are also designed to enhance clear and concise communications among multiple agencies, disciplines, and levels. Public information management and distribution during attacks and disasters, along with pre-event citizen and community education, are other communication facets of the NRF and NIMS partnership.

> **Tip**
>
> The NRF aligns with NIMS; both systems are designed to enhance clear communications among multiple agencies, disciplines, and levels.

Structure of the NRF

The NRF is divided into five major chapters:

1. Roles and responsibilities
2. Response actions
3. Response organization
4. Planning (a critical element of effective response)
5. Additional resources

The NRF organization centers on a core document containing the ESF Annexes, which groups federal resources and capabilities into functional areas that are most frequently needed in a national response (e.g., transportation, firefighting, and mass care).

History of the NRF

Federal planning efforts began with the 1992 Federal Response Plan (FRP). The nascent FRP was severely tested when Hurricane Andrew devastated the Miami/Homestead area. Many federal agencies were unfamiliar with the FRP, resulting in ineffective federal coordination in the Hurricane Andrew response effort. The FRP's foremost deficiency was the intense focus on federal roles instead of local, state, and federal coordination.

In 2004, the NRP replaced the FRP. The NRP addressed all levels of government (not just federal) with an all-encompassing response plan. After Hurricane Katrina, the NRP was modified to include the lessons learned from the 2005 hurricane season. The NRP also addressed the presidential directives—such as HSPD-5, Management of Domestic Incidents, and HSPD-8, National Preparedness—that emerged from shortfalls identified during the 2001 World Trade Center and Pentagon attacks. However, many local and state entities voiced a concern that the NRP was still based on a national-level mindset that failed to incorporate local and regional response issues.

The evolution of the NRF closely parallels the progression of the Incident Command System (ICS) evolving into NIMS. As a result, there is now a close relationship between the NRF and NIMS. The principles of command, logistics, operations, planning, and finance/administration in NIMS provide a UC and operational structure for agencies of all sizes and disciplines to function effectively within the overall NRF. In essence, the NRF and the NIMS are closely aligned and complement each other.

The NRF attempts to address many of the concerns and shortcomings that prevailed in the FRP and NRP. The NRF is not a *plan*; it is a *framework*. This means the NRF document is a template for shared levels and responsibilities among governments, the private sector, and individual citizens. The foundation of this structure begins at the local level and progresses through regional, state, and federal levels as dictated by the needs of the incident.

> **Tip**
>
> The NRF centers on the broad strategy and goal of response and recovery from attacks or disasters.

NRF Strategy

The NRF is a key component in the homeland security strategy of the United States. This strategy incorporates threat analysis, lessons learned from attacks and disasters, and findings from exercises. The broad strategy of homeland security is focused on four goals:

- Prevent and disrupt terrorist attacks.
- Protect the American people and our critical infrastructure and key resources.

- Respond to and recover from incidents that do occur.
- Continue to strengthen the foundation to ensure our long-term success.

The NRF, in alignment with NIMS, centers on the third broad strategy goal of response and recovery from attacks or disaster incidents. The NRF is based on a timely and effective federal response to local attacks or disasters. The response must be fast, effective, and coordinated with local efforts.

The NRF key strategy is described in NIMS as follows:

> A basic premise of both NIMS and the NRF is that incidents typically be managed at the local level first. In the vast majority of incidents, local resources and local mutual aid agreements and assistance agreements provide the first line of emergency management and incident response. If additional or specialized resources or capabilities are needed, Governors may request Federal assistance; however, NIMS is based on the concept that local jurisdictions retain command, control, and authority over response activities for their jurisdictional areas. Adhering to NIMS allows local agencies to better utilize incoming resources.

The community recovery process must ensure a planned and sustainable rebuilding of affected communities and infrastructures. Other strategies are supported by the NRF, including the National Strategy for Combating Terrorism, the National Strategy to Combat Terrorist Travel, the National Strategy for Maritime Security, and the National Strategy for Aviation Security.

Preparedness Cycle

The NRF addresses the three phases of emergency response: preparedness, response, and recovery. The preparedness cycle is planning, organizing, training, equipping, exercising, and evaluating for improvement. This cycle readily integrates with traditional emergency response training and exercising objectives.

Planning

Planning is the all-encompassing process of managing the entire cycle of emergency response beginning with intelligence and threat analysis, policy and procedure development, mutual aid, and strategies.

These plans are written and formal. During response and recovery operations, comprehensive plans evolve into dynamic Incident Action Plans (IAPs) that are developed as needs dictate to guide operational periods.

It is important that entities at all levels develop, maintain, evaluate, and update comprehensive emergency response plans that address all hazards. These plans should include NGOs and relevant private-sector organizations.

Organization, Training, and Equipment

NIMS provides a common organization structure of all agencies and entities in the emergency response continuum. NIMS is the template for a common management system with common terminology for use by all agencies and disciplines. For example, a federal law enforcement agency can effectively coordinate with a local bomb squad, a wildland fire logistics section, and a state aviation unit at a single incident.

NIMS also provides an efficient resource management system. Resources are categorized by kind and type and are deployed, tracked, assigned, supported, and demobilized based on NIMS logistics organization and principles. The ESFs within the NRF align with the NIMS resource management structure to ensure effective support from federal agencies. Many states also use a hybrid of the NRF support functions as a template in their statewide emergency management plan.

Exercising and Training

Training for teams and organizations must be systematic and ongoing to ensure professionalism, qualifications, certification, and compliance with national standards. The primary purpose of exercises is to test plans and evaluate training. It is essential that exercises be realistically evaluated to identify strengths and weaknesses in planning and training. These findings should lead to revisions in emergency planning and training programs. If lessons learned from exercises are not applied, the time and expense of exercise programs become a wasted effort.

Exercises should be interdisciplinary and interjurisdictional to ensure that plans are tested in regional and interagency venues. The US Department of Homeland Security (DHS) has a National Exercise Program with a 5-year national exercise plan that encompasses participation with local and state agencies.

Evaluation and Improvement

Response is based on key actions that deploy personnel and resources to save lives and property and to protect the environment. The key response actions are as follows:

- Gain and maintain situational awareness.
- Activate and deploy key resources.
- Coordinate response actions.
- Demobilize when appropriate.

> **Tip**
>
> The NRF preparedness cycle consists of planning, organizing, training, equipping, exercising, and evaluating for improvement.

Response Cycle

Emergency response agencies must recognize that response actions occur within an interagency scope of operations. This is especially important when considering situational awareness. Situational awareness is an all-inclusive emergency response focus and must include emergency management, fire/rescue, law enforcement, emergency medical, public health, and public works considerations. Interagency situational awareness integrates with a common operational picture (COP) of the incident, which is information shared by all response agencies.

Resource activation and deployment is routinely done at the local level on a minute-by-minute basis every day. Resource management gets complicated in major incidents because resources are deployed for an extended time period over long distances from regional and/or state facilities. Federal resources may be deployed from distances exceeding 1000 miles for periods of weeks or months.

Response actions must be coordinated through a formal process. Assistance may come from communities within a region, from the state, from another state, or from the federal government. The process begins with a local disaster declaration to the state government. States can initiate a disaster declaration that triggers federal assistance. At the federal level, a presidential disaster declaration allows the federal government to support states under the provisions of the Robert T. Stafford Disaster Relief and Emergency Assistance Act. It is notable that federal agencies can provide immediate assistance to local and state governments without a presidential disaster declaration when there is an immediate threat to life.

Demobilization is the safe and orderly return of resources to their original status and location. Resources must be tracked and documented to ensure effective financial reimbursement.

Recovery Cycle

Recovery is a shift in operational tempo from immediate lifesaving and property conservation to assistance for individuals, households, critical infrastructures, and businesses. A short-term recovery is a period that immediately follows response activities. A long-term recovery may take several years and is not within the NRF template.

NRF Roles and Responsibilities

The NRF prescribes key roles and responsibilities for all partners at the local, tribal, state, and federal levels. It is significant that the framework also delineates roles for NGOs and private-sector entities.

Local Roles

At the local level, elected or appointed officials and administrative department heads are responsible for the welfare and safety of the community. These officials are not involved in tactical decisions, but instead are responsible for laws, policies, and budgets that are the foundation of preparedness efforts. These officials must work with their respective community and local businesses to ensure effective decisions are made. During emergency operations, the responsibilities of elected/appointed officials are as follows:

- Clearly state organization/jurisdiction policy.
- Evaluate effectiveness and correct deficiencies.
- Support a multiagency approach.

The emergency manager is a key appointed official responsible for implementing the planning and preparedness policies of senior officials. The emergency manager is responsible for developing and maintaining the local comprehensive emergency plan, maintaining a close relationship with response agencies, and conducting training and exercises that complement and support the community's emergency plan. Developing effective mutual-aid and assistance agreements and conducting public education and awareness programs are additional duties. During emergency operations, the emergency manager serves

as the commander of the local Emergency Operations Center (EOC). Local agency directors are responsible for maintaining their agency capabilities at a high level of readiness and training to ensure an effective response and interagency coordination within the emergency management structure.

Individuals and households have a shared responsibility for emergency preparedness that must complement emergency response efforts. Households should partner with public officials to accomplish the following:

- Remove hazards within homes and surrounding property.
- Maintain a home emergency kit and critical supplies.
- Monitor communications related to public emergencies.
- Serve in volunteer support entities.
- Participate in citizen emergency response training.

> **Tip**
>
> Local roles are a key facet of the NRF and include citizen and local government responsibilities.

State, Tribal, and Territorial Responsibilities

State, tribal, and territorial entities are responsible for supporting local response and recovery activities. The key state official is the governor, who is responsible for the general welfare and safety of the local governments and citizens within a state. The governor commands the National Guard and assigns missions for disaster operations. Governors have a coordination role with other states and the federal government for allocating resources and are responsible for filing a federal disaster declaration to obtain financial assistance. The director of the state emergency management agency works directly with the governor to ensure coordination among state agencies and effective allocation of response resources to local governments needing assistance.

> **Tip**
>
> State roles in the NRF are managed by the governor, who commands the National Guard and has a coordinating role with federal agencies.

Federal Roles

The president of the United States leads the federal response effort. The secretary of DHS, appointed by the president, is responsible for federal response efforts and is the principal federal official for domestic incident management. The NRF provides specific and clear definitions for federal roles and entities as follows:

- *Unified Coordination Group and Staff.* This entity provides coordination in accordance with the NIMS concept of UC.
- *Incident Management Assist Teams (IMAT).* These special interagency response teams are regionally based to provide a rapid federal response. In addition, the Federal Emergency Management Agency (FEMA) provides initial response teams, including the Hurricane Liaison Team (HLT), Urban Search and Rescue (US&R) Task Forces, and Mobile Emergency Response Support (MERS).
- *Principal Federal Official (PFO).* The PFO is a representative of the secretary of DHS and is responsible for the coordination of domestic incidents requiring a federal response.
- *Federal Coordinating Officer (FCO).* As the focal point of coordination in the Unified Coordination Group, this officer ensures integration of federal emergency management activities for Stafford Act incidents.
- *Senior Federal Law Enforcement Official (SFLEO).* This official is appointed by the attorney general to coordinate law enforcement operations related to the incident.
- *Joint Task Force (JTF) Commander.* The JTF is designated by the US Department of Defense to command federal military activities in support of an incident.
- *Joint Field Office (JFO).* The JFO is a temporary federal facility that provides a central location for the coordination of response and recovery activities of federal, state, tribal, and local governments. The JFO is structured and operated using NIMS and ICS as a management template. The JFO does not manage on-scene activities.

National Response Doctrine

The **National Response Doctrine** includes five key principles that support national response operations:

1. *Engaged partnerships.* Local, state, tribal, and federal governments should plan and respond together. This form of incident coordination includes ongoing communication and shared situational awareness. Engaged partnerships begin during the preparedness phase and progress through initial recovery efforts.
2. *Tiered response.* Incidents are managed at the lowest possible level. All incidents begin locally and expand through higher levels of government as needed; only a small number of incidents progress to the federal level.
3. *Scalable, flexible, and adaptable operational capabilities.* The system has the following characteristics:
   - It is scaled up or down to meet the needs of the response effort.
   - It is a flexible, fluid system that changes with each specific incident.
   - It adapts to all hazards or types of incidents.
4. *Unity of effort through UC.* UC is a structure in which diverse agencies and disciplines share responsibilities. All major incidents, and many moderate-level incidents, require diverse agencies from overlapping jurisdictions. Coordination must be accomplished via a unified structure to ensure an effective effort. UC is especially important when military and civilian agencies share operational responsibilities.
5. *Readiness to act.* As previously described, this feature ensures a rapid and timely response.

Tip

The National Response Doctrine includes the five principles of engaged partnership; tiered response; scalable, flexible, and adaptable operations capabilities; unity through UC; and readiness to act.

National Response Structure

The NRF is a template for federal entities that supports local response actions. The **National Operations Center (NOC)** is the primary national hub for situational awareness and operations coordination across the federal government for incident management. It provides the secretary of DHS and other principals with information necessary to make critical national-level incident management decisions.

The NOC is a multiagency operations center that operates on a continuous 24-hour basis. Information related to hazards and threats from throughout the United States and foreign countries is monitored and analyzed by the NOC staff and appropriate agency and private-sector representatives. The NOC includes the following:

- *National Response Coordination Center (NRCC).* The NRCC is FEMA's primary operations management center as well as the focal point for national resource coordination. As a 24/7 operations center, the NRCC monitors potential or developing incidents and supports the efforts of regional and field components.
- *National Infrastructure Coordinating Center (NICC).* The NICC monitors the nation's critical infrastructure and key resources on an ongoing basis. During an incident, the NICC provides a coordinating forum to share information across infrastructure and key resources sectors through appropriate information-sharing entities, such as the Information Sharing and Analysis Centers and the Sector Coordinating Councils.
- *Supporting federal operations centers.* These centers maintain situational awareness within their areas of responsibility and provide relevant and timely information to the NOC. Examples of these centers include the following:
  - *National Military Command Center (NMCC).* The NMCC is the nation's focal point for continuous monitoring and coordination of worldwide military operations.
  - *National Counterterrorism Center (NCTC).* The NCTC serves as the primary federal organization for integrating and analyzing all intelligence pertaining to terrorism and counterterrorism and for conducting strategic operational planning by integrating all instruments of national power.
  - *Strategic Information and Operations Center (SIOC).* The Federal Bureau of Investigation (FBI) SIOC is the focal point and operational control center for all federal intelligence, law enforcement, and investigative law enforcement activities related to domestic terrorist incidents or credible threats, including leading attribution investigations.

- *Other DHS operations centers.* Depending on the type of incident (e.g., National Special Security Events), the operations centers of other DHS operating components may serve as the primary operations management center in support of the secretary of DHS. These operations centers are the US Coast Guard, Transportation Security Administration, US Secret Service, and US Customs and Border Protection operations centers.

Emergency Support Functions

The NRF divides federal support responsibilities into **Emergency Support Functions (ESF)**. Each ESF has a lead federal agency, support agencies, and a defined set of actions and responsibilities. Many state and local governments have adopted ESFs as part of their emergency operations plan (not an NRF requirement). The federal ESFs that are specified in the NRF are as follows, in the indicated order:

- *ESF #1—Transportation:* Department of Transportation
- *ESF #2—Communications:* Department of Homeland Security (National Communications System)
- *ESF #3—Public Works and Engineering:* Department of Defense (US Army Corps of Engineers)
- *ESF #4—Firefighting:* Department of Agriculture (US Forest Service)
- *ESF #5—Emergency Management:* Department of Homeland Security (FEMA)
- *ESF #6—Mass Care, Emergency Assistance, Housing, and Human Services:* Department of Homeland Security (FEMA)
- *ESF #7—Logistics Management and Resource Support:* General Services Administration and Department of Homeland Security (FEMA)
- *ESF #8—Public Health and Medical Services:* Department of Health and Human Services
- *ESF #9—Search and Rescue:* Department of Homeland Security (FEMA)
- *ESF #10—Oil and Hazardous Materials Response:* Environmental Protection Agency
- *ESF #11—Agriculture and Natural Resources:* Department of Agriculture
- *ESF #12—Energy:* Department of Energy
- *ESF #13—Public Safety and Security:* Department of Justice

- *ESF #14—Long-Term Community Recovery:* Department of Homeland Security (FEMA)
- *ESF #15—External Affairs:* Department of Homeland Security

Under this system, local, county, and state emergency management functions are guided by ESF #5—Emergency Management. This function coordinates incident management and response operations, resource management, incident action planning, and financial management. ESF #5 manages EOCs at local, county, and state levels in coordination with federal entities.

Firefighting and rescue functions are guided by ESF #4—Firefighting. These functions include rural, urban, and wildland firefighting, as well as search and rescue operations assisted and supported by federal entities. Operations are managed by Incident or Area Commanders who are supported by local, county, and state operations centers.

Local, regional, and state law enforcement functions are guided by ESF #13—Public Safety and Security. The major law enforcement functions in ESF #13 include facility and resource security, resource planning and technical resource assistance, public safety and security support, support for incident access, and traffic and crowd control. At the local level, ESF #13 is usually under the command of the county sheriff or municipal police chief. At the state level, ESF #13 is usually commanded by the state attorney general. The command and management responsibilities for ESF #13 are dictated by local and state statutes, not the federal NRF.

Health and medical services are guided by ESF #8—Public Health and Medical Services. The primary agency responsible for ESF #8 is the Department of Health and Human Services. Key functions include an incredible collection of tasks ranging from potable water, sanitation, food safety, veterinary services, vector control, emergency medical treatment and transport, medical support for operations personnel, public health, mental health, and mass fatality management. EMS agencies are the key emergency responders at the local and regional levels. Many parties in the medical community and EMS response operations have advocated for an independent ESF that addresses EMS and critical care responsibilities because of the unique and complex response requirements that these individuals face and the time-sensitive functions they perform. To date, the federal government has not acted upon this need.

Public works and engineering functions are guided by ESF #3—Public Works and Engineering. These functions include debris clearing, infrastructure restoration, emergency repairs, and engineering services. Local agencies, private contractors, military units, and state road departments are the key public works organizations.

Scenario Sets and Planning Scenarios

The NRF includes sets of key incident scenarios that are linked with National Planning Scenarios **(Table 15-1)**.

Table 15-1 Key National Planning Scenarios

Key Scenario Set	Scenario Number	Scenario Name
Explosives attack	Scenario 12	Explosives attack—improvised devices
Nuclear attack	Scenario 1	Nuclear detonation—improvised device
Radiological attack	Scenario 11	Radiological attack—dispersal device
Biological attack	Scenario 2	Biological attack—aerosol anthrax
	Scenario 4	Biological attack—plague
	Scenario 13	Biological attack—food contamination
	Scenario 14	Biological attack—foreign animal disease
Chemical attack	Scenario 5	Chemical attack—blister agent
	Scenario 6	Chemical attack—toxic industrial chemicals
	Scenario 7	Chemical attack—nerve agent
	Scenario 8	Chemical attack—chlorine tank explosion
Natural disaster	Scenario 9	Natural disaster—major earthquake
	Scenario 10	Natural disaster—major hurricane
Cyber attack	Scenario 15	Cyber attack
Pandemic influenza	Scenario 3	Biological disease outbreak—influenza

Rural Case Study *Answers*

1. The NRF preparedness cycle was apparently neglected in Smith County and the surrounding cities of Littletown and Stadtown as indicated by the confusion about who was in charge, the lack of UC and unified strategy, and poor resource coordination among local and state agencies. The NRF preparedness cycle includes planning, organizing, training, equipping, exercising, and evaluating for improvement.

2. ESFs are federal (and sometimes local and state) support activities that have a lead agency, support agencies, and a defined set of actions and responsibilities. ESFs for this incident may include the following:
   - ESF #2—Communications
   - ESF #3—Public Works and Engineering
   - ESF #4—Firefighting
   - ESF #5—Emergency Management
   - ESF #6—Mass Care, Emergency Assistance, Housing, and Human Services
   - ESF #8—Public Health and Medical Services
   - ESF #9—Search and Rescue
   - ESF #13—Public Safety and Security
   - ESF #14—Long-Term Community Recovery

Urban Case Study *Answers*

1. The NRF is always in effect as part of the readiness to act strategy and does not require a triggering action by responders. Further, the readiness to act strategy begins at the local level and extends to state, tribal, territorial, and federal agencies. This concept is also described in the NRF as a forward-leaning posture because many incidents have the capability to rapidly expand in size, severity, or complexity.

2. Federal entities that may be involved in this incident per the NRF are as follows:
   - *Unified Coordination Group and Staff.* This entity provides coordination in accordance with the NIMS concept of UC.
   - *Principal Federal Official (PFO).* The PFO is a representative of the secretary of DHS and is responsible for the coordination of domestic incidents requiring a federal response.
   - *Senior Federal Law Enforcement Official (SFLEO).* This official is appointed by the attorney general to coordinate law enforcement operations related to the incident.

3. The NRF is a key component in the homeland security strategy of the United States. The broad strategic goals that align with this incident are as follows: to protect the American people and our critical infrastructures and key resources, and to respond to and recover from incidents that do occur.

Wrap-Up

Summary

- The NRF replaces the NRP and is a response template for the coordinated effort of federal, state, tribal, and local governments, along with NGOs and the private sector.
- The NRF complements the principles in NIMS, such as UC and ICS.
- The emergency response phases of preparedness, response, and recovery are addressed in the NRF document.
- The key doctrine in the NRF includes the following components:
  - Engaged partnerships
  - Tiered response
  - Scalable/flexible operational capabilities
  - Unity of effort through UC
  - Readiness to act
- The NRF framework defines 15 ESFs and specifies a lead federal agency for each support function.
- The NRF includes key scenario sets and 15 national planning scenarios.
- The roles and responsibilities outlined in the framework begin at the individual and household levels and progress through local, tribal, state, and federal levels.
- Roles for NGOs and the private sector are also defined in the NRF.

Glossary

Adaptability: A characteristic of the National Response Framework (NRF) that allows a responsive strategic framework to support local responders' requirements in any type of hazard or attack.

Emergency Support Functions (ESF): Fifteen support functions with a lead federal agency, support agencies, and a defined set of actions and responsibilities.

Flexible coordinating structures: Incident management templates in the National Response Framework (NRF) that provide a common language and organization for agencies and disciplines to integrate effectively.

National Operations Center (NOC): Primary national hub for situational awareness and operations coordination across the federal government during incident management operations.

National Response Doctrine: The five principles of engaged partnership, tiered response, scalability, unity through UC, and readiness to act.

National Response Framework (NRF): A coherent strategic framework (not a series of functional plans) for senior emergency response chiefs, emergency management practitioners, and senior executives in the private sector and NGOs; supersedes the NRP.

Response: Immediate actions to save lives, protect property and the environment, and meet basic human needs.

Scalability: A characteristic of the National Response Framework (NRF) that allows it to contract or expand according to the scope or size of the incident

Wrap-Up Case Study

The 2010 Deepwater Horizon oil spill was the largest hazardous materials incident in history. This long-duration disaster occurred over a period of several months and began as a unique government and private-sector offshore response. As this spill progressed to inland areas, state and local governments in Louisiana, Mississippi, Alabama, and Florida were involved in the response effort. This incident challenged many of the elements in the NRF.

1. What elements in the NRF preparedness cycle were deficient?

   A. Planning for an oil spill of this magnitude and duration was inadequate.

   B. Equipment and training was not sufficient.

   C. An incident of this magnitude was never tested by exercises.

   D. All of the above.

2. List three or more ESFs that played a major role in this incident.

CHAPTER 16

Implementation of NIMS

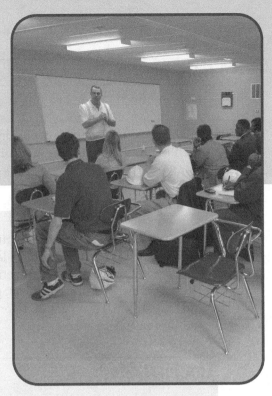

Rural Case Study

Smith County's rural response agencies and resources were quickly overwhelmed by the tornado disaster. One month after the incident, the emergency manager, fire chiefs, and police chiefs in Smith County conducted an after-action review with all the county and regional response agencies to review the response activities and implement corrective measures to ensure improvement. Major issues discussed in the meeting included a lack of Incident Command System (ICS) proficiency and understanding of Unified Command (UC), lack of a resource inventory, ineffective resource allocation, low resource-tracking proficiency, failure to establish an effective public information system, and lack of secondary and tertiary communications capabilities. The county attorney noted that the National Incident Management System (NIMS) was not officially adopted by Stadtown or Smith County. Furthermore, the county administrator and the city manager were only vaguely aware of NIMS.

1. What NIMS innovations should be implemented to address key issues identified in the incident after-action review?
2. What actions should be taken by emergency response leaders to formalize NIMS at the senior executive level?

Urban Case Study

Pleasantville encountered an incident that first appeared as a transportation accident. The incident escalated to a chemical attack that challenged the ICS structure and required intense resource management and public information efforts. There was initial communications confusion because many mutual-aid agencies used noncompatible radio codes instead of plain language. There were major public health issues that were not effectively addressed because the local public health agency did not receive NIMS training and was not included in the comprehensive emergency management plan. Mass sheltering presented a serious food and facilities challenge along with evacuation problems for nursing homes and special-needs evacuees. Local and state agencies did not understand the role of federal agencies that responded to support the incident. In addition, the tornado disaster was the first time in local history that an incident required an Area Command to manage several Incident Commands. The after-action report concluded that the Area Command and Incident Command coordination with the Emergency Operations Center (EOC) was confusing and ineffective.

1. What NIMS tools are available to address the key deficiencies in this incident?
2. What tools are in the National Response Framework (NRF) to assist Pleasantville and Metro in NIMS implementation?

Introduction

Implementing NIMS and getting it right is critically important. At a minimum, agencies and communities risk losing federal preparedness funding if guidelines are not met. A noncompliant community is unprepared to effectively plan for and respond to a disaster or terrorist attack.

At first glance, the NIMS document may seem overwhelming because NIMS is comprehensive, complex, and has far-reaching implications impacting every agency and organizational level in America's emergency response network. Practitioners familiar with ICS have a definite advantage because the command and management component of NIMS is based on the ICS template.

The First Steps

To begin implementing NIMS, lead agencies have to step up to the plate and assume leadership roles. Fire service and emergency management agencies are excellent choices for leading the NIMS implementation effort because they are familiar with ICS and multiagency operations. In some locales, law enforcement and emergency medical services (EMS) may also have ICS proficiency.

> **Tip**
>
> Key agencies must assume leadership roles to ensure an effective NIMS implementation process.

A crucial early goal is to get buy-in from senior executives and elected officials regarding NIMS adoption. Every attempt should be made to convince local and state government leaders that NIMS is an effective tool for the preparation and management of a comprehensive all-hazards response program. The objective is to instill an attitude of proactive acceptance rather than passive compliance. A convincing argument is that NIMS compliance is a condition for receiving federal emergency preparedness funds.

It is important that chief executives and elected officials attend (hopefully with enthusiasm) a NIMS introductory course that includes familiarization with ICS. Chief executive participation in NIMS training sets an example for department heads in nonresponse agencies that may be less than excited about attending a class or an exercise. In many jurisdictions, department heads in areas such as finance,

human resources, and planning do not associate themselves with emergency response issues. The commitment of their leaders to ICS demonstrates the importance of all agencies operating in the ICS mold.

Local legislative adoption of NIMS is an important benchmark. Local legislation ensures that NIMS becomes the legal standard and process for planning and emergency operations within the jurisdiction. NIMS adoption is similar to the process used to adopt and approve emergency management plans or local government policies in the nonemergency arena. The legislative adoption of NIMS is an affidavit to the state and federal government that the NIMS process is local policy. In essence, NIMS gets "teeth" by becoming local law.

> **Tip**
>
> NIMS should be a formalized policy via a local legislative process.

Next, develop a NIMS implementation plan similar to an Incident Action Plan (IAP) format. This format familiarizes agency heads with ICS at an early stage. Basically, the plan is based on milestones and measurable end states.

The following is a hypothetical example of NIMS implementation milestones:

- Milestone I: February 1—Certification of department heads in basic ICS
- Milestone II: March 15—Completion of initial city implementation plans
- Milestone III: April 1—First meeting of the NIMS preparedness committee
- Milestone IV: June 1—Complete NIMS budget requests for budget workshop

Implementing NIMS is an ongoing effort. It is an evaluation and innovation process requiring continuous adjustment to real-world realities.

NIMS Training

Training is paramount when implementing a new and all-encompassing system such as NIMS. Training officers with previous ICS experience are valuable assets in the training effort. The **National Integration Center (NIC)**, formerly known as the NIMS Integration Center, is established at the national level to develop training courses, standards, publications, and training aids.

The initial NIMS training curriculum was based on earlier ICS training developed by the wildland fire service and California's Standard Emergency Management System (SEMS). The training curriculum begins with basic familiarization courses and progresses to advanced courses for field command officers. Many of the ICS training courses are available online from the Federal Emergency Management Agency (FEMA) training Web site (www.training.fema.gov). The online courses are listed in **Table 16–1**. Additional NIMS-related courses that complement ICS training are listed in **Table 16–2**. Advanced ICS courses (such as ICS-300, Intermediate ICS for Expanding Incidents; and ICS-400, Advanced ICS Command and General Staff—Complex Incidents) require active participation in a classroom setting. These courses are administered by each State Emergency Management Agency and are often taught at State Fire Academies.

Table 16-1 Online ICS Training Courses	
Course number	Course title
IS 100.a	Introduction to Incident Command System
IS 100.HC	Introduction of the Incident Command System for Healthcare/Hospitals
IS 100.LEa	Introduction to the Incident Command System for Law Enforcement
IS 100.PWa	Introduction to the Incident Command System for Public Works Personnel
IS 100.SCa	Introduction to the Incident Command System for Schools
IS 200.a	ICS for Single Resources and Initial Action Incidents
IS 200.HC	Applying ICS to Healthcare Organizations

Table 16-2 Courses That Complement ICS Training	
Course number	Course title
IS 700.A	National Incident Management System (NIMS), an Introduction
IS 701	NIMS Multiagency Coordination Systems
IS 702	NIMS Public Information Systems
IS 703	NIMS Resource Management
IS 704	NIMS Communication and Information Management
IS 705	NIMS Preparedness
IS 706	NIMS Intrastate Mutual Aid, an Introduction
IS 800.B	National Response Framework, an Introduction

Members of local organizations should complete a basic ICS introduction. Participating entities should include nonemergency agencies, such as the parks, finance, legal, human resources, and utility departments. Employees in these departments should have a basic overview of ICS and understand their agency's role in the ICS structure. The objective of this introductory class is to present the basic ICS organization and terminology. Students are essentially learning a new language.

Supervisors and managers in nonemergency agencies who have possible EOC assignments need secondary-level training. This training requirement especially applies to new agencies that progressive communities are bringing into ICS. Examples of new players are public works, public health, utilities, and transit authorities.

UC is a specific ICS concept that requires advanced training. Many agency heads, especially fire chiefs and police chiefs, are not inclined to share command with other agencies, such as EMS or public health. UC proficiency requires advanced training and exercises to ensure success in real-world incidents and overcome the reluctance of some response agencies to utilize UC.

Simulations, case studies, and audiovisual aids, such as video, graphics, and incident communications tapes, are effective tools for ICS training. It is important that incidents are utilized that are appropriate for the audience. For example, showing World Trade Center slides and video to an audience in rural Iowa is not effective. Local case studies, such as wildfires for San Diego and hurricanes for Miami, are more relevant. Simulations are effective training interventions because they are readily accepted by trainees and create learned experiences (experiential learning). There are private-sector and government Web sites with emergency incident simulations available for free or a low monthly membership fee. Universities and professional associations have similar Web sites.

Tip
The core of NIMS implementation is a training plan that includes milestones for senior leaders, midlevel managers, responders, and support personnel.

Virtual training expert Roger Schank offers excellent advice that applies to action-oriented NIMS training: "Whatever you do, have people do something." Passive lecture-based training is not as effective as hands-on activities and simulations. As Dr. Frannie Winslow, former director of Emergency Management in San Jose, says, "Teach the gut and heart, not the brain."

Senior emergency response managers, especially those with planning responsibilities, require training on the following aspects of NIMS separate from ICS, including the following:

- Preparedness
- Resource management
- Communications and information management
- Ongoing management and maintenance
- Support technologies

NIMS Five-Year Training Plan

The NIC Incident Management Systems Integration Division developed a NIMS **Five-Year Training Plan** based on several broad objectives:

1. Support NIMS education and training for all stakeholders.
2. Adapt NIMS functions into guidelines and courses for personnel training and credentialing plans.
3. Define minimum personnel qualifications for service in complex multijurisdictional incidents.

The Five-Year Training Plan also sets operational foundations for NIMS training and Personal Qualification Guidelines. These guidelines include core competencies for typical positions, a NIMS core curriculum, training guidance for courses within the core curriculum, and qualification guidelines. Personnel qualifications for specific ICS positions are a final step in the advancement of NIMS training. After completing introductory courses in ICS and NIMS, individuals may progress via a stair-step model beginning with basic positions and ascend to Incident Commander. Practitioners at each ICS level must have on-scene incident experience, documented via task books, before progressing to the next ICS level. The steps in this progression are as follows:

1. Single Resource Leader
2. Unit Leader
3. Branch Director
4. Section Chief
5. Incident Commander

There are established core competencies for positions in the command and management component

Table 16-3 Training Courses for ICS Positions	
Course number	Course title
P400	All-Hazards Incident Commander
P402	All-Hazards Liaison Officer
P403	All-Hazards Public Information Officer
P404	All-Hazards Safety Officer
P430	All-Hazards Operations Section Chief
P440	All-Hazards Planning Section Chief
P450	All-Hazards Logistics Section Chief
P460	All-Hazards Finance Section Chief
P480	All-Hazards Intelligence/Investigations Function

of NIMS. Training courses for specific ICS positions are listed in **Table 16–3**.

The major goals in the NIMS training plan is to have personnel appropriately trained in the following areas:

- NIMS Preparedness
- NIMS Communications and Information Management
- NIMS Resource Management
- NIMS Incident Command System
- NIMS Multiagency Coordination System
- NIMS Public Information

Preparedness Organizations

NIMS defines **preparedness organizations** as "ongoing forums for coordinating preparedness activities in advance of an incident." Preparedness organizations are excellent vehicles for the NIMS implementation process. These organizations may be disaster committees, planning groups or committees, or professional associations. Preparedness organizations are responsible for essential components of NIMS implementation, such as planning, equipping, and training. Preparedness organizations help implement NIMS by developing the following:

- Plans and protocols
- Interoperability procedures
- Common operational picture (COP) capabilities
- Resource support protocols
- Mutual-aid agreements
- Operational security measures
- Force protection procedures

Preparedness organizations should be local and interjurisdictional. All possible disciplines (not just fire and law enforcement) need to be represented. Nonemergency agencies, such as public works and public health, should be included. Additional disciplines should include nongovernmental organizations (NGOs), volunteer organizations, private-sector entities, and professional associations. Preparedness organizations must formally meet on an ongoing basis. Multiple preparedness organizations within a county or region should coordinate their activities. These organizations localize the NIMS implementation process by ensuring that local concerns and issues are addressed. For example, a small town without a SWAT team can collaborate with a regional jurisdiction to incorporate a special team response into a regional plan.

> **Tip**
>
> Preparedness organizations are an effective means to ensure NIMS preparedness among jurisdictions, agencies, private-sector entities, and support organizations.

NIMS in Daily Activities

NIMS is not just for disasters or terrorism events. In fact, NIMS is successfully implemented when it is used daily on every type of incident. Start by using NIMS terminology in everyday language. People learn proper terminology when it is part of their daily conversation. Daily exposure to NIMS terms and the ICS organization results in NIMS procedures permeating the organization. People cannot retain a new vocabulary by hearing a term in a classroom and not hearing it again until the chaos of emergency operations 6 months later. Daily NIMS language means NIMS is part of the organizational culture and becomes second nature.

NIMS is also an effective model for planning major events. Every event requires someone to be in charge (Incident Commander) and have functional requirements that require operations, logistics, planning, intelligence, and finance/administration. For example, a jurisdiction can plan and support a major conference using the ICS component of the NIMS model. ICS ensures that the conference is effectively managed and supported. An added benefit is that participants have an opportunity to use ICS as a learning experience.

The glossary in NIMS should be used as an agency dictionary. Examples of NIMS language include the following:

- Inventory control, call it *resource tracking*
- First alarm assignment, call it a *Task Force*
- Daily plan, call it an *incident action plan* (IAP)
- Leaving the scene, call it *demobilization*

NIMS functions are easily incorporated into meeting agendas. Divide the agenda for a staff meeting or preparedness committee meeting into the five ICS functions of Command, Finance/Administration, Logistics, Planning, and Operations. Any item of business, regardless of the subject, fits into one of the ICS categories. A budget issue is a Finance/Administration topic. A mass-casualty protocol discussion is an Operations topic. Communications issues are listed under Logistics. The same concept applies to memos and documents. For example, on the subject line of an agency memo, state the ICS function in bold type next to the subject. This means that a memo about a new sick leave form is a Finance/Administration subject.

ICS forms are excellent teaching tools. Use ICS forms for as many routine activities as possible. For example, the Unit Log Form (ICS-214) is useful as a sign-in sheet for any meeting; the Incident Briefing Form (ICS-201) can be helpful for meeting agendas; the ICS General Message Form (ICS-213) is good for memos; and the Medical Plan Form (ICS-206) may be used for planning EMS support at the next festival (Appendix D). This system exposes all the players to the NIMS program daily.

Completed forms should be archived, especially forms from emergency incidents because the forms document adherence to NIMS procedures. Official ICS forms also document that a jurisdiction and organization is NIMS compliant.

> **Tip**
>
> Using ICS forms (Appendix D) in daily activities enhances NIMS familiarization and injects NIMS terminology into an agency's everyday language.

Resource Management

The adoption of NIMS resource management procedures is a benchmark in NIMS evolution. Every government and private-sector agency has personnel, supplies, equipment, tools, and vehicles called resources (Chapter 13). Resource management, whether during a disaster or a routine workday, means resources are:

- Acquired
- Inventoried
- Categorized
- Allocated
- Tracked
- Restocked
- Disposed

The NIMS plan covers all of these phases of resource management and should be used 365 days per year in emergency incidents and nonemergency events. It is also important to incorporate resource management problems into NIMS exercises. As a reminder, a disaster is often defined as a *resource-scarce* incident. This is why exercises should test resource capabilities and be based on the assumption that resources are finite. When attacks or disasters occur, resource management is seamless because it is a part of daily organizational activities and exercises. To assist local resource management efforts, FEMA continues to publish Resource Typing Definitions as part of the National Mutual Aid and Resource Management Initiative. This resource guide is part of an ongoing process. The NIC also continually develops and fine-tunes resource tools, including electronic systems for local, state, and federal agencies.

NIMS Exercises

Fortunately, a major disaster or attack is a rare occurrence in most American communities. A full ICS command post staff or a full EOC activation does not happen often enough for key players to get "wartime" experience. Wildland fire incident management teams (overhead teams) are an exception because they are in "combat" every year. Exercises are an effective means to test and practice interagency and interjurisdictional coordination (interoperability and COP). Local agencies need at least one full-scale field exercise with full-scale EOC activation once a year; every 6 months is even better. Quarterly exercises are best.

The NRF complements NIMS by including exercises and evaluation and improvement as key steps in the NRF preparedness cycle. According to the NRF, "exercises assess and validate proficiency levels. They also clarify and familiarize personnel with roles and responsibilities. Well-designed exercises improve interagency coordination and communications, highlight capability gaps, and identify opportunities

for improvement." Exercises should do the following:

- Include multidisciplinary, multijurisdictional incidents.
- Include participation of private-sector organizations and NGOs.
- Cover aspects of preparedness plans, particularly the processes and procedures for activating local, intrastate, or interstate mutual-aid and assistance agreements.
- Contain a mechanism for incorporating corrective actions.

NIMS is the template for the entire exercise process, from planning to demobilization. Exercises should include as many state and federal agency participants as practical, and they should simulate and test measurable objectives. An example of a measurable objective is reducing overall patient triage time to 10 minutes or having a 50 percent response to an off-duty recall within 30 minutes. Exercise plans should include three or four major objectives at most; there is room for discipline-specific subobjectives. The following are examples of major exercise objectives:

1. Test plain language as a replacement for radio codes.
2. Test a mutual aid resource allocation plan.
3. Test UC between the police chief and EMS director.

NIMS exercises should not be choreographed to ensure success. Planners and exercise evaluators should view failure as a learning tool. Exercise controllers should evaluate outcomes as prescribed in NIMS and the NRF and formally suggest changes in procedures, protocols, and training. The ultimate purpose of a NIMS exercise is to implement appropriate interventions that ensure failures will not occur in real-world incidents. Planners should utilize an ICS Safety Officer and have a proactive safety plan for all exercises.

Budget Considerations for NIMS

System-wide implementation of NIMS requires budgeting and fiscal planning. Financial planning for NIMS implementation is important because local agencies often struggle to fund new innovations such as NIMS. Even with federal grants, doing more with less is a given in public safety. Emergency services executives share concerns about the fiscal downside of NIMS because effective budget planning for NIMS must compete with traditional budget priorities. However, NIMS is financially justifiable because NIMS ensures more effective and safer operations in the long run. NIMS budget considerations include the following:

- Exercise funding (development, equipment, and overtime salaries)
- EOC facility upgrading and expansion
- Training costs (facilities and salaries)
- Hardware and software that enhances interoperability and COP

Federal funding fluctuates with the political winds and is tied directly to NIMS compliance (HSPD-5). Therefore, emphasizing compliance with NIMS in grant requests is important in the federal grant process.

Implementation Concepts and Principles

The process for managing and maintaining NIMS ensures that all users and stakeholders, including various levels of government, functional disciplines, NGOs, and private entities, are given the opportunity to participate in NIC activities. To accomplish this goal, the NIC is multijurisdictional and multidisciplinary, and it maintains appropriate interrelationships with private organizations.

The NIMS management and maintenance process relies heavily on lessons learned from actual incidents, incident management training and exercises, and recognized best practices across jurisdictions and functional disciplines.

Rural Case Study *Answers*

1. Several NIMS deficiencies indicated the NIMS implementation process in Smith County was lacking. As a result, implementation steps were identified to correct NIMS deficiencies. Milestones were formally adopted based on budget realities. Implementation steps to correct NIMS shortcomings are as follows:
   - Develop a regional resource inventory using a NIMS kind/type format.
   - Develop a communications failure protocol and test the protocol in a full-scale exercise.
   - Train a Public Information Officer (PIO) and develop a joint information system.
   - Conduct ICS-300 (Intermediate ICS for expanding incidents) and ICS-400 (Advanced ICS for complex incidents) training for all fire, EMS, and law enforcement managers.
   - Establish a formal Emergency Preparedness Committee and include NGOs and private-sector support entities.
2. First, Smith County and the City of Stadtown drafted and adopted legislation mandating NIMS as the formal structure for all emergency response and disaster activities. This legislation also ensured that the local governments continued to receive emergency management funds from the state. Second, a NIMS awareness workshop was conducted for all local government executives and was followed by a NIMS introduction course.

Urban Case Study *Answers*

1. Several NIMS tools are available to correct deficiencies identified after the explosion incident. First, all regional agencies adopted plain language to replace confusing radio codes. The county public health department was included in emergency plans and became a player in future disaster exercises. A 5-year budget plan was developed to address NIMS training and certification for all levels in response agencies and support entities. Last, the Emergency Preparedness Committee, in coordination with NGOs and the private sector, developed a comprehensive mass-sheltering plan including provisions for evacuation and care of special-needs patients.

2. The NRF preparedness cycle includes the key steps of *exercises, evaluation,* and *performance improvement.* The NRF states that well-designed exercises improve interagency coordination and communications, highlight capability gaps, and identify opportunities for improvement. Pleasantville and Metro developed an aggressive 3-year exercise plan for tabletop and full-scale exercises. The exercises include multiple jurisdictions and disciplines along with participation by federal agencies, NGOs, and private-sector entities. A key aspect of the exercise program is a provision for incorporating lessons learned from the exercises into performance improvement with oversight via the Emergency Preparedness Committee and the County Emergency Manager.

Wrap-Up

Summary

- NIMS must be effectively integrated into the everyday operations of a jurisdiction and its agencies.
- NIMS implementation is a continuous and rewarding process because NIMS implementation provides communities with the tools for preparedness, planning, interoperability, a COP, and effective integration with state and federal agencies.
- The important steps of a successful NIMS implementation program are to:
  - Select lead implementation agencies.
  - Ensure buy-in from elected officials and chief executives.
  - Draft a formal plan with milestones and measurable end states.
  - Provide multilevel NIMS and ICS training.
  - Establish a multiagency preparedness organization.
  - Incorporate NIMS into daily activities.
  - Develop a proactive exercise program.
  - Budget for NIMS maintenance and implementation.
  - Utilize the NIC as an implementation tool.

- Training is paramount when implementing a new and all-encompassing system such as NIMS. The NIC Incident Management Systems Integration Division has developed a NIMS Five-Year Training Plan.
- Preparedness organizations are responsible for essential components of NIMS implementation, such as planning, equipping, and training.

Glossary

Five-Year Training Plan: NIMS training plan that sets operational foundations for NIMS training and Personal Qualification Guidelines.

ICS forms: NIMS forms for documenting incident command activities.

National Integration Center (NIC): NIMS center established at the national level to develop training courses, standards, publications, and training aids.

Preparedness organization: Local or regional entity that develops and maintains NIMS competency by developing plans, protocols, resource management, interoperability procedures, COPs, and mutual-aid operations for event and incident response.

The city of Wilshire has a population of 275,000 people. The city has a paid fire department, a third-service EMS system, and a police department. The surrounding county is rural and offers few resources to support incidents within Wilshire. Recently, a commuter jet aircraft crashed on landing during a local thunderstorm. Fourteen passengers and crew members on the aircraft were killed. In addition, 7 people on the ground were killed, 12 people were injured, and 5 structures were destroyed by fire.

An investigation by local and state officials revealed disturbing findings. The after-action report concluded that interagency coordination between the fire and police departments was not effective, there was no ICS in effect, and resource management was uncoordinated and fragmented. Local emergency response officials defended their preparedness efforts by producing documents that implied the ICS had been implemented, but investigators concluded that Wilshire essentially had a "paper plan" that lacked substance. The city manager hired a consultant to develop a NIMS implementation program for all agencies within the city.

1. What should be the core philosophy of the NIMS training program?
    A. Fire fighters should be trained in ICS; police and EMS agencies do not need ICS.
    B. Only emergency responders should receive ICS training because ICS does not apply to support agencies or local officials.
    C. Emergency responders, support agencies, and local officials should be trained in NIMS because emergency response is a partnership among all entities and levels in local government.
    D. Voluntary NIMS training is recommended because mandatory training and certification is not practical.

2. What is the role of formal legislation in NIMS implementation?
    A. Implementing NIMS is a training issue and has no relationship to local legislation.
    B. Local legislation is important to establish NIMS as a formal system and template for managing emergency incidents.
    C. NIMS legislation is used only at the federal level because NIMS is a federal program.
    D. NIMS is implemented by an informal consensus, making legislation irrelevant.

CHAPTER 17

Putting It All Together: NIMS Evaluation and Maintenance

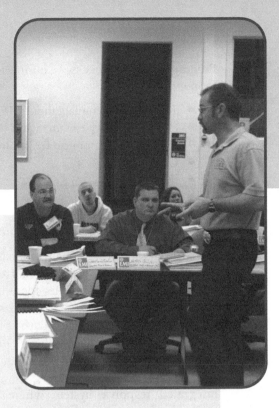

Rural Case Study

Smith County officials considered the tornado disaster a major awakening. However, the data collected after the incident was confusing and presented a formidable challenge. Officials needed a simple and affordable means for evaluating their National Incident Management System (NIMS) capabilities.

1. What is a simple evaluation model (using in-house resources) for agency managers to evaluate their NIMS capabilities and identify challenges?
2. How could a gap analysis in the Human Performance Technology (HPT) model be applied to evaluate NIMS capabilities in Smith County?

Urban Case Study

A review of previous incidents revealed a pattern of close calls and small errors in incident operations and management. These errors created friction points that negatively affected the operational tempo during the terrorism incident. There were also local and regional responders who lacked expertise, training, and credentialing in several NIMS functions. The terrorist attack was the first time in recent Pleasantville history that local agencies had to coordinate with the US Department of Justice and other federal agencies; the role of the federal agencies was confusing.

1. Describe an effective program evaluation process for identifying innovations to correct key deficiencies.
2. How could the National Integration Center (NIC) assist Pleasantville and Metro in NIMS performance improvement?
3. Describe at least one high-reliability organization (HRO) principle to correct deficiencies in the Pleasantville and Metro incident management system.

Introduction

A proactive approach for establishing an organization-wide process of measuring, evaluating, and improv-

ing quality is a critical factor for continued success within a response system. Many organizations have implemented quality management and evaluation programs that provide such a process.

Program and process examples include the following:

- Total quality management (TQM)
- High-reliability organization (HRO)
- Human Performance Technology (HPT)
- Case studies
- Best practices
- Benchmarking
- Best-evidence education
- Performance improvement programs

These programs provide quality management through programmatic evaluation and corrective interventions that remedy deficiencies identified through the evaluation process.

NIMS is following a path of improvement similar to the way the Incident Command System (ICS) changed and improved over the years. The overarching goal of NIMS is to develop a well-integrated response system where all of the elements have a purpose and combine effectively to respond to multihazard incidents with multidisciplinary and multiagency teams. NIMS's ongoing management and maintenance uses best practices and lessons learned as well as information from actual cases to continually refine and enhance NIMS and its response partners. This process requires a proactive and constructive approach for sharing information among NIMS response community partners.

NIMS Program Evaluation Tools

Program evaluation is the process of judging the worth and merit of a program. It is an important process in business and educational organizations and is an applicable concept for determining the effectiveness of NIMS implementation. Several business and academic models can be adapted for ongoing evaluation of NIMS programs for emergency response and support entities. An in-depth discussion of these models is outside the scope of this text; however, a brief overview of SWOT analysis, the HPT model, and HRO is warranted to demonstrate effective NIMS evaluation programs.

Tip
A program evaluation is an organizational management tool that judges the worth and merit of a program such as NIMS.

SWOT Analysis

The SWOT acronym stands for *strengths, weaknesses, opportunities,* and *threats*. A **SWOT analysis** is a management and planning tool for evaluating organizational performance and programs because external and internal forces generate strengths, weaknesses, opportunities, and threats within organizations. The SWOT model begins with a jurisdiction, agency, or organization and candidly evaluates its strengths, weaknesses, opportunities, and threats. An example of an analysis of a hypothetical response agency in a city or county based on the SWOT process is shown in **Table 17–1**.

The SWOT analysis demonstrates that local weaknesses—such as interoperability, common language, and maintenance of a common operational picture (COP)—are addressed by NIMS. NIMS also represents additional opportunities that complement local strengths. Realistically, federal standards and certification requirements mandated to local communities are perceived by some jurisdictions as threats. However, progressive leaders see these changes as opportunities for professionalism.

Table 17-1 Sample SWOT Analysis
Strengths
• ICS experience
• Locals always arrive first
• Knowledge of area
• Culture of dedication and service
Weaknesses
• Inadequate funding
• Interoperability problems
• No common operations picture
• Incompatible equipment
• Low frequency of major incidents
Opportunities
• Multihazard plan
• Public approval
• Standard procedures
• Compatibility
• Efficient and safe operations
Threats
• Federal standards
• Mandated national certification
• Loss of funds for noncompliance
• Unfunded state mandates
• Political changes
• Shifting public opinion
• Economic downturn

Human Performance Technology (HPT) Model

The **Human Performance Technology (HPT) model** developed by the International Society for Performance Improvement is an excellent template for evaluating NIMS effectiveness and determining interventions to close performance gaps. The HPT evaluation process begins with an organizational analysis (internal) and an environmental analysis (external). These steps are important because many program evaluations erroneously focus on work performance and training without considering organizational issues or mitigating factors in the environment. For example, the organizational analysis should consider management structure, senior management commitment, and leadership skills. The environmental analysis factors may include political structure, the economy, and the incident history of a locale or region.

An HPT gap analysis is a key step in evaluating a NIMS program. Gaps are defined as the difference between *desired* performance and *actual* performance. For example, consider the NIMS principle of Unified Command (UC). A desired NIMS implementation goal is having all response agency department heads trained in UC followed by a performance assessment via one or more full-scale exercises. If only half the target participants are trained and an exercise is not conducted, there is a gap.

A determination of the cause(s) of a gap, called a *root cause analysis*, is the next step. Root cause determination is complicated because root causes are often hidden and not as obvious as performance gaps. In the previous UC example, root causes could be funding, lack of senior management support, lack of management follow-up, poor planning, or failure of trainers to meet NIMS implementation milestones.

Interventions that address the root causes of gaps are the next step. Interventions must be identified and implemented to ensure that gaps and root causes have been addressed. In the UC example, a senior staff meeting to explain the gap and root causes followed by a revised training and exercise schedule are interventions to ensure that the UC performance milestones are a reality.

High-Reliability Organization (HRO)

A **high-reliability organization (HRO)** is defined as an entity that encounters numerous unexpected events in a high-tempo and unpredictable environment, yet it has the capability to address surprise events safely and effectively. This is the definition provided by Karl Weick and Kathleen Sutcliffe in their book *Managing the Unexpected*. Many emergency response agencies meet the criteria in the HRO definition and the five characteristics of mindful HROs identified by Weick and Sutcliffe:

1. *Preoccupation with failure.* Small failures and near misses are reported and corrected.
2. *Reluctance to simplify interpretations.* Astute practitioners recognize that many processes are complex, dynamic, and unpredictable; these processes defy simplification.
3. *Sensitivity to operations.* Emergency response agencies must pay attention to operational aspects of a system, especially in areas where humans have direct interface with a process or action.
4. *Commitment to resilience.* The agency must be able to recognize and correct errors without the system failing.
5. *Deference to expertise.* The agency must rely on experts to correct system errors, regardless of each expert's level in the hierarchy.

In an effective NIMS implementation, these characteristics are all applicable. Small errors or near misses should be reported on every incident and appropriately corrected before they become big problems (*preoccupation with failure*). NIMS components such as resource management or UC should not be simplified because they are complex, nonstatic processes prone to unanticipated challenges and surprises (*reluctance to simplify interpretations*). Tactical emergency actions at the NIMS section level should receive mindful attention because errors are likely to occur and create friction points in the response and incident management process (*sensitivity to operations*). NIMS should be used as a flexible framework to detect and recover from inevitable errors during an incident (*commitment to resilience*). NIMS practitioners should rely on experts on the scene rather than a managerial hierarchy for processes that require specialized expertise; for example, a fire fighter who is a high-angle rescue technician should advise a senior Incident Commander on how to execute an elevated rescue operation (*deference to expertise*).

The National Integration Center: An Implementation Tool

The secretary of the Department of Homeland Security (DHS) establishes and administers the NIC. Proposed changes to NIMS are submitted to the NIC for consideration, approval, and publication. The NIC has a delineated set of responsibilities that are prescribed in NIMS. These specified responsibilities include the following:

- Developing and maintaining a national program for NIMS education and awareness, including specific instruction on the purpose and content of NIMS
- Promoting compatibility among national-level standards for NIMS and those developed by other public, private, and professional groups
- Facilitating the establishment and maintenance of a documentation and database system related to qualification, certification, and credentialing of emergency management/response personnel and organizations, which includes reviewing and approving discipline-specific requirements (with input from federal, state, tribal, local, private-sector organizations, nongovernmental organizations [NGOs], and national professional organizations, as appropriate)
- Developing assessment criteria for the various components of NIMS as well as compliance requirements and time lines for federal, state, tribal, and local governments regarding NIMS standards and guidelines
- Integrating into the national research and development (R&D) agenda—in coordination with the DHS Undersecretary for Science and Technology—NIMS-related science and technology needs of departments, agencies, disciplines, NGOs, and private-sector organizations operating within NIMS

NIMS Management and Maintenance

HSPD-5 requires the secretary of DHS to establish a mechanism for ensuring the ongoing management and maintenance of NIMS. To meet HSPD-5 requirements, the secretary has established the multijurisdictional and multidisciplinary NIC. The NIC provides strategic direction for and oversight of NIMS, supporting both routine maintenance and continuous refinement of the system and its components over the long term. The NIC includes mechanisms for direct participation and consultation with other federal departments and agencies; state, local, and tribal incident management entities; emergency responder and incident management professional organizations; and private-sector and nongovernmental organizations.

The NIC is responsible for developing a process for ongoing revisions and updates to NIMS. Revisions to NIMS and other corrective actions can be proposed by local, state, regional, tribal, and federal departments/agencies or entities. Private entities (including business and industry, volunteer organizations, academia, and other nonprofit and nongovernmental organizations) and NIMS-related professional associations can also submit proposed revisions and corrective actions to the NIC.

Concepts and Principles of NIMS Ongoing Management and Maintenance

An essential principle of NIMS management and maintenance is ensuring that every stakeholder in the NIMS response community has an opportunity to participate in NIC programs and activities. Stakeholders include various levels of government, functional disciplines, NGOs, and private entities. The NIC maintains appropriate liaisons with response community partners and private organizations to accomplish ongoing management and maintenance goals.

The NIMS management and maintenance process relies heavily on lessons learned from actual incidents and domestic incident management training and exercises, as well as recognized best practices across jurisdictions and functional disciplines. The NIC Lessons Learned Information Sharing Web site (www.llis.dhs.gov) provides after-action reports and a host of other reports outlining the experiences of other responders and agencies from actual incidents, exercises, and drills. These reports can be accessed by NIMS partners.

Proposed changes to NIMS are submitted to the NIC for consideration, approval, and publication. These changes will likely include new certifications for responders, new or updated training materials, policy and procedural changes, and revisions to the overall system. The secretary of DHS has ultimate authority and responsibility for publishing revisions and modifications to NIMS-related documents. This includes supplementary standards, procedures, and other materials in coordination with all NIMS response community partners with incident management and emergency responder responsibilities, expertise, and experience.

> **Tip**
>
> The Lessons Learned Information Sharing Web site (www.llis. dhs.gov), sponsored by the NIC, provides after-action reports and overviews of the experiences of other responders and agencies during actual incidents, exercises, and drills.

Responsibilities of the National Integration Center

Education and Training

The NIC is responsible for developing a national program for NIMS education and awareness. The education and awareness program includes materials for specific instruction on the purpose and content of the NIMS in general. The NIC guides the definition of general training requirements and the development of national-level training standards and course curricula associated with the NIMS, including the following:

- Modeling and simulation capabilities for training and exercise programs
- Field-based training, specification of mission-essential tasks, and requirements for specialized instruction and instructor training
- Course-completion documentation for all NIMS users
- Facilitation of the development and publication of materials (e.g., training tools, supplementary documentation, and desk guides)

Standards, Protocols, and Guidelines

The NIC also promotes the compatibility of NIMS standards, protocols, and guidelines among national-level agencies and public, private, and professional groups. These standards provide universal templates to support implementation and continuous refinement of NIMS and include guidelines and protocols for incident management training and exercises. The NIC assists in developing assessment criteria for the various components of NIMS as well as compliance requirements and time lines. The NIC is also responsible for the development of national standards and the establishment and maintenance of a publication management system for documents supporting NIMS, including the development or coordination of general publications for all NIMS users and their distribution via a NIMS publication management system.

Certification Standards

The NIC ensures the development and publication of national standards, guidelines, and protocols for the qualification and certification of emergency responder and incident management personnel. This includes reviewing and approving (with the assistance of national professional organizations and with input from federal, state, local, tribal, private-sector, and nongovernmental entities) discipline-specific qualification and certification requirements. The qualification and certification standards are developed based on information submitted by emergency responders and incident management organizations and associations. The NIC also oversees the establishment of a documentation and database system to track the qualification, certification, and credentialing of emergency responders, incident management personnel, and organizations. This database provides incident managers with the detailed qualification, experience, and training information needed to credential personnel for prescribed national incident management positions. This system also provides coordination of minimum professional certification standards and a nationwide credentialing system.

Interoperability Standards

The ability of all agencies and responders to operate in conjunction with one another is a core element for successful incident response and management. Interoperability requires the establishment of standards for the performance, compatibility, and interoperability of incident management and response equipment and communications systems. The NIC is charged with facilitating the development and publication of national standards, guidelines, and protocols for equipment certification, in coordination with standards-making, certifying, and accrediting organizations and NIMS response community partners. This facilitation includes reviewing and approving lists of equipment that meet these established equipment certification requirements and collaborating with organizations responsible for emergency responder equipment evaluation and testing. A final ongoing step is facilitating the development and distribution of national standards for the typing of resources.

Information Sharing

The NIC is responsible for the development and maintenance of an information framework that guides the development of NIMS information systems, including the development of data standards for incident notification and situation reports, status reporting, data analysis, geospatial information, wireless communications, identification and authentication, and incident reports. **Information sharing** is further enhanced by the establishment and maintenance of a repository and clearinghouse for reports and lessons learned from actual incidents, training, exercises, best practices, model structures, and model processes for NIMS-related functions.

Supporting Technology

The NIC coordinates the establishment of technical and technology standards for NIMS users in concert with the DHS Undersecretary for Science and Technology and recognized standards development organizations (SDOs). These standards are integrated into the national research and development agenda for the incident management science and technology needs of departments, agencies, disciplines, private-sector organizations, and NGOs operating within NIMS at all levels.

Rural Case Study *Answers*

1. Smith County conducted an in-house SWOT analysis with help from the local community college. The objective of the analysis was to identify strengths, weaknesses, opportunities, and threats based on data and anecdotal experience from the tornado disaster. A secondary objective of the analysis was the identification of possible future issues that were not identified from the tornado experience.

2. Performance standards, such as NIMS training hours, were compared with actual training hours. When gaps were quantified, root causes for the gaps were identified, and interventions were implemented to close the gaps. In the training example, poor scheduling was identified as the root cause. Training schedules were changed as an intervention to close the training gap.

Urban Case Study *Answers*

1. The cities of Pleasantville and Metro, in a joint venture, utilized a state emergency management planner to conduct a NIMS program evaluation. The planner used an HPT model as the template for the program evaluation. The NIMS program evaluation began with an environmental and organizational analysis, followed by a gap analysis. The follow-up step from the gap analysis was the identification of root causes for key gaps. The planner, in coordination with the emergency preparedness committee, then identified innovations that addressed NIMS deficiencies (closing the gaps). Actual performance improvement will be measured by evaluating future incidents and exercise performance.

2. The NIC sets standards for interoperability, information sharing, and training. The training standards incorporate personal qualification and credentialing mechanisms. The NIC also coordinates science and technology efforts related to emergency response. The NIC also maintains an online information system for lessons learned. This system is a source for real-world case studies and lessons from myriad nationwide emergency incidents.

3. Pleasantville and Metro should adopt the HRO principle of preoccupation with failure. First, a formal near-miss reporting system should be established that mandates the identification, analysis, and correction of close calls or minor system errors. Second, responders from the lowest level to senior managers should report small errors and be rewarded for their reports. Fear of retribution for reporting errors must be eradicated from the organizational culture. Last, reported errors or near misses must be immediately analyzed and corrected.

Wrap-Up

Summary

- NIMS programs should be continuously evaluated through an academically accepted program evaluation model.
- A SWOT analysis is based on assessing the strengths, weaknesses, opportunities, and threats of NIMS.
- The HPT model begins with an organizational and environmental analysis, followed by a gap analysis. Root causes of gaps in the NIMS program are then identified, and interventions are implemented to narrow or close the program gaps.
- The following five HRO principles should be continuously applied to all NIMS response agencies:
  1. Preoccupation with failure
  2. Reluctance to simplify interpretations
  3. Sensitivity to operations
  4. Commitment to resilience
  5. Deference to expertise
- The management and maintenance of NIMS is a continuous process. It is important for all NIMS response community partners to realize that NIMS development is continually changed and refined.
- The NIC is the central national coordinating body that ensures incident response, management, recovery, and planning are efficient and effective across all disciplines, jurisdictions, and agencies.
- The NIMS component of ongoing management and maintenance requires quality management through system-wide assessment and corrective actions that remedy identified deficiencies. Proposed changes to NIMS are submitted to the NIC for consideration, approval, and publication.
- The NIC is responsible for the following:
  - Developing a national program for NIMS education and awareness
  - Ensuring compatibility of standards, protocols, and guidelines
  - Developing and publishing national standards, guidelines, and protocols for the qualification and certification of emergency responders and incident management personnel
  - Establishing standards for the performance, compatibility, and interoperability of incident management and response equipment
  - Developing data standards for incident notification, situation reports, geospatial information, and communications
  - Establishing technical and technology standards for NIMS users
- Ongoing management, maintenance, and continuous quality improvement depend on the input and participation of all NIMS response community members at all jurisdictional, agency, and professional levels.

Glossary

High-reliability organization (HRO): An organization that safely and effectively manages and recovers from unexpected events in dynamic and unpredictable environments.

Human Performance Technology (HPT) model: A program evaluation process that identifies interventions through gap and root cause analyses.

Information sharing: The development of a framework connecting various information systems, including incident notification and situation reports, status reporting, data analysis, geospatial information, wireless communications, and incident reports.

Program evaluation: The process of judging the worth and merit of a program.

SWOT analysis: An evaluation process that identifies organizational strengths, weaknesses, opportunities, and threats.

Market City is an urban community with a population of 2.5 million people. The city has 35 fire stations, and the response time for the first-due paramedic engine company is 9 minutes or less 60 percent of the time. Several community activist groups complained to the city commission about the response time, prompting the fire chief to conduct a SWOT analysis. The analysis confirmed that the response times were a weakness and must be improved.

Fire service leaders suspected that additional paramedic engines had to be established. However, an internal study revealed that antiquated move-up protocols were responsible for long response times in busy areas. An innovative computer-aided move-up system was implemented, and response times were reduced to 8 minutes or less 90 percent of the time, which met the city's new response standard.

1. What organizational evaluation model overarched the gap analysis?
   A. A gap analysis is one of the hallmarks of an HRO.
   B. A gap analysis is a key step in the HPT model.
   C. A gap analysis always follows after weaknesses are identified in a SWOT analysis.
   D. Astute fire service leaders know how to analyze organizational performance without academic models.

2. What steps should follow when performance gaps are identified in an emergency response organization?
   A. Performance gaps should be presented to elected officials because these gaps usually have political solutions.
   B. When performance gaps are identified, the appropriate solution is almost always obvious.
   C. It is not important to close performance gaps because most performance standards are unrealistic and cannot be achieved.
   D. The root cause(s) of a performance gap must be identified because interventions must be structured to correct the cause(s) of the gap.

Homeland Security Presidential Directives

February 28, 2003 Homeland Security Presidential Directive (HSPD)-5

Subject: Management of Domestic Incidents

Purpose

(1) To enhance the ability of the United States to manage domestic incidents by establishing a single, comprehensive national incident management system.

Definitions

(2) In this directive:

(a) the term "Secretary" means the Secretary of Homeland Security.

(b) the term "Federal departments and agencies" means those executive departments enumerated in 5 U.S.C. 101, together with the Department of Homeland Security; independent establishments as defined by 5 U.S.C. 104(1); government corporations as defined by 5 U.S.C. 103(1); and the United States Postal Service.

(c) the terms "State," "local," and the "United States" when it is used in a geographical sense, have the same meanings as used in the Homeland Security Act of 2002, Public Law 107-296.

Policy

(3) To prevent, prepare for, respond to, and recover from terrorist attacks, major disasters, and other emergencies, the United States Government shall establish a single, comprehensive approach to domestic incident management. The objective of the United States Government is to ensure that all levels of government across the Nation have the capability to work efficiently and effectively together, using a national approach to domestic incident management. In these efforts, with regard to domestic incidents, the United States Government treats crisis management and consequence management as a single, integrated function, rather than as two separate functions.

(4) The Secretary of Homeland Security is the principal Federal official for domestic incident management. Pursuant to the Homeland Security Act of 2002, the Secretary is responsible for coordinating Federal operations within the United States to prepare for, respond to, and recover from terrorist attacks, major disasters, and other emergencies. The Secretary shall coordinate the Federal Government's resources utilized in response to or recovery from terrorist attacks, major disasters, or other emergencies if and when any one of the following four conditions applies: (1) a Federal department or agency acting under its own authority has requested the assistance of the Secretary; (2) the resources of State and local authorities are overwhelmed and Federal assistance has been requested by the appropriate State and local authorities; (3) more than one Federal department or agency has become substantially involved in responding to the incident; or (4) the Secretary has been directed to assume responsibility for managing the domestic incident by the President.

(5) Nothing in this directive alters, or impedes the ability to carry out, the authorities of Federal departments and agencies to perform their responsibilities under law. All Federal departments and agencies shall cooperate with the Secretary in the Secretary's domestic incident management role.

(6) The Federal Government recognizes the roles and responsibilities of State and local authorities in domestic incident management. Initial responsibility for managing domestic incidents generally falls on State and local authorities. The Federal Government will assist State and local authorities when their resources are overwhelmed, or when Federal interests are involved. The Secretary will coordinate with State and local governments to ensure adequate planning, equipment, training, and exercise activities. The Secretary will also provide assistance to State and local governments to develop all-hazards plans and capabilities, including those of greatest importance to the security of the United States, and will ensure that State, local, and Federal plans are compatible.

(7) The Federal Government recognizes the role that the private and nongovernmental sectors play in preventing, preparing for, responding to, and recovering from terrorist attacks, major disasters, and other emergencies. The Secretary will coordinate with the private and nongovernmental sectors to ensure adequate planning, equipment, training, and exercise activities and to promote partnerships to address incident management capabilities.

(8) The Attorney General has lead responsibility for criminal investigations of terrorist acts or terrorist threats by individuals or groups inside the United States, or directed at United States citizens or institutions abroad, where such acts are within the Federal criminal jurisdiction of the United States, as well as for related intelligence collection activities within the United States, subject to the National Security Act of 1947 and other applicable law, Executive Order 12333, and Attorney General-approved procedures pursuant to that Executive Order. Generally acting through the Federal Bureau of Investigation, the Attorney General, in cooperation with other Federal departments and agencies engaged in activities to protect our national security, shall also coordinate the activities of the other members of the law enforcement community to detect, prevent, preempt, and disrupt terrorist attacks against the United States. Following a terrorist threat or an actual incident that falls within the criminal jurisdiction of the United States, the full capabilities of the United States shall be dedicated, consistent with United States law and with activities of other Federal departments and agencies to protect our national security, to assisting the Attorney General to identify the perpetrators and bring them to justice. The Attorney General and the Secretary shall establish appropriate relationships and mechanisms for cooperation and coordination between their two departments.

(9) Nothing in this directive impairs or otherwise affects the authority of the Secretary of Defense over the Department of Defense, including the chain of command for military forces from the President as Commander in Chief, to the Secretary of Defense, to the commander of military forces, or military command and control procedures. The Secretary of Defense shall provide military support to civil authorities for domestic incidents as directed by the President or when consistent with military readiness and appropriate under the circumstances and the law. The Secretary of Defense shall retain command of military forces providing civil support. The Secretary of Defense and the Secretary shall establish appropriate relationships and mechanisms for cooperation and coordination between their two departments.

(10) The Secretary of State has the responsibility, consistent with other United States Government activities to protect our national security, to coordinate international activities related to the prevention, preparation, response, and recovery from a domestic incident, and for the protection of United States citizens and United States interests overseas. The Secretary of State and the Secretary shall establish appropriate relationships and mechanisms for cooperation and coordination between their two departments.

(11) The Assistant to the President for Homeland Security and the Assistant to the President for National Security Affairs shall be responsible for interagency policy coordination on domestic and international incident management, respectively, as directed by the President. The Assistant to the President for Homeland Security and the Assistant to the President for National Security Affairs shall work together to ensure that the United States domestic and international incident management efforts are seamlessly united.

(12) The Secretary shall ensure that, as appropriate, information related to domestic incidents is gathered and provided to the public, the private sector, State and local authorities, Federal departments and agencies, and, generally through the Assistant to the President for Homeland Security, to the President. The Secretary shall provide standardized, quantitative reports to the Assistant to the President for Homeland Security on the readiness and preparedness of the Nation— at all levels of government—to prevent, prepare for, respond to, and recover from domestic incidents.

(13) Nothing in this directive shall be construed to grant to any Assistant to the President any authority to issue orders to Federal departments and agencies, their officers, or their employees.

Tasking

(14) The heads of all Federal departments and agencies are directed to provide their full and prompt cooperation, resources, and support, as appropriate and consistent with their own responsibilities for protecting our national security, to the Secretary, the Attorney General, the Secretary of Defense, and the Secretary of State in the exercise of the individual leadership responsibilities and missions assigned in paragraphs (4), (8), (9), and (10), respectively, above.

(15) The Secretary shall develop, submit for review to the Homeland Security Council, and administer a National Incident Management System (NIMS). This system will provide a consistent nationwide approach for Federal, State, and local governments to work effectively and efficiently together to prepare for, respond to, and recover from domestic incidents, regardless of cause, size, or complexity. To provide for interoperability and compatibility among Federal, State, and local capabilities, the NIMS will include a core set of concepts, principles, terminology, and technologies covering the incident command system; multi-agency coordination systems; unified command; training; identification and management of resources (including systems for classifying types of resources); qualifications and certification; and the collection, tracking, and reporting of incident information and incident resources.

(16) The Secretary shall develop, submit for review to the Homeland Security Council, and administer a National Response Plan (NRP). The Secretary shall consult with appropriate Assistants to the President (including the Assistant to the President for Economic Policy) and the Director of the Office of Science and Technology Policy, and other such Federal officials as may be appropriate, in developing and implementing the NRP. This plan shall integrate Federal Government domestic prevention, preparedness, response, and recovery plans into one all-discipline, all-hazards plan. The NRP shall be unclassified. If certain operational aspects require classification, they shall be included in classified annexes to the NRP.

(a) The NRP, using the NIMS, shall, with regard to response to domestic incidents, provide the structure and mechanisms for national level policy and operational direction for Federal support to State and local incident managers and for exercising direct Federal authorities and responsibilities, as appropriate.

(b) The NRP will include protocols for operating under different threats or threat levels; incorporation of existing Federal emergency and incident management plans (with appropriate modifications and revisions) as either integrated components of the NRP or as supporting operational plans; and additional operational plans or annexes, as appropriate, including public affairs and intergovernmental communications.

(c) The NRP will include a consistent approach to reporting incidents, providing assessments, and making recommendations to the President, the Secretary, and the Homeland Security Council.

(d) The NRP will include rigorous requirements for continuous improvements from testing, exercising, experience with incidents, and new information and technologies.

(17) The Secretary shall:

(a) By April 1, 2003, (1) develop and publish an initial version of the NRP, in consultation with other Federal departments and agencies; and (2) provide the Assistant to the President for Homeland Security with a plan for full development and implementation of the NRP.

(b) By June 1, 2003, (1) in consultation with Federal departments and agencies and with State and local governments, develop a national system of standards, guidelines, and protocols to implement the NIMS; and (2) establish a mechanism for ensuring ongoing management and maintenance of the NIMS, including regular consultation with other Federal departments and agencies and with State and local governments.

(c) By September 1, 2003, in consultation with Federal departments and agencies and the Assistant to the President for Homeland Security, review existing authorities and regulations and prepare recommendations for the President on revisions necessary to implement fully the NRP.

(18) The heads of Federal departments and agencies shall adopt the NIMS within their departments and agencies and shall provide support and assistance to the Secretary in the development and maintenance of the NIMS. All Federal departments and agencies will use the NIMS in their domestic incident management and emergency prevention, preparedness, response, recovery, and mitigation activities, as well as those actions taken in support of State or local entities. The heads of Federal departments and agencies shall participate in the NRP, shall assist and support the Secretary in the development and maintenance of the NRP, and shall participate in and use domestic incident reporting systems and protocols established by the Secretary.

(19) The head of each Federal department and agency shall:
  (a) By June 1, 2003, make initial revisions to existing plans in accordance with the initial version of the NRP.
  (b) By August 1, 2003, submit a plan to adopt and implement the NIMS to the Secretary and the Assistant to the President for Homeland Security. The Assistant to the President for Homeland Security shall advise the President on whether such plans effectively implement the NIMS.

(20) Beginning in Fiscal Year 2005, Federal departments and agencies shall make adoption of the NIMS a requirement, to the extent permitted by law, for providing Federal preparedness assistance through grants, contracts, or other activities. The Secretary shall develop standards and guidelines for determining whether a State or local entity has adopted the NIMS.

Technical and Conforming Amendments to National Security Presidential Directive-1 (NSPD-1)

(21) NSPD-1 ("Organization of the National Security Council System") is amended by replacing the fifth sentence of the third paragraph on the first page with the following: "The Attorney General, the Secretary of Homeland Security, and the Director of the Office of Management and Budget shall be invited to attend meetings pertaining to their responsibilities."

Technical and Conforming Amendments to National Security Presidential Directive-8 (NSPD-8)

(22) NSPD-8 ("National Director and Deputy National Security Advisor for Combating Terrorism") is amended by striking "and the Office of Homeland Security," on page 4, and inserting "the Department of Homeland Security, and the Homeland Security Council" in lieu thereof.

Technical and Conforming Amendments to Homeland Security Presidential Directive-2 (HSPD-2)

(23) HSPD-2 ("Combating Terrorism Through Immigration Policies") is amended as follows:
  (a) striking "the Commissioner of the Immigration and Naturalization Service (INS)" in the second sentence of the second paragraph in section 1, and inserting "the Secretary of Homeland Security" in lieu thereof;
  (b) striking "the INS," in the third paragraph in section 1, and inserting "the Department of Homeland Security" in lieu thereof;
  (c) inserting ", the Secretary of Homeland Security," after "The Attorney General" in the fourth paragraph in section 1;
  (d) inserting ", the Secretary of Homeland Security," after "the Attorney General" in the fifth paragraph in section 1;
  (e) striking "the INS and the Customs Service" in the first sentence of the first paragraph of section 2, and inserting "the Department of Homeland Security" in lieu thereof;
  (f) striking "Customs and INS" in the first sentence of the second paragraph of section 2, and inserting "the Department of Homeland Security" in lieu thereof;
  (g) striking "the two agencies" in the second sentence of the second paragraph of section 2, and inserting "the Department of Homeland Security" in lieu thereof;
  (h) striking "the Secretary of the Treasury" wherever it appears in section 2, and inserting "the Secretary of Homeland Security" in lieu thereof;
  (i) inserting ", the Secretary of Homeland Security," after "The Secretary of State" wherever the latter appears in section 3;
  (j) inserting ", the Department of Homeland Security," after "the Department of State," in the second sentence in the third paragraph in section 3;
  (k) inserting "the Secretary of Homeland Security," after "the Secretary of State," in the first sentence of the fifth paragraph of section 3;
  (l) striking "INS" in the first sentence of the sixth paragraph of section 3, and inserting

"Department of Homeland Security" in lieu thereof;

(m) striking "the Treasury" wherever it appears in section 4 and inserting "Homeland Security" in lieu thereof;

(n) inserting ", the Secretary of Homeland Security," after "the Attorney General" in the first sentence in section 5; and

(o) inserting ", Homeland Security" after "State" in the first sentence of section 6.

Technical and Conforming Amendments to Homeland Security Presidential Directive-3 (HSPD-3)

(24) The Homeland Security Act of 2002 assigned the responsibility for administering the Homeland Security Advisory System to the Secretary of Homeland Security. Accordingly, HSPD-3 of March 11, 2002 ("Homeland Security Advisory System") is amended as follows:

(a) replacing the third sentence of the second paragraph entitled "Homeland Security Advisory System" with "Except in exigent circumstances, the Secretary of Homeland Security shall seek the views of the Attorney General, and any other federal agency heads the Secretary deems appropriate, including other members of the Homeland Security Council, on the Threat Condition to be assigned."

(b) inserting "At the request of the Secretary of Homeland Security, the Department of Justice shall permit and facilitate the use of delivery systems administered or managed by the Department of Justice for the purposes of delivering threat information pursuant to the Homeland Security Advisory System." as a new paragraph after the fifth paragraph of the section entitled "Homeland Security Advisory System."

(c) inserting ", the Secretary of Homeland Security" after "The Director of Central Intelligence" in the first sentence of the seventh paragraph of the section entitled "Homeland Security Advisory System".

(d) striking "Attorney General" wherever it appears (except in the sentences referred to in subsections (a) and (c) above), and inserting "the Secretary of Homeland Security" in lieu thereof; and

(e) striking the section entitled "Comment and Review Periods."

GEORGE W. BUSH

December 17, 2003 Homeland Security Presidential Directive (HSPD)-7

Subject: Critical Infrastructure Identification, Prioritization, and Protection

Purpose

(1) This directive establishes a national policy for Federal departments and agencies to identify and prioritize United States critical infrastructure and key resources and to protect them from terrorist attacks.

Background

(2) Terrorists seek to destroy, incapacitate, or exploit critical infrastructure and key resources across the United States to threaten national security, cause mass casualties, weaken our economy, and damage public morale and confidence.

(3) America's open and technologically complex society includes a wide array of critical infrastructure and key resources that are potential terrorist targets. The majority of these are owned and operated by the private sector and State or local governments. These critical infrastructures and key resources are both physical and cyber-based and span all sectors of the economy.

(4) Critical infrastructure and key resources provide the essential services that underpin American society. The Nation possesses numerous key resources, whose exploitation or destruction by terrorists could cause catastrophic health effects or mass casualties comparable to those from the use of a weapon of mass destruction, or could profoundly affect our national prestige and morale. In addition, there is critical infrastructure so vital that its incapacitation, exploitation, or destruction, through terrorist attack, could have a debilitating effect on security and economic well-being.

(5) While it is not possible to protect or eliminate the vulnerability of all critical infrastructure and key resources throughout the country, strategic improvements in security can make it more difficult for attacks to succeed and can lessen the impact of attacks that may occur. In addition to strategic security enhancements, tactical security improvements can be rapidly implemented to deter, mitigate, or neutralize potential attacks.

Definitions

(6) In this directive:

(a) The term "critical infrastructure" has the meaning given to that term in section 1016(e) of the USA PATRIOT Act of 2001 (42 U.S.C. 5195c(e)).

(b) The term "key resources" has the meaning given that term in section 2(9) of the Homeland Security Act of 2002 (6 U.S.C. 101(9)).

(c) The term "the Department" means the Department of Homeland Security.

(d) The term "Federal departments and agencies" means those executive departments enumerated in 5 U.S.C. 101, and the Department of Homeland Security; independent establishments as defined by 5 U.S.C. 104(1); Government corporations as defined by 5 U.S.C. 103(1); and the United States Postal Service.

(e) The terms "State," and "local government," when used in a geographical sense, have the same meanings given to those terms in section 2 of the Homeland Security Act of 2002 (6 U.S.C. 101).

(f) The term "the Secretary" means the Secretary of Homeland Security.

(g) The term "Sector-Specific Agency" means a Federal department or agency responsible for infrastructure protection activities in a designated critical infrastructure sector or key resources category. Sector-Specific Agencies will conduct their activities under this directive in accordance with guidance provided by the Secretary.

(h) The terms "protect" and "secure" mean reducing the vulnerability of critical infrastructure or key resources in order to deter, mitigate, or neutralize terrorist attacks.

Policy

(7) It is the policy of the United States to enhance the protection of our Nation's critical infrastructure and key resources against terrorist acts that could:

(a) cause catastrophic health effects or mass casualties comparable to those from the use of a weapon of mass destruction;

(b) impair Federal departments and agencies' abilities to perform essential missions, or to ensure the public's health and safety;

(c) undermine State and local government capacities to maintain order and to deliver minimum essential public services;

(d) damage the private sector's capability to ensure the orderly functioning of the economy and delivery of essential services;

(e) have a negative effect on the economy through the cascading disruption of other critical infrastructure and key resources; or

(f) undermine the public's morale and confidence in our national economic and political institutions.

(8) Federal departments and agencies will identify, prioritize, and coordinate the protection of critical infrastructure and key resources in order to prevent, deter, and mitigate the effects of deliberate efforts to destroy, incapacitate, or exploit them. Federal departments and agencies will work with State and local governments and the private sector to accomplish this objective.

(9) Federal departments and agencies will ensure that homeland security programs do not diminish the overall economic security of the United States.

(10) Federal departments and agencies will appropriately protect information associated with carrying out this directive, including handling voluntarily provided information and information that would facilitate terrorist targeting of critical infrastructure and key resources consistent with the Homeland Security Act of 2002 and other applicable legal authorities.

(11) Federal departments and agencies shall implement this directive in a manner consistent with applicable provisions of law, including those protecting the rights of United States persons.

Roles and Responsibilities of the Secretary

(12) In carrying out the functions assigned in the Homeland Security Act of 2002, the Secretary shall be responsible for coordinating the overall national effort to enhance the protection of the critical infrastructure and key resources of the United States. The Secretary shall serve as the principal Federal official to lead, integrate, and coordinate implementation of efforts among Federal departments and agencies, State and local governments, and the private sector to protect critical infrastructure and key resources.

(13) Consistent with this directive, the Secretary will identify, prioritize, and coordinate the protection of critical infrastructure and key resources with an emphasis on critical infrastructure and key resources that could be exploited to cause catastrophic health effects or mass casualties comparable to those from the use of a weapon of mass destruction.

(14) The Secretary will establish uniform policies, approaches, guidelines, and methodologies for integrating Federal infrastructure protection and risk management activities within and across sectors along with metrics and criteria for related programs and activities.

(15) The Secretary shall coordinate protection activities for each of the following critical infrastructure sectors: information technology; telecommunications; chemical; transportation systems, including mass transit, aviation, maritime, ground/surface, and rail and pipeline systems; emergency services; and postal and shipping. The Department shall coordinate with appropriate departments and agencies to ensure the protection of other key resources including dams, government facilities, and commercial facilities. In addition, in its role as overall cross-sector coordinator, the Department shall also evaluate the need for and coordinate the coverage of additional critical infrastructure and key resources categories over time, as appropriate.

(16) The Secretary will continue to maintain an organization to serve as a focal point for the security of cyberspace. The organization will facilitate interactions and collaborations between and among Federal departments and agencies, State and local governments, the private sector, academia and international organizations. To the extent permitted by law, Federal departments and agencies with cyber expertise, including but not limited to the Departments of Justice, Commerce, the Treasury, Defense, Energy, and State, and the Central Intelligence Agency, will collaborate with and support the organization in accomplishing its mission. The organization's mission includes analysis, warning, information sharing, vulnerability reduction, mitigation, and aiding national recovery efforts for critical infrastructure information systems. The organization will support the Department of Justice and other law enforcement agencies in their continuing missions to investigate and prosecute threats to and attacks against cyberspace, to the extent permitted by law.

(17) The Secretary will work closely with other Federal departments and agencies, State and local governments, and the private sector in accomplishing the objectives of this directive.

Roles and Responsibilities of Sector-Specific Federal Agencies

(18) Recognizing that each infrastructure sector possesses its own unique characteristics and operating models, there are designated Sector-Specific Agencies, including:
- **(a)** Department of Agriculture—agriculture, food (meat, poultry, egg products);
- **(b)** Health and Human Services—public health, healthcare, and food (other than meat, poultry, egg products);
- **(c)** Environmental Protection Agency—drinking water and water treatment systems;
- **(d)** Department of Energy—energy, including the production refining, storage, and distribution of oil and gas, and electric power except for commercial nuclear power facilities;
- **(e)** Department of the Treasury—banking and finance;
- **(f)** Department of the Interior—national monuments and icons; and
- **(g)** Department of Defense—defense industrial base.

(19) In accordance with guidance provided by the Secretary, Sector-Specific Agencies shall:
- **(a)** collaborate with all relevant Federal departments and agencies, State and local governments, and the private sector, including with key persons and entities in their infrastructure sector;
- **(b)** conduct or facilitate vulnerability assessments of the sector; and
- **(c)** encourage risk management strategies to protect against and mitigate the effects of attacks against critical infrastructure and key resources.

(20) Nothing in this directive alters, or impedes the ability to carry out, the authorities of the Federal departments and agencies to perform their responsibilities under law and consistent with applicable legal authorities and presidential guidance.

(21) Federal departments and agencies shall cooperate with the Department in implementing this directive, consistent with the Homeland Security Act of 2002 and other applicable legal authorities.

Roles and Responsibilities of Other Departments, Agencies, and Offices

(22) In addition to the responsibilities given the Department and Sector-Specific Agencies, there are special functions of various Federal departments and agencies and components of the Executive Office of the President related to critical infrastructure and key resources protection.
- **(a)** The Department of State, in conjunction with the Department, and the Departments of Justice, Commerce, Defense, the Treasury and other appropriate agencies, will work with foreign countries and international organizations to strengthen the protection of United States critical infrastructure and key resources.
- **(b)** The Department of Justice, including the Federal Bureau of Investigation, will reduce domestic terrorist threats, and investigate and prosecute actual or attempted terrorist attacks on, sabotage of, or disruptions of critical infrastructure and key resources. The Attorney General and the Secretary shall use applicable statutory authority and attendant mechanisms for cooperation and coordination, including but not limited to those established by presidential directive.
- **(c)** The Department of Commerce, in coordination with the Department, will work with private sector, research, academic, and government organizations to improve technology for cyber systems and promote other critical infrastructure efforts, including using its authority under the Defense Production Act to assure the timely availability of industrial products, materials, and services to meet homeland security requirements.
- **(d)** A Critical Infrastructure Protection Policy Coordinating Committee will advise the Homeland Security Council on interagency policy related to physical and cyber infrastructure protection. This PCC will be chaired by a Federal officer or employee designated by the Assistant to the President for Homeland Security.
- **(e)** The Office of Science and Technology Policy, in coordination with the Department, will coordinate interagency research and development to enhance the protection of critical infrastructure and key resources.
- **(f)** The Office of Management and Budget (OMB) shall oversee the implementation of government-wide policies, principles, stan-

dards, and guidelines for Federal government computer security programs. The Director of OMB will ensure the operation of a central Federal information security incident center consistent with the requirements of the Federal Information Security Management Act of 2002.

(g) Consistent with the E-Government Act of 2002, the Chief Information Officers Council shall be the principal interagency forum for improving agency practices related to the design, acquisition, development, modernization, use, operation, sharing, and performance of information resources of Federal departments and agencies.

(h) The Department of Transportation and the Department will collaborate on all matters relating to transportation security and transportation infrastructure protection. The Department of Transportation is responsible for operating the national air space system. The Department of Transportation and the Department will collaborate in regulating the transportation of hazardous materials by all modes (including pipelines).

(i) All Federal departments and agencies shall work with the sectors relevant to their responsibilities to reduce the consequences of catastrophic failures not caused by terrorism.

(23) The heads of all Federal departments and agencies will coordinate and cooperate with the Secretary as appropriate and consistent with their own responsibilities for protecting critical infrastructure and key resources.

(24) All Federal department and agency heads are responsible for the identification, prioritization, assessment, remediation, and protection of their respective internal critical infrastructure and key resources. Consistent with the Federal Information Security Management Act of 2002, agencies will identify and provide information security protections commensurate with the risk and magnitude of the harm resulting from the unauthorized access, use, disclosure, disruption, modification, or destruction of information.

Coordination with the Private Sector

(25) In accordance with applicable laws or regulations, the Department and the Sector-Specific Agencies will collaborate with appropriate private sector entities and continue to encourage the development of information sharing and analysis mechanisms. Additionally, the Department and Sector-Specific Agencies shall collaborate with the private sector and continue to support sector-coordinating mechanisms:

(a) to identify, prioritize, and coordinate the protection of critical infrastructure and key resources; and

(b) to facilitate sharing of information about physical and cyber threats, vulnerabilities, incidents, potential protective measures, and best practices.

National Special Security Events

(26) The Secretary, after consultation with the Homeland Security Council, shall be responsible for designating events as "National Special Security Events" (NSSEs). This directive supersedes language in previous presidential directives regarding the designation of NSSEs that is inconsistent herewith.

Implementation

(27) Consistent with the Homeland Security Act of 2002, the Secretary shall produce a comprehensive, integrated National Plan for Critical Infrastructure and Key Resources Protection to outline national goals, objectives, milestones, and key initiatives within 1 year from the issuance of this directive. The Plan shall include, in addition to other Homeland Security-related elements as the Secretary deems appropriate, the following elements:

(a) a strategy to identify, prioritize, and coordinate the protection of critical infrastructure and key resources, including how the Department intends to work with Federal departments and agencies, State and local governments, the private sector, and foreign countries and international organizations;

(b) a summary of activities to be undertaken in order to: define and prioritize, reduce the vulnerability of, and coordinate the protection of critical infrastructure and key resources;

(c) a summary of initiatives for sharing critical infrastructure and key resources information and for providing critical infrastructure and key resources threat warning data to State and local governments and the private sector; and

(d) coordination and integration, as appropriate, with other Federal emergency management and preparedness activities including the National Response Plan and applicable national preparedness goals.

(28) The Secretary, consistent with the Homeland Security Act of 2002 and other applicable legal authorities and presidential guidance, shall establish appropriate systems, mechanisms, and procedures to share homeland security information relevant to threats and vulnerabilities in national critical infrastructure and key resources with other Federal departments and agencies, State and local governments, and the private sector in a timely manner.

(29) The Secretary will continue to work with the Nuclear Regulatory Commission and, as appropriate, the Department of Energy in order to ensure the necessary protection of:

(a) commercial nuclear reactors for generating electric power and non-power nuclear reactors used for research, testing, and training;

(b) nuclear materials in medical, industrial, and academic settings and facilities that fabricate nuclear fuel; and

(c) the transportation, storage, and disposal of nuclear materials and waste.

(30) In coordination with the Director of the Office of Science and Technology Policy, the Secretary shall prepare on an annual basis a Federal Research and Development Plan in support of this directive.

(31) The Secretary will collaborate with other appropriate Federal departments and agencies to develop a program, consistent with applicable law, to geospatially map, image, analyze, and sort critical infrastructure and key resources by utilizing commercial satellite and airborne systems, and existing capabilities within other agencies. National technical means should be considered as an option of last resort. The Secretary, with advice from the Director of Central Intelligence, the Secretaries of Defense and the Interior, and the heads of other appropriate Federal departments and agencies, shall develop mechanisms for accomplishing this initiative. The Attorney General shall provide legal advice as necessary.

(32) The Secretary will utilize existing, and develop new, capabilities as needed to model comprehensively the potential implications of terrorist exploitation of vulnerabilities in critical infrastructure and key resources, placing specific focus on densely populated areas. Agencies with relevant modeling capabilities shall cooperate with the Secretary to develop appropriate mechanisms for accomplishing this initiative.

(33) The Secretary will develop a national indications and warnings architecture for infrastructure protection and capabilities that will facilitate:

(a) an understanding of baseline infrastructure operations;

(b) the identification of indicators and precursors to an attack; and

(c) a surge capacity for detecting and analyzing patterns of potential attacks.

In developing a national indications and warnings architecture, the Department will work with Federal, State, local, and non-governmental entities to develop an integrated view of physical and cyber infrastructure and key resources.

(34) By July 2004, the heads of all Federal departments and agencies shall develop and submit to the Director of the OMB for approval plans for protecting the physical and cyber critical infrastructure and key resources that they own or operate. These plans shall address identification, prioritization, protection, and contingency planning, including the recovery and reconstitution of essential capabilities.

(35) On an annual basis, the Sector-Specific Agencies shall report to the Secretary on their efforts to identify, prioritize, and coordinate the protection of critical infrastructure and key resources in their respective sectors. The report shall be submitted within 1 year from the issuance of this directive and on an annual basis thereafter.

(36) The Assistant to the President for Homeland Security and the Assistant to the President for National Security Affairs will lead a national security and emergency preparedness communications policy review, with the heads of the appropriate Federal departments and agencies, related to convergence and next generation architecture. Within 6 months after the issuance of this directive, the Assistant to the President for Homeland Security and the Assistant to the President for National Security Affairs shall submit for my consideration any recommended changes to such policy.

(37) This directive supersedes Presidential Decision Directive/NSC-63 of May 22, 1998 ("Critical Infrastructure Protection"), and any Presidential directives issued prior to this directive to the extent of any inconsistency. Moreover, the Assistant to the President for Homeland Security and the Assistant to the President for National Security Affairs shall jointly submit for my consideration a Presidential directive to make changes in Presidential directives issued prior to this date that conform such directives to this directive.

(38) This directive is intended only to improve the internal management of the executive branch of the Federal Government, and it is not intended to, and does not, create any right or benefit, substantive or procedural, enforceable at law or in equity, against the United States, its departments, agencies, or other entities, its officers or employees, or any other person.

GEORGE W. BUSH

December 17, 2003 Homeland Security Presidential Directive (HSPD)-8

Subject: National Preparedness

Purpose

(1) This directive establishes policies to strengthen the preparedness of the United States to prevent and respond to threatened or actual domestic terrorist attacks, major disasters, and other emergencies by requiring a national domestic all-hazards preparedness goal, establishing mechanisms for improved delivery of Federal preparedness assistance to State and local governments, and outlining actions to strengthen preparedness capabilities of Federal, State, and local entities.

Definitions

(2) For the purposes of this directive:

  (a) The term "all-hazards preparedness" refers to preparedness for domestic terrorist attacks, major disasters, and other emergencies.

  (b) The term "Federal departments and agencies" means those executive departments enumerated in 5 U.S.C. 101, and the Department of Homeland Security; independent establishments as defined by 5 U.S.C. 104(1); Government corporations as defined by 5 U.S.C. 103(1); and the United States Postal Service.

  (c) The term "Federal preparedness assistance" means Federal department and agency grants, cooperative agreements, loans, loan guarantees, training, and/or technical assistance provided to State and local governments and the private sector to prevent, prepare for, respond to, and recover from terrorist attacks, major disasters, and other emergencies. Unless noted otherwise, the term "assistance" will refer to Federal assistance programs.

  (d) The term "first responder" refers to those individuals who in the early stages of an incident are responsible for the protection and preservation of life, property, evidence, and the environment, including emergency response providers as defined in section 2 of the Homeland Security Act of 2002 (6 U.S.C. 101), as well as emergency management, public health, clinical care, public works, and other skilled support personnel (such as equipment operators) that provide immediate support services during prevention, response, and recovery operations.

  (e) The terms "major disaster" and "emergency" have the meanings given in section 102 of the Robert T. Stafford Disaster Relief and Emergency Assistance Act (42 U.S.C. 5122).

  (f) The term "major events" refers to domestic terrorist attacks, major disasters, and other emergencies.

  (g) The term "national homeland security preparedness-related exercises" refers to homeland security-related exercises that train and test national decision makers and utilize resources of multiple Federal departments and agencies. Such exercises may involve State and local first responders when appropriate. Such exercises do not include those exercises conducted solely within a single Federal department or agency.

  (h) The term "preparedness" refers to the existence of plans, procedures, policies, training, and equipment necessary at the Federal, State, and local level to maximize the ability to prevent, respond to, and recover from major events. The term "readiness" is used interchangeably with preparedness.

  (i) The term "prevention" refers to activities undertaken by the first responder community during the early stages of an incident to reduce the likelihood or consequences of threatened or actual terrorist attacks. More general and broader efforts to deter, disrupt, or thwart terrorism are not addressed in this directive.

  (j) The term "Secretary" means the Secretary of Homeland Security.

  (k) The terms "State," and "local government," when used in a geographical sense, have the same meanings given to those terms in section 2 of the Homeland Security Act of 2002 (6 U.S.C. 101).

Relationship to HSPD-5

(3) This directive is a companion to HSPD-5, which identifies steps for improved coordination in response to incidents. This directive describes the way Federal departments and agencies will prepare for such a response, including prevention activities during the early stages of a terrorism incident.

Development of a National Preparedness Goal

(4) The Secretary is the principal Federal official for coordinating the implementation of all-hazards preparedness in the United States. In cooperation with other Federal departments and agencies, the Secretary coordinates the preparedness of Federal response assets, and the support for, and assessment of, the preparedness of State and local first responders.

(5) To help ensure the preparedness of the Nation to prevent, respond to, and recover from threatened and actual domestic terrorist attacks, major disasters, and other emergencies, the Secretary, in coordination with the heads of other appropriate Federal departments and agencies and in consultation with State and local governments, shall develop a national domestic all-hazards preparedness goal. Federal departments and agencies will work to achieve this goal by:

(a) providing for effective, efficient, and timely delivery of Federal preparedness assistance to State and local governments; and

(b) supporting efforts to ensure first responders are prepared to respond to major events, especially prevention of and response to threatened terrorist attacks.

(6) The national preparedness goal will establish measurable readiness priorities and targets that appropriately balance the potential threat and magnitude of terrorist attacks, major disasters, and other emergencies with the resources required to prevent, respond to, and recover from them. It will also include readiness metrics and elements that support the national preparedness goal including standards for preparedness assessments and strategies, and a system for assessing the Nation's overall preparedness to respond to major events, especially those involving acts of terrorism.

(7) The Secretary will submit the national preparedness goal to me through the Homeland Security Council (HSC) for review and approval prior to, or concurrently with, the Department of Homeland Security's Fiscal Year 2006 budget submission to the Office of Management and Budget.

Federal Preparedness Assistance

(8) The Secretary, in coordination with the Attorney General, the Secretary of Health and Human Services (HHS), and the heads of other Federal departments and agencies that provide assistance for first responder preparedness, will establish a single point of access to Federal preparedness assistance program information within 60 days of the issuance of this directive. The Secretary will submit to me through the HSC recommendations of specific Federal department and agency programs to be part of the coordinated approach. All Federal departments and agencies will cooperate with this effort. Agencies will continue to issue financial assistance awards consistent with applicable laws and regulations and will ensure that program announcements, solicitations, application instructions, and other guidance documents are consistent with other Federal preparedness programs to the extent possible. Full implementation of a closely coordinated interagency grant process will be completed by September 30, 2005.

(9) To the extent permitted by law, the primary mechanism for delivery of Federal preparedness assistance will be awards to the States. Awards will be delivered in a form that allows the recipients to apply the assistance to the highest priority preparedness requirements at the appropriate level of government. To the extent permitted by law, Federal preparedness assistance will be predicated on adoption of Statewide comprehensive all-hazards preparedness strategies. The strategies should be consistent with the national preparedness goal, should assess the most effective ways to enhance preparedness, should address areas facing higher risk, especially to terrorism, and should also address local government concerns and Citizen Corps efforts. The Secretary, in coordination with the heads of other appropriate Federal departments and agencies, will review and approve strategies submitted by the States. To the extent permitted by law, adoption of approved Statewide strategies will be a requirement for receiving Federal preparedness assistance at all levels of government by September 30, 2005.

(10) In making allocations of Federal preparedness assistance to the States, the Secretary, the Attorney General, the Secretary of HHS, the Secretary of Transportation, the Secretary of Energy, the Secretary of Veterans Affairs, the Administrator of the Environmental Protection Agency, and the heads of other Federal departments and agencies that provide assistance for first responder preparedness will base those allocations on assessments of population concentrations, critical infrastructures, and other significant risk factors, particularly terrorism threats, to the extent permitted by law.

(11) Federal preparedness assistance will support State and local entities' efforts including planning, training, exercises, interoperability, and equipment acquisition for major events as well as capacity building for prevention activities such as information gathering, detection, deterrence, and collaboration related to terrorist attacks. Such assistance is not primarily intended to support existing capacity to address normal local first responder operations, but to build capacity to address major events, especially terrorism.

(12) The Attorney General, the Secretary of HHS, the Secretary of Transportation, the Secretary of Energy, the Secretary of Veterans Affairs, the Administrator of the Environmental Protection Agency, and the heads of other Federal departments and agencies that provide assistance for first responder preparedness shall coordinate with the Secretary to ensure that such assistance supports and is consistent with the national preparedness goal.

(13) Federal departments and agencies will develop appropriate mechanisms to ensure rapid obligation and disbursement of funds from their programs to the States, from States to the local community level, and from local entities to the end users to derive maximum benefit from the assistance provided. Federal departments and agencies will report annually to the Secretary on the obligation, expenditure status, and the use of funds associated with Federal preparedness assistance programs.

Equipment

(14) The Secretary, in coordination with State and local officials, first responder organizations, the private sector and other Federal civilian departments and agencies, shall establish and implement streamlined procedures for the ongoing development and adoption of appropriate first responder equipment standards that support nationwide interoperability and other capabilities consistent with the national preparedness goal, including the safety and health of first responders.

(15) To the extent permitted by law, equipment purchased through Federal preparedness assistance for first responders shall conform to equipment standards in place at time of purchase. Other Federal departments and agencies that support the purchase of first responder equipment will coordinate their programs with the Department of Homeland Security and conform to the same standards.

(16) The Secretary, in coordination with other appropriate Federal departments and agencies and in consultation with State and local governments, will develop plans to identify and address national first responder equipment research and development needs based upon assessments of current and future threats. Other Federal departments and agencies that support preparedness research and development activities shall coordinate their efforts with the Department of Homeland Security and ensure they support the national preparedness goal.

Training and Exercises

(17) The Secretary, in coordination with the Secretary of HHS, the Attorney General, and other appropriate Federal departments and agencies and in consultation with State and local governments, shall establish and maintain a comprehensive training program to meet the national preparedness goal. The program will identify standards and maximize the effectiveness of existing Federal programs and financial assistance and include training for the Nation's first responders, officials, and others with major event preparedness, prevention, response, and recovery roles. Federal departments and agencies shall include private organizations in the accreditation and delivery of preparedness training as appropriate and to the extent permitted by law.

(18) The Secretary, in coordination with other appropriate Federal departments and agencies, shall establish a national program and a multi-year planning system to conduct homeland security preparedness-related exercises that reinforces identified training standards, provides for evaluation of readiness, and supports the national preparedness goal. The establishment and maintenance of the program will be conducted in maximum collaboration with State and local governments and appropriate private sector entities. All Federal departments and agencies that conduct national homeland security preparedness-related exercises shall participate in a collaborative, interagency process to designate such exercises on a consensus basis and create a master exercise calendar. The Secretary will ensure that exercises included in the calendar support the national preparedness goal. At the time of designation, Federal departments and agencies will identify their level of participation in national homeland security preparedness-related exercises. The Secretary will develop a multi-year national homeland security preparedness-related exercise plan and submit the plan to me through the HSC for review and approval.

(19) The Secretary shall develop and maintain a system to collect, analyze, and disseminate lessons learned, best practices, and information from exercises, training events, research, and other sources, including actual incidents, and establish procedures to improve national preparedness to prevent, respond to, and recover from major events. The Secretary, in coordination with other Federal departments and agencies and State and local governments, will identify relevant classes of homeland-security related information and appropriate means of transmission for the information to be included in the system. Federal departments and agencies are directed, and State and local governments are requested, to provide this information to the Secretary to the extent permitted by law.

Federal Department and Agency Preparedness

(20) The head of each Federal department or agency shall undertake actions to support the national preparedness goal, including adoption of quantifiable performance measurements in the areas of training, planning, equipment, and exercises for Federal incident management and asset preparedness, to the extent permitted by law. Specialized Federal assets such as teams, stockpiles, and caches shall be maintained at levels consistent with the national preparedness goal and be available for response activities as set forth in the National Response Plan, other appropriate operational documents, and applicable authorities or guidance. Relevant Federal regulatory requirements should be consistent with the national preparedness goal. Nothing in this directive shall limit the authority of the Secretary of Defense with regard to the command and control, training, planning, equipment, exercises, or employment of Department of Defense forces, or the allocation of Department of Defense resources.

(21) The Secretary, in coordination with other appropriate Federal civilian departments and agencies, shall develop and maintain a Federal response capability inventory that includes the performance parameters of the capability, the timeframe within which the capability can be brought to bear on an incident, and the readiness of such capability to respond to domestic incidents. The Department of Defense will provide to the Secretary information describing the organizations and functions within the Department of Defense that may be utilized to provide support to civil authorities during a domestic crisis.

Citizen Participation

(22) The Secretary shall work with other appropriate Federal departments and agencies as well as State and local governments and the private sector to encourage active citizen participation and involvement in preparedness efforts. The Secretary shall periodically review and identify the best community practices for integrating private citizen capabilities into local preparedness efforts.

Public Communication

(23) The Secretary, in consultation with other Federal departments and agencies, State and local governments, and non-governmental organizations, shall develop a comprehensive plan to provide accurate and timely preparedness information to public citizens, first responders, units of government, the private sector, and other interested parties and mechanisms for coordination at all levels of government.

Assessment and Evaluation

(24) The Secretary shall provide to me through the Assistant to the President for Homeland Security an annual status report of the Nation's level of preparedness, including State capabilities, the readiness of Federal civil response assets, the utilization of mutual aid, and an assessment of how the Federal first responder preparedness assistance programs support the national preparedness goal. The first report will be provided within 1 year of establishment of the national preparedness goal.

(25) Nothing in this directive alters, or impedes the ability to carry out, the authorities of the Federal departments and agencies to perform their responsibilities under law and consistent with applicable legal authorities and presidential guidance.

(26) Actions pertaining to the funding and administration of financial assistance and all other activities, efforts, and policies in this directive shall be executed in accordance with law. To the extent permitted by law, these policies will be established and carried out in consultation with State and local governments.

(27) This directive is intended only to improve the internal management of the executive branch of the Federal Government, and it is not intended to, and does not, create any right or benefit, substantive or procedural, enforceable at law or in equity, against the United States, its departments, agencies, or other entities, its officers or employees, or any other person.

GEORGE W. BUSH

Letter from the Department of Homeland Security

Secretary

U.S. Department of Homeland Security
Washington, DC 20528

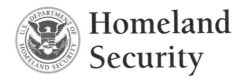

Homeland
Security

December 18, 2008

Dear NIMS Stakeholders:

Homeland Security Presidential Directive (HSPD)-5, *Management of Domestic Incidents*, directed the development and administration of the National Incident Management System (NIMS). Originally issued on March 1, 2004, by the Department of Homeland Security (DHS), NIMS provides a consistent nationwide template to enable Federal, State[1], tribal, and local[2] governments, nongovernmental organizations (NGOs), and the private sector to work together to prevent, protect against, respond to, recover from, and mitigate the effects of incidents, regardless of cause, size, location, or complexity.

HSPD-5 also required DHS to establish a mechanism for ongoing coordination to provide strategic direction for, and oversight of, NIMS. The National Integration Center's (NIC) Incident Management Systems Integration Division (IMSI)—formerly the NIMS Integration Center—was established to support both routine maintenance and the continuous refinement of NIMS.

Since 2006, the NIMS document has been revised to incorporate best practices and lessons learned from recent incidents. The NIMS revision also clarifies concepts and principles, and refines processes and terminology throughout the document. A wide range of feedback was incorporated while maintaining the core concepts of NIMS and no major policy changes were made to the document during the revision. Below is a summary of changes to the NIMS document:

- Eliminated redundancy;
- Reorganized document to emphasize that NIMS is more than the Incident Command System (ICS);
- Clarified ICS concepts;
- Increased emphasis on planning and added guidance on mutual aid;
- Clarified roles of private sector, NGOs, and chief elected and appointed officials;
- Expanded the Intelligence/Investigation function; and
- Highlighted relationship between NIMS and National Response Framework.

I ask for your continued assistance as we implement NIMS. I look forward to continuing our collective efforts to better secure the homeland and protect our citizens. Thank you for your hard work in this important endeavor.

Sincerely,

Michael Chertoff

---

[1] As defined in the Homeland Security Act of 2002 P.L. 107-296, the term "State" means "any State of the United States, the District of Columbia, the Commonwealth of Puerto Rico, Guam, American Samoa, the Commonwealth of the Northern Mariana Islands, and any possession of the United States." 6 U.S.C. 101 (14)

[2] As defined in the Homeland Security Act of 2002, Section 2 (10): the term "local government" means "(A) county, municipality, city, town, township, local public authority, school district, special district, intrastate district, council of governments . . . regional or interstate government entity, or agency or instrumentality of a local government: an Indian tribe or authorized tribal organization, or in Alaska a Native village or Alaska Regional Native Corporation: and a rural community, unincorporated town or village, or other public entity." 6 U.S.C. 101 (10)

Homeland Security Terror Alert Chart

The US Department of Homeland Security Advisory System is posted daily to heighten awareness of the current terrorist threat. The threat levels are color coded as follows:

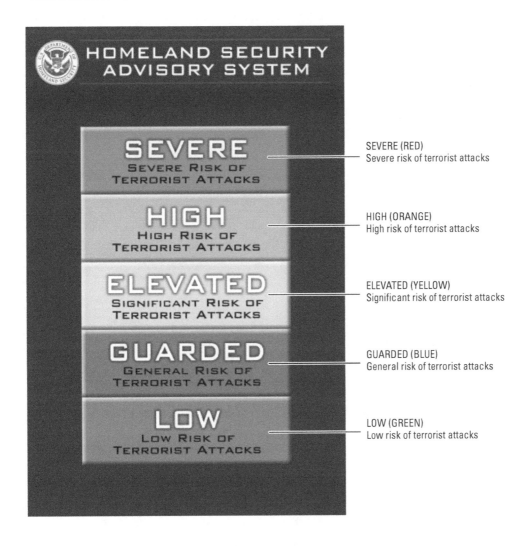

209

ICS Forms

Initial Briefing

ICS 201
Cover Page

Incident Name:		Date Prepared:	Time Prepared:

Operational Period Date: From: To:	Operational Period Time: From: To:

Required Forms: (Checked Required Forms are Attached)

☐ Incident Map ICS 201-1   ☐ Current Organization ICS 201-3
☐ Summary of Current Actions ICS 201-2   ☐ Resources Summary ICS 201-4

Support Forms: (Checked Support Forms are Attached)

☐ Fire & Safety Control Analysis ICS 201-5   ☐ Site Assessment ICS 201-7
☐ Meteorological Data ICS 201-6   ☐ Tanker Information ICS 201-8
☐ _____   ☐ _____

Weather Forecast for Operational Period:

_____

_____

Projected Wind Chill	Tides		Daylight		Air Temperature		Wind	
Degrees (°F):	High(s):	Low(s):	Sunrise:	Sunset:	High(s):	Low(s):	Speed:	Direction:

Cooling Power of Wind Expressed as "Equivalent Chill Temperature"

Wind	Speed	Temperature (°F)																				
Knots	MPH																					
Calm	Calm	40	35	30	25	20	15	10	5	0	–5	–10	–15	–20	–25	–30	–35	–40	–45-	–50	–55	–60
		Equivalent Chill Temperature																				
3–6	5	35	30	25	20	15	10	5	0	–5	–10	–15	–20	–25	–30	–35	–40	–45	–50	–55	–65	–70
7–10	10	30	20	15	10	5	0	–10	–15	–20	–25	–35	–40	–45	–50	–60	–60	–70	–75	–80	–90	–95
11–15	15	25	15	10	0	–5	–10	–20	–25	–30	–40	–45	–50	–60	–65	–70	–80	–85	–90	–100	–105	–110
16–19	20	20	10	5	0	–10	–15	–25	–30	–35	–45	–50	–60	–65	–75	–80	–85	–95	–100	–110	–115	–120
20–32	25	15	10	0	–5	–20	–20	–30	–35	–45	–50	–60	–65	–75	–80	–90	–95	–105	–110	–120	–125	–135
24–28	30	10	5	0	–10	–25	–25	–30	–40	–50	–55	–65	–70	–80	–85	–95	–100	–110	–115	–125	–130	–140
29–32	35	10	5	–5	–10	–30	–30	–35	–40	–50	–60	–65	–75	–80	–90	–100	–105	–115	–120	–130	–135	–145
33–36	40	10	0	–5	–10	–20-	–30	–35	–45	–55	–60	–70	–75	–85	–95	–100	–110	–115	–125	–130	–140	–150

Winds above 40°F have little additional effect	Little Danger	Increasing Danger (Flesh may freeze within 1 minute)	Great Danger (Flesh may freeze within 30 seconds)

Comments:

Prepared By:	Company Name:	ICS Position:
Approved By:	Company Name:	ICS Position:

Incident Briefing

ICS 201

Incident Name:	Date Prepared:	Time Prepared:
Operational Period:	Operational Period Date/Time: From:	To:

INCIDENT LOCATION:

MAP ATTACHED?   Yes _____   No _____

BRIEF SUMMARY OF INCIDENT:

CURRENT/COMPLETED ACTIONS:

CURRENT ORGANIZATION:

RESOURCES SUMMARY: (Type, Number, ETA, Location/Assignment) (Leave Blank if ICS 204 Attached)

Prepared By: **(Name/Title)**	**Approved by** **EOC Director:**

ICS 201 (07/25/2005)

212   NATIONAL INCIDENT MANAGEMENT SYSTEM: Principles and Practice, Second Edition

Initial Briefing

Incident Name:		Date Prepared:	Time Prepared:

Operational Period Date: From: To:	Operational Period Time: From: To:

Describe Incident:

_____

_____

_____

_____

_____

_____

_____

_____

_____

_____

_____

_____

_____

Preliminary Incident Objectives:

_____

_____

_____

_____

_____

_____

_____

_____

_____

_____

_____

_____

_____

_____

_____

_____

_____

Prepared By:	Company Name:	ICS Position:
Approved By:	Company Name:	ICS Position:

ICS 201-2 (9/95)

Initial Briefing

Incident Name:		Date Prepared	Time Prepared:

| Operational Period Date:
From: To: | | Operational Period Time:
From: To | |

```
                    ┌──────────────┐   ┌────────────────────┐   ┌──────────────┐
                    │    State     │   │ Incident Commander │   │   Federal    │
                    │              │   │                    │   │              │
                    └──────────────┘   └────────────────────┘   └──────────────┘

            ┌─────────────────────┐                    ┌──────────────────────────┐
            │    Legal Officer    │                    │ Public Information Officer │
            │                     │                    │                            │
            └─────────────────────┘                    └──────────────────────────┘

            ┌─────────────────────┐                    ┌──────────────────────────┐
            │    Safety Officer   │                    │      Liaison Officer       │
            │                     │                    │                            │
            └─────────────────────┘                    └──────────────────────────┘

                    ┌──────────────────────────┐       ┌──────────────────────────┐
                    │ Deputy Incident Commander │       │      Security Officer      │
                    │                           │       │                            │
                    └──────────────────────────┘       └──────────────────────────┘

    ┌─────────────────┐  ┌─────────────────┐  ┌─────────────────┐  ┌─────────────────┐
    │ Operations Chief│  │   Plans Chief   │  │ Logistics Chief │  │  Finance Chief  │
    │                 │  │                 │  │                 │  │                 │
    └─────────────────┘  └─────────────────┘  └─────────────────┘  └─────────────────┘
```

Prepared By:	Company Name:	ICS Position:
Approved By:	Company Name:	ICS Position:

Initial Briefing

Incident Name:				Date Prepared:	Time Prepared:

Operational Period Date: From: To:				Operational Period Time: From: To:	

Local Resources Ordered/Source	Quantity	Time Ordered	ETA Day/Hour	Current Location/Assignment

Prepared By:	Company Name:	ICS Position:
Approved By:	Company Name:	ICS Position:

ICS 201-4 (9/95)

Initial Briefing

ICS 201-5
Site Safety and Control Analysis

Incident Name:	Date Prepared:	Time Prepared:

Operational Period Date: From: To:	Operational Period Time: From: To:

1. Wind Direction Across Incident: ❏ Towards Your Position ❏ Away From Your Position

2. Are people injured or trapped? Injured ❏ Yes ❏ No   Trapped ❏ Yes ❏ No

3. Are people involved as unorganized observers or involved in rescue attempts? Observers ❏ Yes ❏ No   Rescuers ❏ Yes ❏ No

4. Are there any immediate signs of potential hazards:

   a. Electrical line down or overhead? ❏ Yes ❏ No

   b. Unidentified liquid or solid products visible? ❏ Yes ❏ No

   c. Colored vapors visible? ❏ Yes ❏ No

   d. Smells which are not natural noted? ❏ Yes ❏ No

   e. Fire, sparks nearby, sources of ignition present? ❏ Yes ❏ No

   f. Holes, caverns, deep ditches, fast moving water, cliffs nearby? ❏ Yes ❏ No

   g. Is local traffic a potential problem? ❏ Yes ❏ No

   h. Signs, placards, or color codes indicating danger? ❏ Yes ❏ No

   i. Spill zone ❏ Dry ❏ Yes ❏ No

5. As you approach the scene from the upwind side, do you note a change in status of any of the above? ❏ Yes ❏ No

6. Have you established control of the area involved in the incident? ❏ Yes ❏ No

7. Have you determined the necessity for any of the following:

   a. Security? ❏ Yes ❏ No

   b. Hazardous material identified. Being monitored? ❏ Yes ❏ No

   c. Protective gear and to what level of protection? _____ ❏ Yes ❏ No

   d. Site for decontamination center? ❏ Yes ❏ No

   e. Site for command center? ❏ Yes ❏ No

   f. Safety equipment you will need to eliminate the problems? ❏ Yes ❏ No

   g. Placement of the warning sign? (i.e., benzene, no smoking, etc.) ❏ Yes ❏ No

   h. Number of personnel needed to control the situation? _____ ❏ Yes ❏ No

8. Entry Objectives: | Description:

9. a. Decontamination Equipment and Materials Required: | Description:

   b. Emergency Decontamination Instructions:

   c. Personal Protective Equipment:

   ❏ A. To be selected when greatest level of skin, respiratory, and eye protection is needed.
   ❏ B. To be selected when highest level of respiratory protection is needed, but lesser level of skin protection is needed (SCBA).
   ❏ C. To be selected when concentrations and types of airborne substances are known and the criteria for using air purifying respirators are met.
   ❏ D. To be selected when the atmosphere contains no known hazard; and work functions preclude splashes, immersion, or potential for unexpected inhalation of or contact with hazardous levels of any chemicals.

Page 1 of 2

216 NATIONAL INCIDENT MANAGEMENT SYSTEM: Principles and Practice, Second Edition

Initial Briefing

Incident Name:	Date Prepared:	Time Prepared:
Operational Period Date: From: To:	Operational Period Time: From: To:	

10. Emergency Escape Route:	Description:	
11. a. Sampling Equipment Listed:	(Combustible gas indicator, O_2 monitor, colonmetric tubes (type) HNU/OVA, etc.)	
b. Sample Frequency:	(Indicate continuous, hourly, daily, other)	
12. Personal Monitoring:	(Describe any personal sampling programs being carried out on site personnel)	
13. Medical Monitoring:	(Describe procedures in effect, i.e., monitoring body temperature, body weight, pulse rate, etc.)	

14. Remarks

_____

_____

_____

_____

_____

_____

_____

_____

_____

_____

1. Before entering a potentially hazardous work environment, IT MUST BE EVALUATED BY A COMPETENT PERSON to establish safe work practices, personal protective equipment, and other control procedures. As a minimum lower explosive limit (LEL), Oxygen and Benzene levels must be evaluated.
2. Spill cleanup areas shall be controlled as "regulated areas." If Benzene vapors are or may be expected to equal the action level of 0.5 ppm, then the area must be posted with the following warning:

Danger
Benzene Cancer Hazard
Flammable—No Smoking
Authorized Personnel Only
Respirator Required

Prepared By:	Company Name:	ICS Position: On-Site Safety Unit Leader
Approved By:	Company Name:	ICS Position:

Initial Briefing

Incident Name:	Date Prepared:	Time Prepared:

Operational Period Date: From: To:	Operational Period Time: From: To:

State of the Weather:
Visibility:
Waves Height and Period:
Surface Current:
Weather Forecast for Next 24 Hours:
Latitude/Longitude of Weather Station:
Sea Temperature:
Air Temperature:
Tide Movement:
Ice Problems:
Sunrise/Sunset:

General Information

Prepared By:	Company Name:	ICS Position:
Approved By:	Company Name:	ICS Position:

ICS 201-6 (9/95)

Initial Briefing

ICS 201-7
Initial Site Assessment

Incident Name:	Date Prepared:	Time Prepared:

Operational Period Date: From: To: | **Operational Period Time:** From: To:

Safe Approach Possible?
☐ Yes ☐ No

Injuries?
☐ Yes ☐ No | **Description of Injuries:**

Spill Location:

Type of Substance:

Source of Spill: (Valve, break in line, rupture, truck, and/or vessel)

_____

_____

Estimated Spill Volume:	Estimated Spill Rate:
Weather:	Wind Speed:	Wind Direction:

Cause: (Unknown, accident, sabotage, corrosion and/or other)

_____

_____

Current Situation Narrative: (Brief)

Direction of oil movement _____

Description of contaminated area _____

Proximity to sensitive areas _____

Nearest access _____

Equipment involved _____

Additional information _____

Suggested Response Equipment:

_____

_____

Response Action Taken:

_____

_____

Reconnaissance Boxes:

Prepared By:	Company Name:	ICS Position:
Approved By:	Company Name:	ICS Position:

ICS 201-7 (9/95)

Incident Objectives, ICS Form 202

INCIDENT OBJECTIVES	1. INCIDENT NAME	2. DATE	3. TIME

4. OPERATIONAL PERIOD (DATE/TIME)

5. GENERAL CONTROL OBJECTIVES FOR THE INCIDENT (INCLUDE ALTERNATIVES)

6. WEATHER FORECAST FOR OPERATIONAL PERIOD

7. GENERAL SAFETY MESSAGE

8. Attachments (☑ if attached)

☐ Organization List (ICS 203)   ☐ Medical Plan (ICS 206)   ☐ Weather Forecast

☐ Assignment List (ICS 204)   ☐ Incident Map   ☐ _____

☐ Communications Plan (ICS 205)   ☐ Traffic Plan   ☐ _____

9. PREPARED BY (PLANNING SECTION CHIEF)	10. APPROVED BY (INCIDENT COMMANDER)

Organization Assignment List, ICS Form 203

ORGANIZATION ASSIGMENT LIST		1. INCIDENT NAME	2. DATE PREPARED	3. TIME PREPARED
POSITION	**NAME**	**4. OPERATIONAL PERIOD (DATE/TIME)**		

5. INCIDENT COMMAND AND STAFF		**9. OPERATIONS SECTION**	
INCIDENT COMMANDER		CHIEF	
DEPUTY		DEPUTY	
SAFETY OFFICER		a. BRANCH I- DIVISION/GROUPS	
INFORMATION OFFICER		BRANCH DIRECTOR	
LIAISON OFFICER		DEPUTY	
		DIVISION/GROUP	
6. AGENCY REPRESENTATIVES		DIVISION/ GROUP	
AGENCY	**NAME**	DIVISION/ GROUP	
		DIVISION/GROUP	
		DIVISION /GROUP	
		b. BRANCH II- DIVISIONS/GROUPS	
		BRANCH DIRECTOR	
		DEPUTY	
		DIVISION/GROUP	
7. PLANNING SECTION		DIVISION/GROUP	
CHIEF		DIVISION/GROUP	
DEPUTY		DIVISION/GROUP	
RESOURCES UNIT			
SITUATION UNIT		c. BRANCH III- DIVISIONS/GROUPS	
DOCUMENTATION UNIT		BRANCH DIRECTOR	
DEMOBILIZATION UNIT		DEPUTY	
TECHNICAL SPECIALISTS		DIVISION/GROUP	
		DIVISION/GROUP	
		DIVISION/GROUP	
8. LOGISTICS SECTION		d. AIR OPERATIONS BRANCH	
CHIEF		AIR OPERATIONS BR. DIR.	
DEPUTY		AIR TACTICAL GROUP SUP.	
		AIR SUPPORT GROUP SUP.	
		HELICOPTER COORDINATOR	
a. SUPPORT BRANCH		AIR TANKER/FIXED WING CRD.	
DIRECTOR			
SUPPLY UNIT			
FACILITIES UNIT			
GROUND SUPPORT UNIT		**10. FINANCE/ADMINISTRATION SECTION**	
		CHIEF	
		DEPUTY	
b. SERVICE BRANCH		TIME UNIT	
DIRECTOR		PROCUREMENT UNIT	
COMMUNICATIONS UNIT		COMPENSATION/CLAIMS UNIT	
MEDICAL UNIT		COST UNIT	
FOOD UNIT			

PREPARED BY (RESOURCES UNIT)

Assignment List, ICS Form 204

1. BRANCH	2. DIVISION/GROUP	**ASSIGNMENT LIST**

3. INCIDENT NAME	4. OPERATIONAL PERIOD
	DATE _____ TIME _____

5. OPERATIONAL PERSONNEL

OPERATIONS CHIEF _____ DIVISION/GROUP SUPERVISOR _____

BRANCH DIRECTOR _____ AIR TACTICAL GROUP SUPERVISOR _____

6. RESOURCES ASSIGNED TO THIS PERIOD

STRIKE TEAM/TASK FORCE/ RESOURCE DESIGNATOR	EMT	LEADER	NUMBER PERSONS	TRANS. NEEDED	PICKUP PT./TIME	DROP OFF PT./TIME

7. CONTROL OPERATIONS

8. SPECIAL INSTRUCTIONS

9. DIVISION/GROUP COMMUNICATIONS SUMMARY

FUNCTION		FREQ.	SYSTEM	CHAN.	FUNCTION		FREQ.	SYSTEM	CHAN.
COMMAND	LOCAL				SUPPORT	LOCAL			
	REPEAT					REPEAT			
DIV./GROUP TACTICAL					GROUND TO AIR				

PREPARED BY (RESOURCE UNIT LEADER)	APPROVED BY (PLANNING SECT. CH.)	DATE	TIME

EOC REQUEST / TASK ASSIGNMENT

ICS 204-1

Incident Name:	OP #:	24 Hr. Time:	Date:

REQUEST FOR SUPPORT	Completed by Request Handler	Forward to EOC Director

Name/Title:

Contact Information: (Telephone / fax, e-mail, etc.)

Organization:

Details of Request   *(Who, what, where, when, why, and how)*   *(Initial Actions and Coordination)*

Request Handler (Name/Position):

OBJECTIVE / ASSIGNMENT	Completed by EOC Director or Designee	Original to Assignee / Duplicate to Planning Section

Work Unit Information   *(Section, Unit, Branch, Agency)*

Assigned to:

Coordinate with:

Control Operations   *(Include Special Instructions)*

Prepared By: (Name/Title)	**Approved by EOC Director:**

IMPLEMENTATION	**NUMBER**	Completed by Work Unit / Assignee	Forward to EOC Director Upon Completion

(Date/Time & Initial All Entries) (Attach all coordination documents)

FINAL DISPOSITION / CLOSEOUT	Completed by EOC Director	Forward to Planning Section Upon Completion

Date / Time Closed: **EOC Director Signature:**

ICS 204-1 (07/25/2005)

Incident Action Plan

ICS 204-2
Task Force/Strike Teams Personnel

Incident Name:		Date Prepared:	Time Prepared:
Operational Period Date: From: To:		Operational Period Time: From: To:	
Division: (Alpha/Numeric Designation)	Group: (Alpha/Numeric Designation)	❐ Air Ops ❐ Nearshore ❐ Offshore ❐ Onshore ❐ On Land	

Operation Personnel Assigned This Period

Operations Chief:	Division/Group Leader:
Branch Director:	Location Assigned:

Resources Assigned This Period (Task Force and Strike Teams)

	Personnel				
Task Force Strike Team	Name	Badge No.	Transportation Needed Yes No	Drop Off/Pick Up Time	Pick Up/Drop Off Time

Prepared By:	Company Name:	ICS Position:
Approved By:	Company Name:	ICS Position:

ICS 204-2 (9/95)

Incident Communications Plan, ICS Form 205

INCIDENT RADIO COMMUNICATIONS PLAN	1. Incident Name	2. Date/Time Prepared	3. Operational Period Date/Time

4. Basic Radio Channel Utilization					
System/Cache	Channel	Function	Frequency/Tone	Assignment	Remarks

5. Prepared by (Communications Unit)

Incident Action Plan

EOC Positions/Phone Numbers

ICS 205-1

Incident Name:		Date Prepared:		Time Prepared:	
Operational Period:		Operational Period Date/Time: From:		To:	

Position	Name	Phone	Pager	Email
EOC Director				
Public Information Officer				
Alternate Public Information Officer				
Operations Section Chief				
Deputy Operations Chief				
Planning Section Chief				
Situation Unit Leader				
Technical Specialist				
Logistics Section Chief				
Support Branch				
Communications Center				
Communications Center				
Communications Center				
Finance Section Chief				
Recovery Unit Leader				

Prepared By: (Name/Title)	Approved by EOC Director:

ICS 205-1 (07/25/2005)

Incident Action Plan

Incident Name:	Date Prepared:	Time Prepared:
Operational Period Date: From: To:	Operational Period Time: From: To:	

Incident Medical Aid Stations

Medical Aid Station	Telephone/Radio	Location	EMT	ETT

Transportation (Assigned/Stanby Ambulance Services)

Name	Telephone/Radio	Address	Ground	Air	Doctor	Nurse	EMT	ETT

Ambulance Services In Addition to Above				
Name	Telephone/Radio	Location	EMT	ETT

Hospitals

Name	Telephone/Radio	Address	Travel Time		Helipad (Y/N)	Burn Center (Y/N)
			Ground	Air		

Medical Emergency Procedures

Prepared By:	Company Name:	ICS Position: **Medical Unit Leader**
Approved By:	Company Name:	ICS Position: **Safety Officer**

ICS 206 (9/95)

Incident Organization Chart

ICS 207

Incident Name:	Date Prepared:	Time Prepared:
Operational Period:	Operational Period Date/Time:	From:	To:

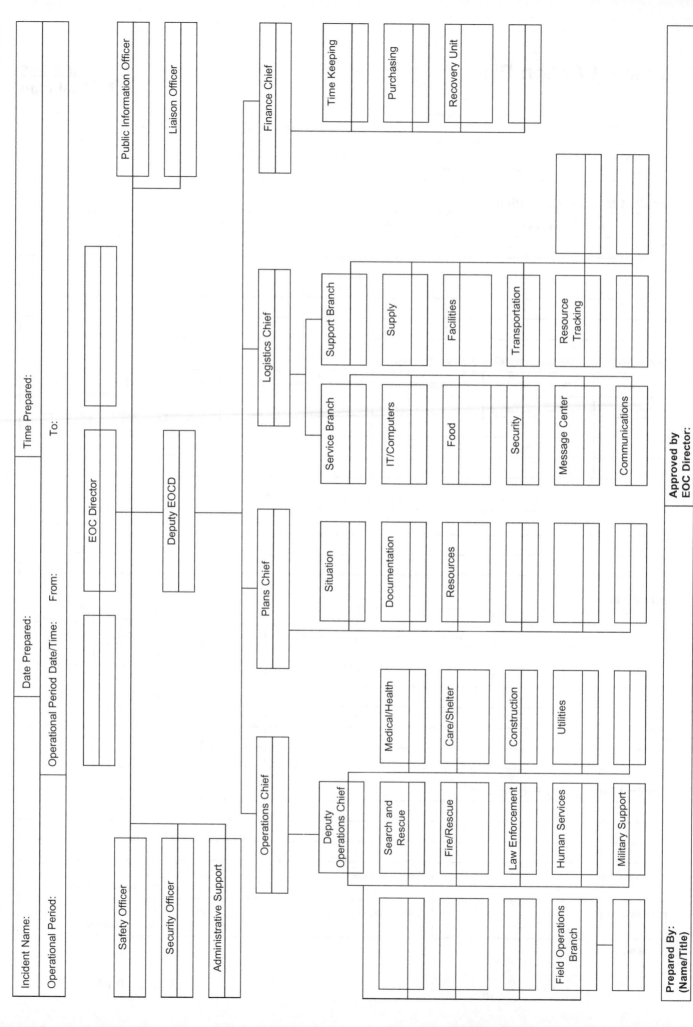

- EOC Director
  - Public Information Officer
  - Liaison Officer
  - Safety Officer
  - Security Officer
  - Administrative Support
- Deputy EOCD
  - Operations Chief
    - Deputy Operations Chief
      - Search and Rescue
      - Fire/Rescue
      - Law Enforcement
      - Human Services
      - Military Support
      - Medical/Health
      - Care/Shelter
      - Construction
      - Utilities
      - Field Operations Branch
  - Plans Chief
    - Situation
    - Documentation
    - Resources
  - Logistics Chief
    - Service Branch
      - IT/Computers
      - Food
      - Security
      - Message Center
      - Communications
    - Support Branch
      - Supply
      - Facilities
      - Transportation
      - Resource Tracking
  - Finance Chief
    - Time Keeping
    - Purchasing
    - Recovery Unit

Prepared By:
(Name/Title)

Approved by
EOC Director:

ICS 207 (07/25/2005)

Incident Schedule of Meetings/Events

ICS 208

Incident Name:		Date Prepared:	Time Prepared:

Operational Period:	Operational Period Date/Time:	From:	To:

Time	Meeting/Event	Location	Attendance
0000			
0100			
0200			
0300			
0400			
0500			
0600			
0700			
0800			
0900			
1000			
1100			
1200			
1300			
1400			
1500			
1600			
1700			
1800			
1900			
2000			
2100			
2200			
2300			
2400			

Prepared By: (Name/Title)	Approved by EOC Director:

ICS 208 (07/25/2005)

Incident Action Plan

Incident Name:		Date Prepared:		Time Prepared:

Operational Period Date: From: To:		Operational Period Time: From: To:	

Incident Commander		Cost Center	
Location		Spiller	
Type of Incident (P/L, Marine, Terminal, Tundra, etc.)		Vessel Name	
Incident Start Date/Time		Cause	

Oil Status (Estimated)

Disposition	Previous Total +	Last 12 Hr. =	Total
Total Oil Lost			
Recovered Liquids			
Evaporation			
Natural Dispersion			
Chemical Dispersion			
Burned			
Uncontained			
OnShore			
Offshore			

Offshore Equipment Resources

Type	Previous Total +	Last 12 Hr. =	Total
Boom Deployed (Field)			
Pressure Washers			
Vacuum Trucks			
Bioremediation (Sq. Feet)			
Booms (Total Feet)			
Snare Boom (Total Feet)			
Skimmers (Total)			
Vessels/Boats (Total)			

Waste Management (List Quantities in BBLS./Yards)

Type	Recovered	Stored	Recovered
Oil			
Oily Liquids			
Liquids			
Oily Solids			
Solids			
Hazardous			

Manpower Resources

Affiliation	Inc. Command Post	Field
Response Spec.		
Contract		
Others		
Total		

Shoreline Impacts

Degree of Oiling	Total Miles Affected	Total Miles Treated
Response Spec.		
Contract		
Others		
Total		

Meteorology Forecast: Next Operational Period

Wind Direction & Speed	
Temperature	
Wind Chill	
High Tide/Time	
Low Tide/Time	
Long./Lat. of Weather Station	

Companies or Regional Response Centers Commiting Additional Resources

Company/Response Center									Totals
Helicopters									
Aircraft									
Boom									
Skimmers									

Prepared By:		Company Name:		ICS Position:	
Approved By:		Company Name:		ICS Position:	

ICS 209 (9/95)

ICS 209-1
Situation Status Update

Incident Name:	Date Prepared:	Time Prepared:

Operational Period Date: From: To:	Operational Period Time: From: To:

Temperature:	Wind Speed:	Wind Chill:	Visibility:	Water Flow:	Sunrise:	Sunset:

Division:	Task Force:	Division:	Task Force:	Division:	Task Force:
Time:		Time:		Time:	
Progress Summary:		Progress Summary:		Progress Summary:	
Boom Deployed:		Boom Deployed:		Boom Deployed:	
Oil Collected:		Oil Collected:		Oil Collected:	
Safety Concerns:		Safety Concerns:		Safety Concerns:	
Personnel Discrepancies:		Personnel Discrepancies:		Personnel Discrepancies:	
Equipment Discrepancies:		Equipment Discrepancies:		Equipment Discrepancies:	
Task Force Leader:		Task Force Leader:		Task Force Leader:	
Channel No.:		Channel No.:		Channel No.:	

Prepared By:	Company Name:	ICS Position: **Situation Status Unit**
Approved By:	Company Name:	ICS Position:

ICS 209-1 (9/95)

Original: Documents, Copies: OSC, UC's or IC, PIO Liaison Office, and LSC

Incident Action Plan

ICS 209-2 Marine
Situation Status Summary

Incident Name:		Date Prepared:	Time Prepared:

Operational Period Date:
  From: To:
		Operational Period Time:
		  From: To:	

Oil Status Condition

% Emulsion:		Viscosity:	

Estimated Amounts, bbls

Location	Site A	Site B	Total
Total Oil Loss			
Recov'd Liquids			
Dispersed			
Burned			
Slick Size			
Oil Onshore			
Uncontained			
Natural Dispersion			
Chemical Dispersion			
Evaporated Dispersion			

Weather	Current	12 Hr. Frcst	24 Hr. Frcst
Wind Speed			
Wind Direction			
Temperature			
Visibility			
Ceiling			
Tide Time			
Tide Height			
Sunrise/Sunset			
Sea Status			

Resources/Type	Assigned	Available	Arriving, O/S
ERV's			
Tugs			
Fishing Vessels			
Tenders			
Helicopters			
Aircraft			
Boom			
Barges			
Storage Cap Mbbl			
Skimmers			
Skm Cap Mbbl/hr.			
Landing Craft			
Lightering Craft			
Adds Pack			

General Remarks

Pipeline Operations Status

	Yes/No	Current	24 Hr. Frcst
Shipping Lanes Open			
Port Valdez Open			
Tank Space			
Berths in Service			
Berths Occupied			
Taps Flow			
		Time	Date
Shutdown Projected			

People

Affiliation	VEOC	Field	Enroute
Shipper			
Alyeska			
Agencies			
Public/Government			
Observer/Other			
Fish Vessel Crew			
Contractor			
RCAC			
CG			
ADEC			
Shoreline Cleanup			
Total			

Wildlife

Source:			
Type	Dead	Srv'd	Total
Birds			
Sea Lions			
Sea Otters			
Harbor Seals			

Beach Impact	Class	Amount
Light		
Medium		
Heavy		
Total		

Disposal	Amount
Oily Liquids	
Oily Solids	

Tanker Status	
Location:	Activity:

Prepared By:	Company Name:	ICS Position:
Approved By:	Company Name:	ICS Position:

ICS 209-2 (9/95)

RESOURCE STATUS CHANGE (ICS 210)

1. Incident Name:		2. Operational Period: Date From: Date To: Time From: Time To:			
3. Resource Number	**4. New Status** (Available, Assigned, O/S)	**5. From** (Location and Status):	**6. To** (Location and Status):	**7. Time and Date of Location and Resource Status Change:**	

8. Comments:

9. Prepared by: Name: _____   Position/Title: _____ Signature: _____

ICS 210   Date/Time: _____

ICS 210
Resource Status Change

Purpose. The Resource Status Change (ICS 210) is used by the Incident Communications Center Manager to record status change information received on resources assigned to the incident. This information could be transmitted with a General Message (ICS 213). The form could also be used by Operations as a worksheet to track entry, etc.

Preparation. The ICS 210 is completed by radio/telephone operators who receive status change information from individual resources, Task Forces, Strike Teams, and Division/Group Supervisors. Status information could also be reported by Staging Area and Helibase Managers and fixed-wing facilities.

Distribution. The ICS 210 is maintained by the Resources Unit, and a second copy is retained by the Communications Unit.

Notes:
- The ICS 210 is essentially a message form that can be used to update Resource Status Cards or T-Cards (ICS 219) for incident-level resource management.
- If additional pages are needed, use a blank ICS 210 and repaginate as needed.

Block Number	Block Title	Instructions
1	**Incident Name**	Enter the name assigned to the incident.
2	**Operational Period** • Date and Time From • Date and Time To	Enter the start date (month/day/year) and time (using the 24-hour clock) and end date and time for the operational period to which the form applies.
3	**Resource Number**	Enter the resource identification (ID) number (this may be a letter and number combination) assigned by either the sending unit or the incident.
4	**New Status** (Available, Assigned, Out of Service)	Indicate the current status of the resource: • Available—Indicates resource is available for incident use immediately. • Assigned—Indicates resource is checked in and assigned a work task on the incident. • Out of Service—Indicates resource is assigned to the incident but unable to respond for mechanical, rest, or personnel reasons. If space permits, indicate the estimated time of return (ETR). It may be useful to indicate the reason a resource is out of service (e.g., "O/S—Mech" (for mechanical issues), "O/S—Rest" (for off shift), or "O/S—Pers" (for personnel issues).
5	**From** (Location and Status)	Indicate the current location of the resource (where it came from) and the status. When more than one Division, Staging Area, or Camp is used, identify the specific location (e.g., Division A, Staging Area, Incident Command Post, Western Camp).
6	**To** (Location and Status)	Indicate the assigned incident location of the resource and status. When more than one Division, Staging Area, or Camp is used, identify the specific location.
7	**Time and Date of Location and Resource Status Change**	Enter the time and location of the status change (24-hour clock). Enter the date as well if relevant (e.g., out of service).
8	**Comments**	Enter any special information provided by the resource or dispatch center. This may include details about why a resource is out of service, or individual identifying designators (IDs) of Strike Teams and Task Forces.
9	**Prepared by** • Name • Position/Title • Signature • Date/Time	Enter the name, ICS position/title, and signature of the person preparing the form. Enter date (month/day/year) and time prepared (24-hour clock).

Check In/Out Log

ICS 211

| Incident Name: | | Date Prepared: | | Time Prepared: |
| Operational Period: | | Operational Period Date/Time: | From: | To: |

Print Name	Agency	EOC Position	Date	Time In	Time Out

ICS 211 (07/25/2005)

Incident Demobilization Vehicle Safety Inspection

Vehicle Operator: Complete items above double lines prior to inspection

Incident Name		Order No.	
Vehicle: License No.	Agency		Reg/Unit
Type (Eng., Bus., Sedan)	Odometer Reading		Veh. ID No.

Inspection Items	Pass	Fail	Comments
1. Gauges and lights. See back*			
2. Seat belts. See back *			
3. Glass and mirrors. See back *			
4. Wipers and horn. See back *			
5. Engine compartment. See back			
6. Fuel system. See back *			
7. Steering. See back *			
8. Brakes. See back *			
9. Drive line U-joints. Check play			
10. Springs and shocks. See back			
11. Exhaust system. See back *			
12. Frame. See back *			
13. Tire and wheels. See back *			
14. Coupling devices. * Emergency exit (Buses)			
15. Pump Operation			
16. Damage on Incident			
17. Other			

* Safety Item - Do not Release Until Repaired

Additional Comments:

		HOLD FOR REPAIRS				RELEASE	
Date		Time			Date		Time

Inspector Name (Print)	Operator Name (Print)
Inspector Signature	Operator Signature

This form may be photocopied, but three copies must be completed.
Distribution: Original to Inspector, copy to vehicle operator, copy to Incident Documentation Unit

ICS 212

2/96

INSPECTION ITEMS

(REF: FEDERAL MOTOR CARRIER SAFETY REGULATIONS)

HOLD FOR REPAIRS IF:

1.	Gauges & Lights	- Speedometer inoperative. (Federal Motor Carrier Safety Regulation ([FMCSR] 393.82) - All required lighting devices, reflectors and electrical equipment must be properly positioned, colored, and working. (FMCSR 393.9)
2.	Seat Belts	- Any driver's or right outboard seat belt missing or inoperative. (FMCSR 393.93) - Passenger carrying have missing or inoperative seat belts in passenger seats, buses excepted.
3.	Glass & Mirrors	- Any windshield crack over 1/4" wide. - Any damage 3/4" or greater in diameter. - Any 2 damaged areas are closer than 3" to each other. - Any crack less than 1/4" wide intersects with any other crack. (FMCSR 393.60) - Any crack or discoloration in the windshield area lying within the sweep of the wiper on either side of the windshield. (FMCSR Appendix G, Sub. B) - Any required mirror missing. One on each side, firmly attached to the outside of the vehicle, and so located as to reflect to the driver a view of the highway to the rear along both sides of the vehicle. See Exceptions. (FMCSR 393.80) - Any required mirror broken.
4.	Wipers & Horn	- Wiper blade(s) fail to clean windshield within 1" of windshield sides. (FMCSR 393.78) - Horn, missing, inoperative, or fails to give an adequate and reliable warning signal. (FMCSR 393.81)
5.	Engine Compartment	- Low fluid levels. - Loose or leaking battery. - Excessive leaks. - Cracked or deteriorated belts or hoses. - Any condition of impending or probable failure.
6.	Fuel System	- Visible leak at any point. - Fuel tank cap missing. - Fuel tank not securely attached to vehicle by reason of loose, broken, or missing mounting bolts or brackets. (FMCSR Appendix G, Sub. B)
7.	Steering	- Steering wheel does not turn freely, has any spokes cracked, loose spokes, or missing parts. - Steering lash not within parameters, see chart in FMCSR 393.209. - Steering column is not secure. - Steering system; any U-joints worn, faulty, or repaired by welding. - Steering gear box is loose, cracked, or missing mounting bolts. - Pitman arm loose. - Power steering; any components inoperative. Any loose, broken, or missing parts. Belts frayed, cracked, or slipping. - Any fluid leaks, fluid reservoir not full. (FMCSR 393.209)
8.	Brakes	- Brake system has any missing, loose, broken, out of adjustment, or worn out components. - Brake system has any air or fluid leaks. (FMCSR Appendix G, Sub. B) - Brake system has any other deficiencies as described in FMCSR Appendix G, Sub. B.
10.	Springs & Shocks	- Any U-bolt, spring, spring hanger, or any other axle positioning part is cracked, broken, loose, or missing resulting in any shifting of an axle from its normal position. (FMCSR Appendix G, Sub. B)
11.	Exhaust	- Any leaks at any point forward of or directly below the driver and/or sleeper compartment. - Bus exhaust leaks or discharge forward of the rearmost part of the bus in excess of 6' for gasoline powered or 15" for other than gasoline powered, or forward of any door or window designed to be opened on other than gasoline-powered bus. (Exception: emergency exit) - Any part of the exhaust system so located as would be likely to result in burning, charring, or damaging the wiring, fuel supply or any combustible part of the vehicle. (FMCSR Appendix G, Sub. B)
12.	Frame	- Any cracked, broken, loose, or sagging frame member. - Any loose or missing fasteners including those attaching engine, transmission, steering gear, suspension, body, or frame to contact the tire or wheel assemblies. - Adjustable axle assemblies with locking pins missing or not engaged. (FMCSR Appendix G, Sub. B)
13.	Tires & Tread	- Tread depth less than 4/32" on steering axle. - Less than 2/32" on any other axle. - Any body ply or belt material exposed through tread or sidewall. - Any tread or sidewall separation. - Any cut exposing ply or belt material. - Any tire marked "Not for highway use." - A tube-type radial tire without radial tube stem markings. - Any mixing of bias and radial tires on the same axle. - Any tire not properly inflated or overloaded. - Any bus with recapped tires. (FMCSR Appendix G, Sub. B) - Lock or slide rings; any bent, broken, cracked, improperly seated, sprung, or mismatched ring(s). - Wheels and rims; any cracked or broken or has elongated bolt holes. - Fasteners (both spoke and disc wheels). Any loose, missing, broken, cracked, stripped, or otherwise ineffective fasteners. - Any cracks in welds attaching disc wheel disc to rim. - Any crack in welds attaching tubeless demountable rim to adapter. - Any welded repair on aluminum wheel(s) on a steering axle or any welded repair other than disc to rim attachment on steel disc wheel(s) on steering axle. (FMCSR Appendix G, Sub. B)

GENERAL MESSAGE FORM

ICS 213

Incident Name:	Date Prepared:	Time Prepared:

Operational Period:	Operational Period Date/Time:	From:	To:

TO:	**POSITION:**
FROM:	**POSITION:**
Subject:	

Message:

Disposition:

Date and Time:	Name/Position:

ROUTING

SENDER: Retain Bottom (Pink) Copy	**RECIPIENT:** Retain Middle (Yellow) Copy	Return <u>Top Copy</u> (White) to Sender for review then to Planning Section (DOCU)

ICS 213 (07/25/2005)

Unit Log

ICS 214

Incident Name:		Date/Time Prepared:	Page _____ of _____
Operational Period #:	Operational Period Date/Time:	From:	To:
Unit Name/Designator:		Unit Leader (Name & Position):	

Time	Activity/Events

Prepared By:	Agency Name:	EOC Position:

ICS 214 (07/25/2005)

Unit Name:	Unit Leader:	Date Prepared:

Activity Log (Continued)

Time	Major Events

ICS 214-1 (9/95)

Page: of:

ICS 215

Operational Planning Summary

	Incident Name:	Date Prepared:	Time Prepared:	Operational Period Date: From: To:	Operational Period Time: From: To:

Division/Group Or Other Location — **Work Assignments**

Resource	Req. / Have / Need	Equipment	Personnel	Reporting Location	Requested Arrival Time

(Rows, each with Req. / Have / Need)

- Req. / Have / Need
- Req. / Have / Need
- Req. / Have / Need
- Req. / Have / Need
- Req. / Have / Need
- Req. / Have / Need
- Req. / Have / Need
- Req. / Have / Need
- Req. / Have / Need
- Req. / Have / Need

Total Resources Required:

Total Resources on Hand:

Total Resources Needed:

Prepared By:	Company Name:	ICS Position:	Approved By:	Company Name:	ICS Position:

Prepared By: (Name & Position) _____ Company Name: _____ ICS Position: _____

ICS 215 (9/95)

Note: this page is a summary of the 215-1 worksheets.

Incident Name:	Date Prepared:	Time Prepared:

Operational Period Date: From: To:	Operational Period Time: From: To:

Resources Required

R: Required
H: Have
N: Need

	Division:	Task Force:		Division:	Task Force:		Division:	Task Force:		Division:	Task Force:		Divison:	Task Force:		Totals

Assignment:

Reporting Location:

Reporting Time:

1 Personnel	R	H	N	R	H	N	R	H	N	R	H	N	R	H	N	
Laborers																
Operators																
Teamsters																
Fitters																
Welders																

2 Backhoes																
JD450 w/Hoe																
Rubber Tire Hoe																
235/245 Backhoe																

ICS 215-1 (9/95)   Page 1 of 6

Resources Required

	Division: Task Force:			Division: Task Force:			Division: Task Force:			Division: Task Force:			Divison: Task Force:			Totals
3 Dozers	R	H	N	R	H	N	R	H	N	R	H	N	R	H	N	
D6																
D8/9																
4 Loaders																
930 w/Forks & Bucket																
966/980/988 w/Forks & Bucket																
977 Truck Loader																
5 Cranes																
18–40 Ton Rubber Tire Crane																
6 Trenchers																
Ditchwitch																

ICS 215-1 (9/95)   Page 2 of 6

Resources Required

	Division:	Task Force:		Division:	Task Force:		Division:	Task Force:		Division:	Task Force:		Divison:	Task Force:		Totals	
7 Trucks	R	H	N	R	H	N	R	H	N	R	H	N	R	H	N		
Truck Tractor																	
45–48' Float																	
50–75 Ton Lowboy																	
Flatbed																	
Rollback																	
End Dump																	
Fire Truck																	
Fuel Truck																	
Vacuum Truck																	
Water Truck																	
8 Boats																	
Aiboat																	
Riverboat																	

ICS 215-1 (9/95)   Page 3 of 6

Resources Required

	Division:	Task Force:		Division:	Task Force:		Division:	Task Force:		Division:	Task Force:		Divison:	Task Force:		Totals	
9 ATVs	R	H	N	R	H	N	R	H	N	R	H	N	R	H	N			
Truck Bombadier																		
4-Wheeler																		
Snowmachine																		
10 Pallets																		
Small Tools																		
Ice																		
Helicopter Slings																		
Emergency Shelter																		
Protective Clothing																		
Decon																		

ICS 215-1 (9/95)   Page 4 of 6

Resources Required

		Division:	Task Force:		Division:	Task Force:		Division:	Task Force:		Division:	Task Force:		Divison:	Task Force:		Totals	
11	**Skimmers**	R	H	N	R	H	N	R	H	N	R	H	N	R	H	N		
	Acme																	
	Komara																	
	Manta																	
	Pedco																	
	Rope Mop Pallet w/Gen.																	
12	**Storage**																	
	55 Gal. Drum																	
	1000/3000 Fold-A-Tank																	
	7000 Modu Tank																	
	2400 Fast Tank																	
	10,000 Tanker																	
	Bladder																	

ICS 215-1 (9/95)   Page 5 of 6

Resources Required

	Division:	Task Force:		Division:	Task Force:		Division:	Task Force:		Division:	Task Force:		Division:	Task Force:		Totals	
13 Sorbents	R	H	N	R	H	N	R	H	N	R	H	N	R	H	N			
Pads (Carton)																		
Rolls (Roll)																		
Boom (Bundle)																		
14 Misc.																		
Lite Tower/Generator																		
Fresh Air Heater																		
Helicopter																		
Pumps																		
Hose																		

Prepared By:		ICS Position:
Approved By:	Company Name:	ICS Position:

ICS 215-1 (9/95)   Page 6 of 6

Resource Status & Dispatch Request

ICS 216

Incident Name:	Date Prepared:	Time Prepared:

Operational Period:	Operational Period Date/Time:	From:	To:

Date/Time of Dispatch:		Notification Target: (i.e. OESS staff, agencies)	

	Notification Target	√	Pager number	Home number	Status[1]	Comments
1.						
2.						
3.						
4.						
5.						
6.						
7.						
8.						
9.						
10.						
11.						
12.						
13.						
14.						
15.						
16.						
17.						
18.						
19.						
20.						
21.						
22.						
23.						
24.						
25.						
26.						
27.						
28.						
29.						
30.						

Prepared By: (Name/Title)	Approved by: (Name/Title)	Page _____ of _____

Notes: 1. Show status as Assigned/responding, Available, De-Mob, or Out-of-Service.

ICS 216 (07/25/2005)

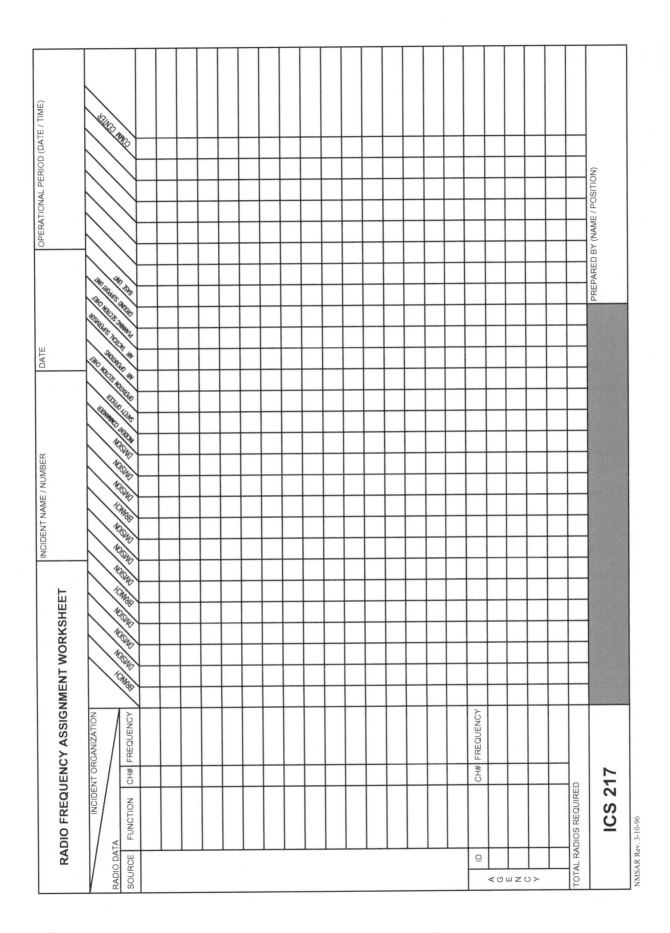

RADIO FREQUENCY ASSIGNMENT WORKSHEET

INCIDENT NAME / NUMBER

DATE

OPERATIONAL PERIOD (DATE / TIME)

INCIDENT ORGANIZATION

COMM CENTER

BASE UNIT

GROUND SUPPORT UNIT

PLANNING SECTION CHIEF

AIR TACTICAL SUPERVISOR

AIR OPERATIONS

OPERATION SECTION CHIEF

SAFETY OFFICER

INCIDENT COMMANDER

DIVISION

DIVISION

DIVISION

BRANCH

DIVISION

DIVISION

DIVISION

BRANCH

DIVISION

DIVISION

DIVISION

BRANCH

RADIO DATA

SOURCE

FUNCTION

CH#

FREQUENCY

ID

CH#

FREQUENCY

AGENCY

TOTAL RADIOS REQUIRED

PREPARED BY (NAME / POSITION)

ICS 217

NMSAR Rev. 3-10-96

ICS 218
Support Vehicle Inventory

Incident Name:		Operational Period Date:		Operational Period Time:	
		From:	To:	From:	To:

Vehicle Information (Use separate sheet for each vehicle category)

Type	Make	Capacity/Size	Agency/Owner APSC/Rental	I.D. Number	Location	Released To	Time

Prepared By:	Company Name:	ICS Position: **Ground Support Unit**	Approved By:	Company Name:	ICS Position:

ICS 218 (9/95)

Incident Action Plan

ICS 220
Air Operations Summary

Incident Name:	Date Prepared:	Time Prepared:	Operational Period Date: From: To:	Operational Period Time: From: To:

Personnel & Communications

Position	Name	Radio Freq.	Phone	Fax
Air Operations Director				
Helicopter Coordinator				
Fixed Wing Coordinator				
Airborne Dispersant Coord.				
Ground Support Coord.				
Aviation Safety Officer				

Helibase Locations:

Landing Strip Locations:

Assignment		Time Available	Takeoff Time	Return Time	Remarks
Base/Function	Fixed Wing (No. & Type)	Helicopter (No. & Type)			
Totals					

Prepared By:	Company Name:	ICS Position:	Approved By:	Company Name:	ICS Position:

ICS 220 (9/95)

DEMOBILIZATION CHECKOUT

ICS-221

1. INCIDENT NAME/NUMBER	2. DATE/TIME	3. DEMOB NO.

4. UNIT/PERSONNEL RELEASED

5. TRANSPORTATION TYPE/NO.

6. ACTUAL RELEASE DATE/TIME

7. MANIFEST   YES   NO

NUMBER _____

8. DESTINATION

_____

9. AREA/AGENCY/REGION NOTIFIED

NAME _____

DATE _____

10. UNIT LEADER RESPONSIBLE FOR COLLECTING PERFORMANCE RATING

11. UNIT/PERSONNEL   YOU AND YOUR RESOURCES HAVE BEEN RELEASED SUBJECT TO SIGNOFF FROM THE FOLLOWING:

(DEMOB. UNIT LEADER CHECK ✔ APPROPRIATE BOX)

LOGISTICS SECTION

☐ SUPPLY UNIT _____

☐ COMMUNICATIONS UNIT _____

☐ FACILITIES UNIT _____

☐ GROUND SUPPORT UNIT LEADER _____

PLANNING SECTION

☐ DOCUMENTATION UNIT _____

FINANCE/ADMINISTRATION SECTION

☐ TIME UNIT _____

OTHER

☐ _____   _____

☐ _____   _____

12. REMARKS

_____

_____

221 ICS 1/83

INSTRUCTIONS FOR COMPLETING THE DEMOBILIZATION CHECKOUT
(ICS FORM 221)

Prior to actual demobilization, Planning Section (Demobilization Unit) should check with the Command Staff (Liaison Officer) to determine any agency specific needs related to demobilization and release. If any, add to line Number 11.

Item Number	Item Title	Instructions
1.	Incident Name/No.	Print Name and/or Number of incident.
2.	Date/Time	Enter Date and Time prepared.
3.	Demob No.	Enter Agency Request Number, Order Number, or Agency Demobilization Number if applicable.
4.	Unit/Personnel Released	Enter appropriate vehicle or Strike Team/Task Force I.D. Number(s) and Leader's name or individual overhead or staff personnel being released.
5.	Transportation Type/No.	Method and vehicle I.D. Number for transportation back to home unit. Enter N/A if own transportation is provided. *Additional specific details should be included in Remarks, block #12.
6.	Actual Release Date/time	To be completed at conclusion of demobilization at time of actual release from incident. Would normally be last item of form to be completed.
7.	Manifest	Mark appropriate box. If yes, enter manifest number. Some agencies require a manifest for air travel.
8.	Destination	Location to which Unit or personnel have been released, i.e., Area, Region, Home base, Airport, Mobilization Center, etc.
9.	Area/Agency/ Region Notified	Identify Area, Agency, or Region notified and enter date & time of notification.
10.	Unit Leader Responsible for Collecting Performance Ratings	Self-explanatory. Note, not all agencies require these ratings.
11.	Unit/Personnel	Demobilization Unit Leader will identify with a check in the box to the left of those units requiring check-out. Identified Unit Leaders are to initial to the right to indicate release. Blank boxes are provided for any additional check (unit requirements as needed), i.e., Safety Officer, Agency Representative, etc.
12.	Remarks	Any additional information pertaining to demobilization or release.

*GPO 1985-0-593-005/14032

ICS 222
Supply/Materials Request

Unit Distribution: ☐ Finance ☐ Purchasing ☐ Planning ☐ Personnel ☐ Housing ☐ Food

Incident Name:	Date Prepared:	Time Prepared:

Operational Period Date:

From: To:

Operational Period Time:

From: To:

Requested By: Title:

Mark For: Date Required: Time Required:

Date: Time:

ETA Date: ETA Time:

Delivery Location:

Prepared By:

Item	Quantity	Unit	Description	Vendor	M.R. No.	P.O. No.	MFG PN	Unit Cost	Total Cost	Status	Date	Time
1												
2												
3												
4												
5												

Action Taken:

Comments:

Prepared By:	Company Name:	ICS Position:
Approved By:	Company Name:	ICS Position: Unit Leader
Approved By:	Company Name:	ICS Position: Logistics Section Chief

ICS 222 (9/95)

Incident Action Plan

Incident Name:	Date Prepared:	Time Prepared:

Operational Period Date:
        From: To:
	Operational Period Time:
	        From: To:

Major Hazards and Risks:

Narrative:

Prepared By:	Company Name:	ICS Position: **Safety Officer**
Approved By:	Company Name:	ICS Position:

ICS 223 (9/95)

Incident Action Plan

Incident Name:	Date Prepared:	Time Prepared:

Operational Period Date: From: To:	Operational Period Time: From: To:

Area Environmental Data:

_____
_____
_____
_____

Priorities for Mitigating Environmental and Cultural Impacts:

_____
_____
_____
_____

Wildlife Assessments and Rehabilitation:

_____
_____
_____
_____

Permits: (Dispersants, Burning, and/or Other)

_____
_____
_____
_____

Waste Management:

_____
_____
_____
_____

Other Environmental Concerns:

_____
_____

Logistical Support Needs:

_____

Prepared By:	Company Name:	ICS Position:
Approved By:	Company Name:	ICS Position:

ICS 224 (9/95)

INCIDENT PERSONNEL PERFORMANCE RATING	INSTRUCTIONS: The immediate job supervisor will prepare this form for each subordinate. It will be delivered to the planning section before the rater leaves the fire. Rating will be reviewed with employee who will sign at the bottom.

THIS RATING IS TO BE USED ONLY FOR DETERMINING AN INDIVIDUAL'S PERFORMANCE

1. Name	2. Fire Name and Number

3. Home Unit (address)	4. Location of Fire (address)

5. Fire Position	6. Date of Assignment From: To:	7. Acres Burned	8. Fuel Type(s)

9. Evaluation

Enter **X** under appropriate rating number and under proper heading for each category listed. Definition for each rating number follows:

0 - Deficient. Does not meet minimum requirements of the individual element.

    DEFICIENCIES MUST BE IDENTIFIED IN REMARKS.

1 - Needs to improve. Meets some or most of the requirements of the individual element.

    IDENTIFY IMPROVEMENT NEEDED IN REMARKS.

2 - Satisfactory. Employee meets all requirements of the individual element.

3 - Superior. Employee consistently exceeds the performance requirements.

Rating Factors	Hot Line				Mop-Up				Camp				Other (specify)			
	0	1	2	3	0	1	2	3	0	1	2	3	0	1	2	3
Knowledge of the job																
Ability to obtain performance																
Attitude																
Decisions under stress																
Initiative																
Consideration for personnel welfare																
Obtain necessary equipment and supplies																
Physical ability for the job																
Safety																
Other (specify)																

10. Remarks

11. Employee (signature) This rating has been discussed with me	12. Date

13. Rated By (signature)	14. Home Unit (address)	15. Position of Fire	16. Date

ICS 225

NFES 1576

Incident Name:		Date Prepared:	Time Prepared:
Operational Period Date: From: To:		Operational Period Time: From: To:	

Initial Actions

Activity	Activity Name	Position Responsibility
Notifications	Federal	
	State	
	Local	
Site Safety and Control	Air Monitoring	
	Fire/Explosion	
	Identify Unsafe Conditions	
	Identify Health Hazards	
	Identify Biological Hazards	
Spill Assessment Report	Complete Report	
Initial Briefing	Complete ICS 201 Briefing Packet	
Source Control	Flow Control/Mitigation	
	Contact Source Supervisor	
	Repair	
	Salvage	

Response

Activity	Activity Name	Position Responsibility
Containment	Natural (Earth/Snow Berming)	
	Exclusion Booming	
	Diversion Booming	
	Absorbent Booming	
	Passive Collection	
	Onshore Response	
	Offshore Response	
Recovery	Mechanical	
	Skimming	
	Transport	
	Sorbents	
	Onshore Response	
	Offshore Response	
Chemical Control	Permitting	
	Dispersants	
	Collecting Agents	
	Gelling Agents	

ICS 226 (9/95)

Page 1 of 3

Response (cont.)

Activity	Activity Name	Position Responsibility
Decontamination	Establish Decontamination Unit	
Insitu Burning	Permitting	
	Fire Boom Transport	
	Deployment	
Surveillance/Tracking	Aerial Reconnaissance	
	Perimeter Mapping	
	Trajectory Modeling	
	Weather Forecasting	
	Weather Monitoring	
	Protection Priorities	
	Environmental Impacts	
	Cultural Impacts	
Shoreline Protection	Assessment/Cultural Impacts	
	Entrapment Booming	
	Cleanup	
	Booming/Sorbents	
	Debris Removal	
Oil Storage	Store Recovered Debris	
Communications	Communications Plan	
	Frequency Assignments	
	Equipment Assignments	

Environmental

Activity	Activity Name	Position Responsibility
Environmental Sensitivity Ident.	Identify Critical Areas	
Wildlife Response	Hazing	
	Capture	
	Stabilization	
	Rehabilitation	
Permitting	Burn Permitting	
	Dispersant Permitting	
	Chemical Permitting	
	Wildlife Permitting	
	Waste Management Permitting	

ICS 226 (9/95)

Environmental (cont.)

Activity	Activity Name	Position Responsibility
Waste Management	Storage	
	Transport	
	Disposal	
	Incineration	
Nat. Resource Damage Assess.	Documentation	

Ancillary Activities

Activity	Activity Name	Position Responsibility
Public Relations	Initial Press Briefing	
	Media Release	
Security	Establish At Scene	
	Establish At Site Entrace	
	Establish At Incident Command Post	
Logistical Support	Housing Ordering	
	Food Ordering	
	Heavy Equipment Ordering	
	Vessels/Boat Ordering	
	Mutual Aid	
	Contractors Ordering	
Organization Transition	Transition to Owner	
	Transition to Co-op	
	Transition to Contractor	

Spill Project Closure

Activity	Activity Name	Position Responsibility
Demobilizaiton Plan	Prepare Plan	
	Initiate Plan	
	Contract Closures	
	Personnel Debriefing	
	Surplus Material Handling	
Site Restoration	Bioremediation	

Prepared By:	Company Name:	ICS Position:
Approved By:	Company Name:	ICS Position:

ICS 226 (9/95)

Participating in the National Incident Management System: A Checklist for NIMS Implementation

If your agency, organization, or association has decided to implement the NIMS within your community, a good start is to assess your organization's current status and develop new policies. The following questions and/or checklists have been developed to guide your organization in implementing the NIMS. Remember, the NIMS is a flexible and adjustable system; you can add questions to this checklist as your program develops.

1. Establishing the NIMS
   - ☐ Develop a NIMS policy statement.
   - ☐ Develop a NIMS multiagency committee or task force.
   - ☐ Make sure all public, private, and nongovernmental organizations (NGOs) are invited to participate in the program.
   - ☐ Set clear deadlines.
   - ☐ Assign project management personnel to coordinate NIMS project activities.
   - ☐ Assign appropriate time and funding resources for the NIMS project.
   - ☐ Collect all current disaster or emergency planning policies, directives, plans, manuals, and so on for your current disaster and preparedness programs. These materials will be very helpful during the development stages.
   - ☐ Collect past critiques, historical documents, and lessons learned from incidents within your jurisdiction and neighboring jurisdictions.

2. Command and Management
   - ☐ The Incident Command System (ICS) is in place.
   - ☐ The ICS is modular and scalable.
   - ☐ The ICS has interactive management components.
   - ☐ The ICS has established common ICS terminology, standards, and procedures that enable diverse organizations to work with your program effectively.
   - ☐ The ICS incorporates measurable objectives.
   - ☐ The implementation of the ICS will have the least possible disruption on existing systems and processes.
   - ☐ The ICS is user-friendly and is applicable across a wide spectrum of emergency response and incident management disciplines.
   - ☐ Define organizational functions.
   - ☐ Identify and define Command and General Staff responsibilities.
   - ☐ The ICS is applicable across a wide spectrum of emergency response and incident management disciplines, including private-sector and nongovernmental organizations.
   - ☐ ICS terminology is being used.
   - ☐ ICS organizational functions (Divisions, Branches, Units, etc.) are clearly identified, defined, and standardized.
   - ☐ Major resources used to support incident management activities (including personnel, facilities, equipment, supplies, materials, and rental equipment) have common names and are typed to avoid confusion and enhance interoperability.
   - ☐ All incident facilities have been identified.
   - ☐ The management-by-objectives approach is used throughout the ICS.
   - ☐ The Incident Action Plan (IAP) communicates the overall incident objectives.

- ☐ Predetermined incident locations and facilities have been identified.
- ☐ The resource management process has been identified and resources are typed and up to date.
- ☐ The integrated communication system has been tested and is interoperable.
- ☐ An established policy and procedure is in place for the establishment and transfer of command.
- ☐ A clearly established chain of command and line of authority has been defined and identified.
- ☐ Unified Command (UC) involving multiple jurisdictions has been defined.
- ☐ Accountability at all jurisdictions has been identified and described, including check-in, the IAP, unity of command, span of control, and resource tracking.
- ☐ Authority has been identified and defined for the deployment and management of resources.
- ☐ A clear plan outlines the methods of collecting and managing information and intelligence.
- ☐ The responsibilities of the Area Command have been identified and defined.
- ☐ The responsibilities of the Emergency Operations Center (EOC) have been identified and defined.
- ☐ EOC multiagency coordination responsibilities have been identified and defined.

3. Intelligence/Investigations Functions
- ☐ A process has been developed for sharing information and intelligence, including security and classified information and operational information, to identify risk.
- ☐ Key medical intelligence factors have been identified.
- ☐ Surveillance needs have been identified.
- ☐ Vulnerability and risk assessments have been conducted.
- ☐ Security procedures are in place to share information and intelligence with Command Staff, Operations Staff, Planning Staff, and General Staff.
- ☐ A plan is in place to identify the level of security for information and intelligence.
- ☐ Methods are in place to collect and use:
  - ☐ Weather information data
  - ☐ Geospatial and census data
  - ☐ Infrastructure design data
  - ☐ Toxic contamination levels data
  - ☐ Utilities and public works data
  - ☐ Syndromic surveillance data
  - ☐ Communication infrastructure data and backup systems

4. Public Information
- ☐ The responsibilities of the Public Information Officer (PIO) have been identified and defined.
- ☐ The job actions of the PIO are clearly defined and identified.
- ☐ A list of all press and media outlets and key contacts is available.
- ☐ Media and public inquiry policies and procedures are in place.
- ☐ Procedures are in place to address rumors and false information.
- ☐ HIPAA issues (what can be released and not released to the media) have been addressed.
- ☐ A procedure is in place for issuing public service announcements (PSAs) or public service alerts.
- ☐ Procedures and protocols are in place to communicate and coordinate effectively with the Joint Information Center (JIC) and components of the ICS organization.
- ☐ Procedures and protocols are in place for coordinating information across integrated jurisdictions and functional agencies, private-sector entities, and NGOs.
- ☐ Plans are in place for interagency coordination and integration.
- ☐ Protocols for standardized messages and message delivery systems are in place.

5. Preparedness
- ☐ Identify the agency or organization responsible for the management and coordination of incident preparedness.
- ☐ Identify responsible persons, agencies, and organizations that should be involved in the preparedness planning and development process.
- ☐ Identify key personnel to oversee the NIMS implementation.
- ☐ Document all NIMS-compliance meetings.
- ☐ Define the roles and responsibilities of the preparedness agency.
- ☐ Identify Emergency Operations Plan (EOP) team members and their responsibilities, authority, and mission.
- ☐ Identify the levels of capabilities to include training, equipment, exercising, evaluating, and action to mitigate.

☐ Establish standardized guidelines and protocols for planning, training, personnel qualifications and certification, equipment certification, and publication management.

☐ Ensure mission integration and interoperability across functional and jurisdictional lines, as well as with public and private organizations.

☐ Establish public education and outreach activities designed to reduce loss of life and destruction of property.

☐ Ensure code enforcement.

☐ Establish an ongoing process for the maintenance of preparedness organizations.

☐ Establish mutual-aid agreements or letters of understanding.

☐ Establish interoperability standards and procedures.

☐ Identify and establish corrective action plans and mitigation plans.

☐ Identify and establish recovery plans.

☐ Identify and outline operational involvements with county, state, and federal agencies.

☐ Identify and outline operational involvements with private-sector and nongovernmental organizations.

☐ Develop and maintain training drills and exercises.

☐ Establish a qualification and certification program for all personnel involved in the NIMS program.

☐ Establish an equipment certification program.

☐ Manage all NIMS publications, training, and supplies used for training and educating personnel. This includes all job aids, forms, ICS materials, computer programs, training course materials, guides, and so on.

6. Resource Management

☐ Identify and type all resources.

☐ Establish guidelines, protocols, and procedures for certifying, credentialing, and maintaining personnel.

☐ Establish guidelines, protocols, and procedures for categorizing resources.

☐ Establish systems and programs for inventorying resources.

☐ Identify resource requirements.

☐ Establish processes and guidelines for ordering and acquiring resources.

☐ Establish guidelines, protocols, and procedures for mobilizing resources.

☐ Establish guidelines, protocols, and procedures for tracking and reporting resource activities.

☐ Establish guidelines, protocols, and procedures for recovering and recalling resources.

☐ Establish guidelines, protocols, and procedures for reimbursement of resources used.

☐ Establish a plan to obtain resources in advance of an incident to allow for management and employment of resources for any all-hazards incident.

☐ Establish guidelines, protocols, procedures, and advance agreements with mutual-aid agencies, private-sector groups, NGOs, and local businesses to obtain resources during an incident.

☐ Establish guidelines, protocols, and procedures for acquisition processes.

☐ Establish guidelines, protocols, and procedures for resources needed in specific operations within each division of the ICS.

☐ Identify resources needed if all electronic communications fail.

☐ Identify the facilities to be used during an incident.

☐ Identify risk factors in mobilizing resources.

7. Communications and Information Management

☐ Identify all individual jurisdictions that must adhere to national interoperability communications standards.

☐ Identify and develop incident communications standards under the NIMS and ICS.

☐ Establish guidelines, protocols, and procedures for all entities involved in the incident to use the common terminology identified in the NIMS.

☐ Identify all communication equipment and specifications for interoperability.

☐ Establish guidelines, protocols, and procedures for information management.

☐ Establish guidelines, protocols, and procedures for preincident information, information management, networks, and technology usage.

☐ Establish guidelines, protocols, and procedures for interoperability standards.

☐ Establish guidelines, protocols, and procedures for incident notifications and situations reporting.

☐ Establish guidelines, protocols, and procedures for incident status reporting.

- ☐ Establish guidelines, protocols, and procedures for analytical data collection.
- ☐ Establish guidelines, protocols, and procedures for the collection of geospatial data.
- ☐ Establish guidelines, protocols, and procedures for wireless communication infrastructures and systems used during an incident.
- ☐ Establish guidelines, protocols, and procedures for identification and authentication of information.
- ☐ Establish guidelines, protocols, and procedures for the collection of incident data for the national database and incident reporting systems managed by the National Integration Center.

8. Supporting Technologies
- ☐ Establish guidelines, protocols, and procedures for interoperability and compatibility of data standards, digital data formats, equipment standards, and design standards.
- ☐ Establish guidelines, protocols, and procedures for technology support and maintenance.
- ☐ Establish guidelines, protocols, and procedures for technology standards.
- ☐ Establish guidelines, protocols, and procedures for broad-based requirements.
- ☐ Establish guidelines, protocols, and procedures for strategic incident management planning and research and development (R&D).

- ☐ Establish guidelines, protocols, and procedures for operational scientific support for incident management activities.
- ☐ Establish guidelines, protocols, and procedures for technical standards support among various systems and equipment to ensure they perform consistently, effectively, and reliably together without disrupting one another.
- ☐ Establish guidelines, protocols, and procedures for performance measurements.
- ☐ Establish guidelines, protocols, and procedures for consensus-based performance standards.
- ☐ Establish guidelines, protocols, and procedures for testing and evaluating equipment standards by objective experts.
- ☐ Establish guidelines, protocols, and procedures for technical guidelines and emergency responder training and equipment used at incidents.
- ☐ Establish guidelines, protocols, and procedures for further R&D to solve operations problems.

9. Ongoing Management and Maintenance
- ☐ Establish an ongoing working relationship between the US Department of Homeland Security (DHS) National Integration Center and support agencies.
- ☐ Establish guidelines, protocols, and procedures for ongoing testing, evaluation, and updating the NIMS.

Planning Responsibilities Checklist

The following is a checklist and description of planning responsibilities and specific planning activities:

1. General Responsibilities

   The general responsibilities associated with the planning meeting and the development of the Incident Action Plan (IAP) are described in the following list. The Planning Section Chief should review these with the General Staff prior to the planning meeting.

   a. Planning Section Chief
   - Conduct the planning meeting and coordinate preparation of the IAP.

   b. Incident Commander
   - Provide overall control objectives and strategy.
   - Establish procedures for off-incident resource ordering.
   - Establish procedures for resource activation, mobilization, and employment.
   - Approve completed IAP plan by signature.

   c. Financial/Administration Section Chief
   - Provide cost implications of control objectives, as required.
   - Evaluate facilities being used to determine if any special arrangements are needed.
   - Ensure the IAP is within the financial limits established by the Incident Command (IC).

   d. Operations Section Chief
   - Determine division work assignments and resource requirements.

   e. Logistics Section Chief
   - Ensure that incident facilities are adequate.
   - Ensure that the resource ordering procedure is understood by the appropriate agency dispatch center(s).
   - Develop a transportation system to support operational needs.
   - Ensure that the section can logistically support the IAP.
   - Place order(s) for resources.

2. Preplanning Steps: Understanding the Problem and Establishing Objectives and Strategy

   The Planning Section Chief should take the following actions prior to the initial planning meeting (if possible, obtain a completed ICS-201, Incident Briefing Form):
   - Evaluate the current situation and decide whether the current planning is adequate for the remainder of the operational period (i.e., until the next plan takes effect).
   - Advise the IC and the Operations Section Chief of any suggested revisions to the current plan, as necessary.
   - Establish a planning cycle for the IC.
   - Determine planning meeting attendees in consultation with the IC. For major incidents, attendees should include the following:
     - Incident Commander
     - Command Staff members
     - General Staff members
     - Resources Unit Leader
     - Situation Unit Leader
     - Air Operations Branch Director (if established)
     - Communications Unit Leader
     - Technical specialists (as required)
     - Agency representatives (as required)
   - Establish the location and time for the planning meeting.
   - Ensure that planning boards and forms are available.
   - Notify necessary support staff about the meeting and their assignments.
   - Ensure that a current situation and resource briefing will be available for the meeting.
   - Obtain an estimate of regional resource availability from agency dispatch for use in planning for the next operational period.
   - Obtain the necessary agency policy, legal, or fiscal constraints for use in the planning meeting.

3. Conducting the Planning Meeting

The planning meeting is normally conducted by the Planning Section Chief. The following checklist provides a basic sequence of steps to aid the Planning Section Chief in developing the IAP. The planning checklist is used with the ICS Planning Matrix Board and/or form ICS-215, Operational Planning Worksheet (the worksheet is laid out in the same manner as the Planning Matrix Board). Every incident must have an action plan. However, not all incidents require written plans. The need for written plans and attachments is based on the requirements of the incident and the decision of the IC. The planning meeting checklist is as follows:

- Give briefing on situation and resource status (Planning Section).
- Set control objectives (IC).
- Plot control lines and division boundaries (Operations Section).
- Specify tactics for each Division or Group (Operations Section).
- Specify resources needed by Division or Group (Operations Section, Planning Section).
- Specify facilities and reporting locations and plot on map (Operations Section, Planning Section, Logistics Section).
- Place resource and overhead personnel order (Logistics Section).
- Consider communications, medical, and traffic plan requirements (Planning Section, Logistics Section).
- Finalize, approve, and implement IAP (IC, Planning Section, Operations Section).

4. Brief on Situation and Resource Status

The Planning Section Chief and/or Resources and Situation Unit Leaders should provide an up-to-date briefing on the situation. Information for this briefing may come from any or all of the following sources:

- Initial Incident Commander
- Incident Briefing Form (ICS-201)
- Field observations
- Operations reports
- Regional resources and situation reports

5. Set Control Objectives

This step is accomplished by the IC. The control objectives are not limited to any single operational period but will consider the total incident situation. The IC establishes the general strategy; states major policy, legal, or fiscal constraints on accomplishing the objectives; and offers appropriate contingency considerations.

6. Plot Control Lines and Division Boundaries on Map

This step is normally accomplished by the Operations Section Chief (for the next operational period) in conjunction with the Planning Section Chief, who will determine control line locations, establish division and branch boundaries for geographical divisions, and determine the need for functional group assignments for the next operational period. These will be plotted on the map.

7. Specify Tactics for Each Division

After determining division geographical assignments, the Operations Section Chief will establish the specific work assignments to be used for each division for the next operational period. (Note that it may be necessary or desirable to establish a functional group in addition to geographical divisions.) Tactics (work assignments) must be specific and must be within the boundaries set by the IC's general control objectives (strategies). These work assignments should be recorded on the planning matrix. At this time, the IC, Operations Section Chief, and Logistics Section Chief should consider the need for any alternative strategies or tactics and ensure that they are properly noted on the planning matrix.

8. Specify Resources Needed by Division

After specifying tactics for each division, the Operations Section Chief, in conjunction with the Planning Section Chief, determines the division resource needs to accomplish the work assignments. Resource needs are recorded on the planning matrix. Resource needs are considered on the basis of the type of resources required to accomplish the assignment.

9. Specify Operations Facilities and Reporting Locations and Plot on Map

The Operations Section Chief, in conjunction with the Planning and Logistics Section Chiefs, should designate and make available the facilities and reporting locations required to accomplish Operations Section work assignments. At this time, the Operations Section Chief should also indicate the reporting time requirements for the resources and any special resource assignments.

10. Place Resource and Personnel Order

At this time, the Planning Section Chief should assess resource needs using the needs indicated by the Operations Section Chief and resources data available from the Planning Section's Resources Unit. The planning matrix, when properly completed, will show resource requirements and the resources available to meet those requirements. Subtracting the resources available from those required will indicate any additional resource needs. From this assessment, a new resource order can be developed and provided to the IC for approval and then placed through normal dispatch channels by the Logistics Section.

11. Consider Security, Communications, Medical, and Traffic Plan Requirements

The IAP will normally consist of the Incident Objectives (ICS-202), Organization Chart (ICS-203), Division Assignment List (ICS-204), and a map of the incident area. Larger incidents may require additional supporting attachments, such as a separate Communications Plan (ICS-205), a Medical Plan (ICS-206), and a law enforcement security plan. (For examples of ICS forms, see Appendix D.) The Planning Section Chief must determine the need for these attachments and ensure that the appropriate units prepare such attachments. For major incidents, the IAP and attachments will normally include the items listed in Table 5-1.

Prior to the completion of the plan, the Planning Section Chief should review the division and group tactical work assignments for any changes due to lack of resource availability.

The Resources Unit may then transfer division assignment information, including alternatives from the Planning Matrix Board or form ICS-215, onto the Division Assignment Lists (ICS-204).

12. Finalize, Approve, and Implement the Incident Action Plan

The Planning Section is responsible for seeing that the IAP is completed, reviewed, and distributed. The following is the sequence of steps for accomplishing this:

1. Set the deadline for completing IAP attachments.

2. Obtain plan attachments and review them for completeness and approvals.

3. Determine the number of IAPs required.

4. Arrange with the Documentation Unit to reproduce the IAP.

5. Review the IAP to ensure it is up to date and complete prior to the operations briefing and plan distribution.

6. Provide the IAP briefing plan, as required, and distribute the plan prior to the beginning of the new operational period.

Summary of Major ICS Positions

Table G-1 Summary Table of Major ICS Positions*

Major ICS Position	Primary Functions
Incident Commander or Unified Command	• Have clear authority and know agency policy. • Ensure incident safety. • Establish the ICP. • Set priorities, and determine incident objectives and strategies to be followed. • Establish ICS organization needed to manage the incident. • Approve the IAP. • Coordinate Command and General Staff activities. • Approve resource requests and use of volunteers and auxiliary personnel. • Order demobilization as needed. • Ensure after-action reports are completed. • Authorize information release to the media.
Public Information Officer	• Determine, according to direction from IC, any limits on information release. • Develop accurate, accessible, and timely information for use in press/media briefings. • Obtain the IC's approval of news releases. • Conduct periodic media briefings. • Arrange for tours and other interviews or briefings that may be required. • Monitor and forward media information that may be useful to incident planning. • Maintain current information summaries and/or displays on the incident. • Make information about the incident available to incident personnel. • Participate in Planning Meetings. • Implement methods to monitor rumor control.
Safety Officer	• Identify and mitigate hazardous situations. • Create a Safety Plan. • Ensure safety messages and briefings are made. • Exercise emergency authority to stop and prevent unsafe acts. • Review the IAP for safety implications. • Assign assistants qualified to evaluate special hazards. • Initiate preliminary investigation of accidents within the incident area. • Review and approve the Medical Plan. • Participate in Planning Meetings to address anticipated hazards associated with future operations.
Liaison Officer	• Act as a point of contact for Agency Representatives. • Maintain a list of assisting and cooperating agencies and Agency Representatives. • Assist in setting up and coordinating interagency contacts. • Monitor incident operations to identify current or potential interorganizational problems. • Participate in Planning Meetings, providing current resource status, including limitations and capabilities of agency resources. • Provide agency-specific demobilization information and requirements.

(Continues)

Operations Section Chief	• Ensure safety of tactical operations. • Manage tactical operations. • Develop operations portions of the IAP. • Supervise execution of operations portions of the IAP. • Request additional resources to support tactical operations. • Approve release of resources from active operational assignments. • Make or approve expedient changes to the IAP. • Maintain close contact with the IC, subordinate Operations personnel, and other agencies involved in the incident.
Planning Section Chief	• Collect and manage all incident-relevant operational data. • Supervise preparation of the IAP. • Provide input to the IC and Operations in preparing the IAP. • Incorporate Traffic, Medical, and Communications Plans and other supporting material into the IAP. • Conduct/facilitate Planning Meetings. • Reassign out-of-service personnel within the ICS organization already on scene, as appropriate. • Compile and display incident status information. • Establish information requirements and reporting schedules for Units (e.g., Resources Unit, Situation Unit). • Determine need for specialized resources. • Assemble and disassemble Task Forces and Strike Teams not assigned to Operations. • Establish specialized data collection systems as necessary (e.g., weather). • Assemble information on alternative strategies. • Provide periodic predictions on incident potential. • Report significant changes in incident status. • Oversee preparation of the Demobilization Plan.
Logistics Section Chief	• Provide all facilities, transportation, communications, supplies, equipment maintenance and fueling, food, and medical services for incident personnel, and all off-incident resources. • Manage all incident logistics. • Provide logistics input to the IAP. • Brief Logistics staff as needed. • Identify anticipated and known incident service and support requirements. • Request additional resources as needed. • Ensure and oversee development of Traffic, Medical, and Communications Plans as required. • Oversee demobilization of Logistics Section and associated resources.
Finance/Administration Section Chief	• Manage all financial aspects of an incident. • Provide financial and cost analysis information as requested. • Ensure compensation and claims functions are being addressed relative to the incident. • Gather pertinent information from briefings with responsible agencies. • Develop an operational plan for the Finance/Administration Section and fill Section supply and support needs. • Determine the need to set up and operate an incident commissary. • Meet with assisting and cooperating Agency Representatives as needed. • Maintain daily contact with agency(s) headquarters on finance matters. • Ensure that personnel time records are completed accurately and transmitted to home agencies. • Ensure that all obligation documents initiated at the incident are properly prepared and completed. • Brief agency administrative personnel on all incident-related financial issues needing attention or followup. • Provide input to the IAP.

* The Intelligence/Investigations Function may be under the direction of a separate General Staff position.

APPENDIX H

Examples of Resources for Which Typing Has Been Completed

As an illustration of how national resource typing is used, **Table H-1** shows a single resource that has been completely typed, a Track Dozer. **Table H-2** is an example of a team resource that has been completely typed, a Swiftwater/Flood and Rescue Team.

Table H-1 Single Resource (Track Dozer) That Has Been Typed

Resource: Track Dozer

Category:	Public Works and Engineering (ESF #3)		Kind:	Equipment	
Minimum Capabilities:		Type I	Type II	Type III	Type IV	Other
Component	Measures					
Equipment	Example	D10R—Cat 3412E Turbo Charged Diesel	D6N—Cat 3126B Diesel	D3G—Cat 3046 Diesel		D10R WHA (Waste Handling)—Cat 3412E Turbo Charged Diesel
Gross Power	RPM	1,900	2,100	2,400		1,900
Gross Power	kW/hp	457/613	127/170	57/77		457/613
Operating Weight	lb	144,191	34,209	16,193		144,986
Height	ft/in.	6' 11"	4' 1"	3' 0.8"		10' 5"
Ground Clearance	ft/in.	4' 11"	3' 2.7"			4' 10"
Total Tilt	ft/in.	3' 3"	2' 2.2"	1' 2.5"		3' 6.3"
Width Over End Bits	ft/in.	15' 11"	10' 6"	8' 0.9"		17' 3"
Blade Lift Height	in.			27.1		
Digging Depth	in.			21.8		
Multishank Arrangements		1 to 3	3			1 to 3
Ground Clearance Under Tip	in.	35	19.9	16.2		35
Machine Ground Clearance	in.			14.7		
Max. Penetration	in.		14.2			37
Max. Reach at Ground Line	in.		29.1	29.1		
Width	ft/in.	9' 7"	7' 2.7"	8' 0.9"		9' 7"
Winch-Drum Capacity	ft	226	371	371		226
Fuel Capacity	gal.	293	79	43.6		293
Max. Line Pull Bare Drum	lb			40,000		
Full Drum	lb			25,000		
Comments:	The major difference for D10R WHA (Waste Handling)—Cat 3412E Turbo Charged Diesel is that it contains a larger blade and protection guards to prevent landfill-type debris from tangling its drives.					

Table H-2 Team Resource (Swiftwater/Floor Search and Rescue Team) That Has Been Typed

Resource: Swiftwater/Floor Search and Rescue Team

Category:	Search and Rescue		Kind:	Team	

Minimum Capabilities:		Type I	Type II	Type III	Type IV
Component	Measure				
Personnel	Team Composition	14-member team: 2 managers 2 squad leaders 10 personnel	6-member team: 1 squad leader 5 personnel	4-member team: 1 squad leader 3 personnel	3-member team: 1 squad leader 2 personnel
Personnel	Minimum number: Technical Animal Rescue	2	1	1	
Personnel	Minimum number: ALS Certified	2			
Personnel	Minimum number: Helicopter/ Aquatic Rescue Operations	4	2		
Personnel	Minimum number: Powered Boat Operators	4	2		
Personnel	Minimum number: SCUBA-trained Support Personnel with Equipment				
Personnel	Number and level EMTs	14 EMTs—B 2 EMTs—P	Same as Type III	Same as Type IV	1 EMT—B
Team	Sustained Operations	Same as Type II	24-hour operations	Same as Type IV	18-hour operations
Team	Capabilities	• Manage search operations • Power vessel operations • Helicopter rescue operations • Animal rescue • HazMat • ALS • Communications • Logistics	• Manage search operations • Power vessel operations • Helicopter rescue operations • Animal rescue • HazMat • BLS	• Assist in search operations • Nonpowered watercraft • Animal rescue • HazMat • BLS	• Low-risk operations • Land-based operations • HazMat • BLS
Team	Specialty S&R Capabilities	Same as Type II	Same as Type III plus: Technical rope systems	• In-water contact rescue • Dive rescue	

(Continues)

Table H-2 Team Resource (Swiftwater/Floor Search and Rescue Team) That Has Been Typed (Continued)

Resource: Swiftwater/Floor Search and Rescue Team

Category:	Search and Rescue		Kind:	Team	
Minimum Capabilities:		Type I	Type II	Type III	Type IV
Component	**Measure**				
Team	Training	Same as Type II except: Divers to have 80 hours of formal public safety diver training	Same as Type III plus: • Helicopter operations awareness • Technical rope rescue	Same as Type IV plus: Divers to have 60 hours of formal public safety diver training	• Class 3 paddle skills • Contact and self-rescue skills • HazMat • ICS • Swiftwater rescue technician
Team	Certifications	• ALS • Advanced First Aid & CPR	Same as Type IV	Same as Type IV	• BLS • Advanced First Aid & CPR
Equipment	Transportation Resources	Equipment trailer, personnel support vehicle			
Personnel	Team Composition	14-member team: 2 managers 2 squad leaders 10 personnel	6-member team: 1 squad leader 5 personnel	4-member team: 1 squad leader 3 personnel	3-member team: 1 squad leader 2 personnel
Equipment	Communication	Same as Type II	Same as Type III plus: Aircraft radio	Same as Type IV plus: Headset	• Batteries • Portable radios • Cell phone
Equipment	Medical	• ALS medical kit • Blankets • Spineboard • Litter	Same as Type III plus: Spineboard	Same as Type IV plus: Litter	• BLS medical kil • Blankets
Equipment	Personal	Same as Type II	Same as Type III plus: • Life vests • HEED except: PFD Type V	Same as Type IV plus: • Fins • Lamps	• Light sticks • Flares • Markers • Flashlights • Bags • Helmets • Gloves • Knives • PFD Type III/IV • Shoes • Whistles

(Continues)

Resource: Swiftwater/Floor Search and Rescue Team

Category:	Search and Rescue		Kind:		Team	
Minimum Capabilities:		Type I	Type II		Type III	Type IV
Component	Measure					
Equipment	SCUBA	Same as Type III	Same as Type III		• SCUBA cylinder • Buoyancy compensator • Weight belt • 2 cutting tools • Chest harness & snap shackle • Full face mask • Underwater communication • Dry suit • Search line • Spare SCUBA cylinder	
Vehicle	Rescue Boat	2—Fueled	1—Fueled		1—Nonpowered 4-person	
Comments:	Conduct search and rescue operations in all water environments, including swiftwater and flood conditions. Water rescue teams come with all team equipment required to conduct operations safely and effectively. For a complete list of recommended training, skills, and equipment, please refer to the FIRESCOPE Swiftwater/Flood Search and Rescue definition at www.firescope.org/ics-usar/ICS-SF-SAR-020-1.pdf.					

Note: HEED = helicopter emergency egress device; PFD = personal flotation device

Answers to Wrap-Up Case Study Questions

Chapter 1
1. B
2. C
3. B

Chapter 2
1. D
2. A
3. D

Chapter 3
1. C
2. A
3. B

Chapter 4
1. C
2. A
3. B
4. D

Chapter 5
1. D
2. A
3. D

Chapter 6
1. C
2. D
3. D

Chapter 7
1. B
2. D
3. C

Chapter 8
1. B
2. C
3. C

Chapter 9
1. D
2. D
3. A

Chapter 10
1. B
2. D
3. B

Chapter 11
1. D
2. C
3. D

Chapter 12
1. D
2. D
3. D

Chapter 13
1. B
2. D
3. D
4. A

Chapter 14
1. C
2. A
3. B

Chapter 15

1. D

2. Any three of the following:
- ESF #3—Public Works and Engineering
- ESF #4—Firefighting
- ESF #5—Emergency Management
- ESF #7—Logistics Management and Resource Support
- ESF #8—Public Health and Medical Services
- ESF #10—Oil and Hazardous Materials Response
- ESF #14—Long-Term Community Recovery
- ESF #15—External Affairs

Chapter 16

1. C

2. B

Chapter 17

1. B

2. D

Acronym Glossary

ALOHA	Areal locations of hazardous atmospheres
ALS	Advanced Life Support
ANSI	American National Standards Institute
ASTM	American Society for Testing and Materials
BLS	Basic Life Support
CAD	Computer-aided dispatch
CAMEO	Computer-aided management of emergency operations
CBRNE	Chemical, biological, radiological, nuclear, or explosive material
CEPPO	Chemical Emergency Preparedness and Prevention Office
CIKR	Critical infrastructure and key resources
COP	Common operational picture
CQI	Continuous quality improvement
CTO	Chief Technology Officer
DARPA	Defense Advanced Research Projects Agency
DHS	US Department of Homeland Security
DMAT	Disaster medical assistance team
DOC	Department Operations Centers
DTRIM PCC	Domestic Threat Reduction and Incident Management Policy Coordination Center
EMAC	Emergency Management Assistance Compact
EMS	Emergency medical services
EMT	Emergency Medical Technician
ENS	Emergency Notification System
EOC	Emergency Operations Center
EOP	Emergency Operations Plan
ESF	Emergency Support Functions
FAA	Federal Aviation Administration
FBI	Federal Bureau of Investigation
FCC	Federal Communications Commission
FCO	Federal Coordinating Officer
FEMA	Federal Emergency Management Agency
FOG	Field operations guide
FRP	Federal Response Plan
GAEMS	Georgia Association of Emergency Medical Services
GIS	Geographical information systems
GPS	Global positioning system
HIPAA	Health Insurance Portability and Accountability Act of 1996
HLT	Hurricane Liaison Team

HPT	Human Performance Technology
HRO	High-reliability organization
HSI	Homeland Security Institute
HSPD	Homeland Security Presidential Directive
IAEMSC	International Association of Emergency Medical Services Chiefs
IAP	Incident Action Plan
IC	Incident Command
ICP	Incident Command Post
ICS	Incident Command System
IMAT	Incident Management Assist Team
IMT	Incident Management Team
INFOSEC	Information security
JFO	Joint Field Office
JIC	Joint Information Center
JIS	Joint Information System
JTF	Joint Task Force
LNO	Liaison Officer
MACS	Multiagency Coordination System
MERS	Mobile Emergency Response Support
MMRS	Metropolitan medical response system
MOU	Memorandum of understanding
MVA	Motor vehicle accident
NAEMSP	National Association of EMS Physicians
NAEMT	National Association of Emergency Medical Technicians
NCP	National Oil and Hazardous Substances Pollution Contingency Plan
NCTC	National Counterterrorism Center
NFPA	National Fire Protection Association
NGO	Nongovernmental organization
NIC	National Integration Center
NICC	National Infrastructure Coordinating Center
NIJ	National Institute of Justice
NIOSH	National Institute for Occupational Safety and Health
NIMS	National Incident Management System
NIST	National Institute of Standards and Technology
NMCC	National Military Command Center
NOAA	National Oceanic and Atmospheric Administration
NRCC	National Response Coordination Center
NREMT	National Registry of Emergency Medical Technicians
NRF	National Response Framework
NRP	National Response Plan
NRP-CIA	National Response Plan Catastrophic Incident Annex
NRP-CIS	National Response Plan Catastrophic Incident Supplement
OIC	Office for Interoperability and Compatibility
OPS	Operations Section Chief
OPSEC	Operational security
PDD	Presidential Decision Directive
PFO	Principal Federal Official
PIO	Public Information Officer
POLREP	Pollution Report
POTEE	Plan, organize, train, exercise, evaluate
PPE	Personal protective equipment
PSA	Public service announcement

PSC	Planning Section Chief
R&D	Research and development
ROC	Regional operations center
SDO	Standards development organization
SEMS	Standard Emergency Management System (California)
SFLEO	Senior Federal Law Enforcement Official
SIOC	Strategic Information and Operations Center
SITREP	Situation Report
SO	Safety Officer
SOP	Standard operating procedure
SWOT	Strengths, weaknesses, opportunities, and threats
TQM	Total quality management
UC	Unified Command
UP	Unified Planning
USAR	Urban Search and Rescue Team
USFA	United States Fire Administration
WMD	Weapons of mass destruction

GLOSSARY

For online access to the NIMS December 2008 Glossary of Key Terms, go to www.fema.gov/nimscast/Glossary.do.

Action messages: Information that prompts the public to take immediate action.

Adaptability: A characteristic of the National Response Framework (NRF) that allows a responsive strategic framework to support local responders' requirements in any type of hazard or attack.

Advisories and warnings: Information that informs the public and provides specific instructions.

Air Operations Branch: The component of the ICS responsible for all air resources. This includes both fixed- and rotor-wing aircraft, their support personnel, and landing areas.

Air Support Group: Component of the Air Operations Branch that is responsible for all record keeping related to the aviation assets at an incident site.

Air Tactical Group Supervisor: The individual responsible for the coordination of all airborne activity at an incident site.

Air-to-air nets: Networks for communications among aviation units.

Area Command: An organization established to oversee the management of either multiple incidents that are each being handled by an Incident Command System organization or one large incident that has multiple Incident Management Teams assigned to it.

Area Command Logistics Chief: Provides logistics support to the Area Commander and the related Incident Commander.

Area Command Planning Chief: Provides planning support for the Area Commander and the related Incident Commanders.

Area Commander: Responsible for the direction of incident management teams in a given area.

Assigned resources: Resources that are engaged in supporting an incident.

Available resources: Resources that are immediately capable of being assigned to a mission to support incident management operations.

Aviation Coordinator: Coordinates aviation activities, including airspace management and resource prioritization, with the Area Commander.

Branches: Areas of incident management established to delegate an appropriate span of control under the Operations Section Chief.

Command net: Network for communications among Command Staff, Section Chiefs, Branch Directors, and Division and Group Supervisors.

Common operational picture (COP): A broad-based view of critical information from multiple sources that is processed by the Planning Section. It gives an overview of an incident, including resource status and situation status.

Communications failure protocol: Procedures for identifying major communication infrastructures and backup procedures in the case of system failures.

Communications Unit: Plans the effective use of communications equipment and facilities assigned to an incident.

Compensation/Claims Unit: A functional unit within the Finance/Administration Section that oversees and handles injury compensation and claims. This unit coordinates activities with the Medical Unit for on-scene care.

Corrective action plans: Implemented solutions that result in the reduction or elimination of an identified problem.

Cost Unit: A functional unit within the Finance/Administration Section that is responsible for collecting, analyzing, and reporting all costs related to the management of an incident.

Demobilization Unit: The unit in the Planning Section that develops the specific plan related to the release and return of resources to their original status.

Department Operations Center (DOC): An agency-specific center that coordinates with the EOC Operations Section.

Director of Emergency Management: The senior manager of a local, county, or state emergency management agency.

Division: A geographic area of an incident. Divisions are created to maintain span of control at large incident sites.

Documentation Unit: The unit in the Planning Section that is responsible for all event documentation and administrative functions (copying, filing, etc.).

Emergency Operations Center (EOC): A facility that serves as an incident support center. It displays a common operational picture of an incident or event.

Emergency Operations Plan (EOP): A systematic process to initiate, manage, and recover from any emergency in a similar manner to improve preparation and response.

Emergency Support Functions (ESF): Fifteen support functions with a lead federal agency, support agencies, and a defined set of actions and responsibilities.

Expendable resources: Equipment, supplies, or tools that are normally used up or consumed in service or those that are easier to replace than rescue, salvage, or protect.

Facilities Unit: Sets up, maintains, and demobilizes all facilities used in support of incident operations.

Finance/Administration Section: The functional section of the ICS responsible for financial reimbursement and administrative services to support an incident.

Finance/Administration Section Chief: A member of the General Staff who provides cost estimates and ensures that the Incident Action Plan (IAP) is within the financial limits established by the Incident Commander.

Five-Year Training Plan: NIMS training plan that sets operational foundations for NIMS training and Personal Qualification Guidelines.

Flexible coordinating structures: Incident management templates in the National Response Framework (NRF) that provide a common language and organization for agencies and disciplines to integrate effectively.

Food Unit: Plans food operations for facilities and sheltering operations.

Force protection: Protection of key personnel and facilities to prevent losses in the event of an attack.

General Staff: Consists of the following Incident Command System positions: the Operations Section Chief, the Logistics Section Chief, the Planning Section Chief, the Finance/Administration Section Chief, and possibly an Intelligence/Investigations Section Chief.

Ground Support Unit: Maintains and repairs primary tactical equipment, vehicles, and mobile ground support equipment. Supplies fuel and provides transportation support.

Ground-to-air net: Network for communications among ground and aviation units.

Groups: Functional areas of an incident. Groups are usually labeled according to their assigned job (e.g., law enforcement or intelligence). Groups are not limited by geographic boundaries.

High-reliability organization (HRO): An organization that safely and effectively manages and recovers from unexpected events in dynamic and unpredictable environments.

Human Performance Technology (HPT) model: A program evaluation process that identifies interventions through gap and root cause analyses.

ICS forms: NIMS forms for documenting incident command activities.

Incident Action Plan (IAP): A formal document that includes several components and provides a coherent means of communicating overall incident objectives in the contexts of both operational and support activities. The most important section is the incident objectives. An IAP is often verbal during fast-moving tactical events.

Incident Command (IC): The Incident Command System position responsible for overall incident management. This person establishes all strategic incident objectives and ensures that those objectives are carried out effectively.

Incident Command Post: The location from which Incident Command manages the incident. The command post should be easily identified and its location known to all responding resources.

Incident Command System (ICS): A system for domestic incident management that is based on an expandable, flexible structure and that uses common terminology, positions, and incident facilities.

Incident traffic plan: A plan that specifies traffic routes and procedures for vehicles entering and departing an incident site, command post, or support area.

Information sharing: The development of a framework connecting various information systems, including incident notification and situation reports, status reporting, data analysis, geospatial information, wireless communications, and incident reports.

Intelligence/Investigations: Responsible for the collection and analysis of information related to the incident. Usually exists as part of the Command Staff, a section, a unit within the Planning Section, or as part of the Situation Unit, depending upon the scope and nature of the incident and the need for intelligence.

Intelligence/Investigations Function: The component of NIMS that strives to provide the IC/UC with accurate and timely knowledge about a potential adversary and the surrounding operational environment.

Interoperability: The ability of diverse organizations to effectively coordinate and integrate command and support functions during routine incidents, events, or disasters.

Joint Information Center (JIC): The office within NIMS responsible for ensuring that all public information released about an incident is consistent; also responsible for screening any inappropriate facts that may damage an investigation.

Joint Information System (JIS): An integrated and coordinated mechanism to ensure the delivery of timely and accurate information.

Liaison Officer (LNO): The Command Staff position responsible for providing a method of communication between the Incident Command/Unified Command and other supporting organizations.

Logistics Section: Responsible for all support requirements needed to facilitate effective incident management.

Management information systems: Tools used to collect, update, and process data; track resources; and display readiness status.

Marine nets: Networks for communications among marine units and land-based agencies.

Medical Unit: Develops the Incident Medical Plan and manages medical operations.

Mitigation: Reduction of harshness or hostility.

Mitigation plans: Proposals to reduce or alleviate potentially harmful impacts. Any sustained action taken to reduce or eliminate the long-term risk to human life and property from hazards.

Multiagency Coordination (MAC) Group: Committee that manages incident-related decision support information, such as tracking critical resources, situation status, and intelligence or investigative information. Also provides public information to the news media and public.

Multiagency Coordination System (MACS): A combination of facilities, equipment, personnel, procedures, and communications integrated into a common system for incident coordination and support. Usually located at an EOC and structured via the ICS template.

Mutual-aid agreements: Intergovernmental or interagency agreements that provide shared and common assistance when requested by member agencies. The equipment and personnel provided by a mutual-aid request may be predetermined for a particular type of incident or it may be determined at the time of the request in consideration of available resources.

Narrative information: General information that informs the public about the nature and progress of an incident or event.

National Integration Center (NIC): NIMS center established at the national level to develop training courses, standards, publications, and training aids.

National Operations Center (NOC): Primary national hub for situational awareness and operations coordination across the federal government during incident management operations.

National Response Doctrine: The five principles of engaged partnership, tiered response, scalability, unity through UC, and readiness to act.

National Response Framework (NRF): A coherent strategic framework (not a series of functional plans) for senior emergency response chiefs, emergency management practitioners, and senior executives in the private sector and NGOs; supersedes the NRP.

New normalcy: Developed by the Advisory Panel to Assess Domestic Response Capabilities for Terrorism Involving Weapons of Mass Destruction (commonly known as the Gilmore Commission), this concept calls upon the United States to develop a new, higher level of preparedness and attentiveness.

Nonexpendable resources: Equipment that is not normally used up or consumed in service or that can be easily recovered and made ready for continued service.

Operational security (OPSEC): The protection of information that would compromise security or tactical operations.

Operations Section: Component of the ICS responsible for tactical operations at the incident site. The goal of the Operations Section is to reduce the immediate hazard, save lives and property, establish situational control, and restore normal conditions.

Operations Section Chief (OPS): The member of the general staff who directly manages all incident tactical activities and implements the IAP. This individual usually has the greatest technical and tactical expertise with the incident problem.

Out-of-service resources: Resources that are unavailable.

Physical resources: Personnel, teams, facilities, supplies, and major items of equipment available for assignment or employment during incidents.

Planning Section: One of the major components of the ICS. This section collects, evaluates, and disseminates incident situation information and intelligence to the IC/UC and incident management personnel, prepares status reports, displays situation information, maintains the status of resources assigned to the incident, and develops and documents the IAP based on guidance from the IC/UC.

Planning Section Chief (PSC): The supervisor of the Planning Section.

Policy Group: Elected officials and senior executives who give policy advice to the EOC Command.

Preparedness organization: Local or regional entity that develops and maintains NIMS competency by developing plans, protocols, resource management, interoperability procedures, COPs, and mutual-aid operations for event and incident response.

Procurement Unit: A functional unit within the Finance/Administration Section that is responsible for the purchase of goods or services.

Program evaluation: The process of judging the worth and merit of a program.

Public Information Officer (PIO): The position within NIMS responsible for gathering and releasing incident information to the media and other appropriate agencies.

Pull logistics: Ordering of personnel, supplies, and equipment from outside local response or support agencies.

Push logistics: Initial response equipment and supplies transported by responding units.

Recovery plans: Guides for the activities to be undertaken by federal, state, or private entities to direct recovery efforts in areas affected by disasters.

Research and development (R&D): The collection of information about a particular subject to create an action, process, tool, or result.

Resource management: The coordination and oversight of assets that provide incident managers with timely and appropriate mechanisms to accomplish operational objectives during an incident.

Resources: Personnel, supplies, and equipment needed for incident operations.

Resources Unit: The component of the Planning Section (in the ICS structure) that serves as the primary manager of all assigned personnel or other resources that have checked in at an incident site.

Resources Unit Leader: The individual responsible for maintaining the status of all resources at an incident.

Response: Immediate actions to save lives, protect property and the environment, and meet basic human needs.

Safety Officer (SO): The Command Staff position responsible for the management of the incident safety plan. This person has the authority to immediately stop any on-scene activity that is deemed to be unsafe.

Scalability: A characteristic of the National Response Framework (NRF) that allows it to contract or expand according to the scope or size of the incident.

Service Branch: Provides communications, food, water, and medical services. Consists of the Communications Unit, Food Unit, and Medical Unit.

Single command: The Command structure in which a single individual is responsible for all of the strategic objectives of the incident. Typically used when an incident is within a single jurisdiction and is managed by a single discipline.

Single resource: An individual response unit that is employed at or during an incident (e.g., a helicopter, water tanker, police vehicle, etc.).

Situation Unit: This unit collects, processes, and organizes ongoing situation information; prepares situation summaries; and develops projections and forecasts of future events related to the incident. The Situation Unit also prepares maps and gathers and disseminates information and intelligence for use in the IAP.

Situation Unit Leader: Monitors the status of objectives for each incident.

Situational awareness: The ability to access all required information for effectively managing an incident. It is similar to the common operational picture (COP).

Staging area: The location at which resources assigned to an incident are held until they are assigned to a specific function.

Standard operating procedures (SOPs): Detailed written procedures for the uniform performance of a function.

Standards development organizations (SDOs): Organizations with long-standing interest or expertise on existing approaches to establish standards for equipment and systems. Examples include the National Institute of Standards and Technology (NIST), the National Institute for Occupational Safety and Health (NIOSH), the American National Standards Institute (ANSI), and the National Fire Protection Association (NFPA).

Strike Team: A set number of the same type of resources operating under one leader.

Supply Unit: Orders, receives, and processes all incident-related resources, personnel, and supplies.

Support Branch: Provides services that assist incident operations by providing supplies, facilities, transport, and equipment maintenance. Consists of the Supply Unit, Facilities Unit, and Ground Support Unit.

Support net: Communications network that supports logistics requests, resource status changes, and other nontactical functions.

SWOT analysis: An evaluation process that identifies organizational strengths, weaknesses, opportunities, and threats.

Tactical net: Communication network that connects operating agencies and functional units.

Task Force: A combination of resources that work together to complete a specific mission.

Technical specialists: Personnel activated on an as-needed basis who bring specific skills or knowledge to the incident management effort.

Technical Unit: A unit within the Planning Section that can be set up to house technical specialists who will have long-term commitments to the incident and who will provide ongoing information to the incident management effort.

Time Unit: A functional unit within the Finance/Administration Section that is responsible for ensuring the proper daily recording of personnel time. This unit also may track equipment usage time.

Treatment area: An incident facility that is used as a location for the collection and treatment of patients prior to transport; typically organized according to patient status.

Unified Area Command: An Area Command that spans multiple jurisdictions and gives each jurisdiction appropriate representation.

Unified Command (UC): The command structure in which multiple individuals are cooperatively responsible for all the strategic objectives of the incident; typically used when an incident is within multiple jurisdictions and/or is managed by multiple disciplines.

Unified logistics: Utilization and coordination of two or more agencies or jurisdictions to manage diverse logistics functions.

Unified Planning (UP): The utilization of two or more planners from different agencies, disciplines, or jurisdictions who function as a coordinated planning section (similar to the UC concept).

Unit: A component of the ICS that is subordinate to a section.

US Department of Homeland Security (DHS): The federal agency tasked with all aspects of domestic incident management.

Figures and tables are indicated with f and t following the page numbers.

Section 1 Opener, page 1 © Robert A. Mansker/ShutterStock, Inc.

Section 2 Opener, page 159 Courtesy of Jocelyn Augustino/FEMA

Chapter 1
Opener Courtesy of Dave Silva/ United States Coast Guard

Chapter 2
Opener Courtesy of Captain David Jackson, Saginaw Township Fire Department

Chapter 3
Opener Courtesy of Bob McMillan/FEMA

Chapter 4
Opener Courtesy of Journalist 1st Class Mark D. Faram/U.S. Navy

Chapter 5
Opener Courtesy of Jocelyn Augustino/FEMA

Chapter 6
Opener Courtesy of FEMA

Chapter 7
Opener Courtesy of Jocelyn Augustino/FEMA

Chapter 8
Opener Courtesy of Leif Skoogfors/FEMA

Chapter 9
Opener Courtesy of FEMA

Chapter 10
Opener © Karin Hildebrand Lau/ShutterStock, Inc.

Chapter 11
Opener Courtesy of Jocelyn Augustino/FEMA

Chapter 12
Opener Courtesy of Robert Kaufmann/FEMA

Chapter 13
Opener Courtesy of Bob McMillan/FEMA

Chapter 14
Opener Courtesy of Jocelyn Augustino/FEMA

Chapter 15
Opener Courtesy of Jocelyn Augustino/FEMA

Chapter 16
Opener Courtesy of Marvin Nauman/FEMA

Chapter 17
Opener Courtesy of Jocelyn Augustino/FEMA